# LEARNING FROM SARS

## Preparing for the Next Disease Outbreak

Workshop Summary

Stacey Knobler, Adel Mahmoud, Stanley Lemon, Alison Mack,
Laura Sivitz, and Katherine Oberholtzer, *Editors*

Forum on Microbial Threats

Board on Global Health

INSTITUTE OF MEDICINE
*OF THE NATIONAL ACADEMIES*

THE NATIONAL ACADEMIES PRESS
Washington, D.C.
**www.nap.edu**

**THE NATIONAL ACADEMIES PRESS  500 Fifth Street, N.W.  Washington, DC  20001**

NOTICE: The project that is the subject of this report was approved by the Governing Board of the National Research Council, whose members are drawn from the councils of the National Academy of Sciences, the National Academy of Engineering, and the Institute of Medicine.

Support for this project was provided by the U.S. Department of Health and Human Services' National Institutes of Health, Centers for Disease Control and Prevention, and Food and Drug Administration; U.S. Agency for International Development; U.S. Department of Defense; U.S. Department of State; U.S. Department of Veterans Affairs; U.S. Department of Agriculture; American Society for Microbiology; Burroughs Wellcome Fund; Pfizer; GlaxoSmithKline; and The Merck Company Foundation. The views presented in this report are those of the editors and attributed authors and are not necessarily those of the funding agencies.

This report is based on the proceedings of a workshop that was sponsored by the Forum on Microbial Threats. It is prepared in the form of a workshop summary by and in the name of the editors, with the assistance of staff and consultants, as an individually authored document. Sections of the workshop summary not specifically attributed to an individual reflect the views of the editors and not those of the Forum on Microbial Threats. The content of those sections is based on the presentations and the discussions that took place during the workshop.

**Library of Congress Cataloging-in-Publication Data**

Learning from SARS : preparing for the next disease outbreak : workshop summary / Stacey Knobler ... [et al.], editors ; Forum on Microbial Threats, Board on Global Health.
    p. ; cm.
  Includes bibliographical references.
  ISBN 0-309-09154-3 (pbk.)  ISBN 0-309-53034-2 (PDF)
  1. SARS (Disease)
  [DNLM: 1. Severe Acute Respiratory Syndrome—prevention & control—Congresses.
2. Severe Acute Respiratory Syndrome—transmission—Congresses. 3. Disease Outbreaks—prevention & control—Congresses. 4. SARS Virus—isolation & purification—Congresses.
5. SARS Virus—pathogenicity—Congresses. 6. Socioeconomic Factors—Congresses.
WC 505 L438 2004] I. Knobler, Stacey. II. Institute of Medicine (U.S.). Forum on Microbial Threats. III. Institute of Medicine (U.S.). Board on Global Health. IV. Title.

  RA644.S17L43 2004
  614.5'92—dc22

                                        2004007115

Additional copies of this report are available from the National Academies Press, 500 Fifth Street, N.W., Lockbox 285, Washington, DC 20055; (800) 624–6242 or (202) 334–3313 (in the Washington metropolitan area); Internet, http://www.nap.edu.

For more information about the Institute of Medicine, visit the IOM home page at: **www.iom.edu.**

The serpent has been a symbol of long life, healing, and knowledge among almost all cultures and religions since the beginning of recorded history. The serpent adopted as a logotype by the Institute of Medicine is a relief carving from ancient Greece, now held by the Staatliche Museum in Berlin.

**COVER:** The background for the cover of this workshop summary is a photograph of a batik designed and printed specifically for the Malaysian Society of Parasitology and Tropical Medicine. The print contains drawings of various parasites and insects; it is used with the kind permission of the Society.

*"Knowing is not enough; we must apply.*
*Willing is not enough; we must do."*
—Goethe

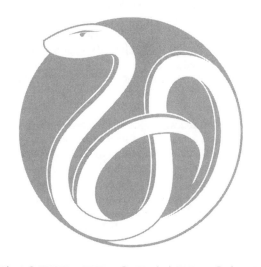

# INSTITUTE OF MEDICINE
## *OF THE NATIONAL ACADEMIES*

**Adviser to the Nation to Improve Health**

# THE NATIONAL ACADEMIES
*Advisers to the Nation on Science, Engineering, and Medicine*

The **National Academy of Sciences** is a private, nonprofit, self-perpetuating society of distinguished scholars engaged in scientific and engineering research, dedicated to the furtherance of science and technology and to their use for the general welfare. Upon the authority of the charter granted to it by the Congress in 1863, the Academy has a mandate that requires it to advise the federal government on scientific and technical matters. Dr. Bruce M. Alberts is president of the National Academy of Sciences.

The **National Academy of Engineering** was established in 1964, under the charter of the National Academy of Sciences, as a parallel organization of outstanding engineers. It is autonomous in its administration and in the selection of its members, sharing with the National Academy of Sciences the responsibility for advising the federal government. The National Academy of Engineering also sponsors engineering programs aimed at meeting national needs, encourages education and research, and recognizes the superior achievements of engineers. Dr. Wm. A. Wulf is president of the National Academy of Engineering.

The **Institute of Medicine** was established in 1970 by the National Academy of Sciences to secure the services of eminent members of appropriate professions in the examination of policy matters pertaining to the health of the public. The Institute acts under the responsibility given to the National Academy of Sciences by its congressional charter to be an adviser to the federal government and, upon its own initiative, to identify issues of medical care, research, and education. Dr. Harvey V. Fineberg is president of the Institute of Medicine.

The **National Research Council** was organized by the National Academy of Sciences in 1916 to associate the broad community of science and technology with the Academy's purposes of furthering knowledge and advising the federal government. Functioning in accordance with general policies determined by the Academy, the Council has become the principal operating agency of both the National Academy of Sciences and the National Academy of Engineering in providing services to the government, the public, and the scientific and engineering communities. The Council is administered jointly by both Academies and the Institute of Medicine. Dr. Bruce M. Alberts and Dr. Wm. A. Wulf are chair and vice chair, respectively, of the National Research Council

**www.national-academies.org**

# FORUM ON MICROBIAL THREATS

**ADEL MAHMOUD** *(Chair)*, President, Merck Vaccines, Whitehouse Station, New Jersey

**STANLEY LEMON** *(Vice-Chair)*, Dean, School of Medicine, University of Texas Medical Branch, Galveston, Texas

**DAVID ACHESON,** Chief Medical Officer, Center for Food Safety and Applied Nutrition, Food and Drug Administration, Rockville, Maryland

**STEVEN BRICKNER,** Research Advisor, Pfizer Global Research and Development, Pfizer Inc., Groton, Connecticut

**DENNIS CARROLL,** U.S. Agency for International Development, Washington, DC

**NANCY CARTER-FOSTER,** Director, Program for Emerging Infections and HIV/AIDS, U.S. Department of State, Washington, DC

**GAIL CASSELL,** Vice President, Scientific Affairs, Eli Lilly & Company, Indianapolis, Indiana

**JESSE GOODMAN,** Director, Center for Biologics Evaluation and Research, Food and Drug Administration, Rockville, Maryland

**EDUARDO GOTUZZO,** Director, Instituto de Medicina Tropical "Alexander von Humbolt," Universidad Peruana Cayetano Heredia, Lima, Peru

**MARGARET HAMBURG,** Vice President for Biological Programs, Nuclear Threat Initiative, Washington, DC

**CAROLE HEILMAN,** Director, Division of Microbiology and Infectious Diseases, National Institute of Allergy and Infectious Diseases, National Institutes of Health, Bethesda, Maryland

**DAVID HEYMANN,** Director, Polio Eradication Program, World Health Organization, Geneva, Switzerland

**JAMES HUGHES,** Assistant Surgeon General and Director, National Center for Infectious Diseases, Centers for Disease Control and Prevention, Atlanta, Georgia

**LONNIE KING,** Dean, College of Veterinary Medicine, Michigan State University, East Lansing, Michigan

**JOSHUA LEDERBERG,** Raymond and Beverly Sackler Foundation Scholar, The Rockefeller University, New York, New York

**JOSEPH MALONE,** Director, Department of Defense Global Emerging Infections System, Walter Reed Army Institute of Research, Silver Spring, Maryland

**LYNN MARKS,** Global Head of Infectious Diseases, GlaxoSmithKline, Collegeville, Pennsylvania

**STEPHEN MORSE,** Director, Center for Public Health Preparedness, Columbia University, New York, New York

**MICHAEL OSTERHOLM,** Director, Center for Infectious Disease Research and Policy and Professor, School of Public Health, University of Minnesota, Minneapolis, Minnesota

**GEORGE POSTE,** Director, Arizona BioDesign Institute, Arizona State University, Tempe, Arizona
**GARY ROSELLE,** Program Director for Infectious Diseases, VA Central Office, Veterans Health Administration, Department of Veterans Affairs, Washington, DC
**JANET SHOEMAKER,** Director, Office of Public Affairs, American Society for Microbiology, Washington, DC
**P. FREDERICK SPARLING,** J. Herbert Bate Professor Emeritus of Medicine, Microbiology, and Immunology, University of North Carolina, Chapel Hill, North Carolina

**Liaisons**

**ENRIQUETA BOND,** President, Burroughs Wellcome Fund, Research Triangle Park, North Carolina
**EDWARD McSWEEGAN,** National Institute of Allergy and Infectious Diseases, National Institutes of Health, Bethesda, Maryland

**Staff**

**STACEY KNOBLER,** Director, Forum on Microbial Threats
**KARL GALLE,** Research Associate
**KATHERINE OBERHOLTZER,** Research Assistant
**LAURA SIVITZ,** Research Associate

*vii*

# Reviewers

All presenters at the workshop have reviewed and approved their respective sections of this report for accuracy. In addition, this workshop summary has been reviewed in draft form by independent reviewers chosen for their diverse perspectives and technical expertise, in accordance with procedures approved by the National Research Council's Report Review Committee. The purpose of this independent review is to provide candid and critical comments that will assist the Institute of Medicine (IOM) in making the published workshop summary as sound as possible and to ensure that the workshop summary meets institutional standards. The review comments and draft manuscript remain confidential to protect the integrity of the deliberative process.

The Forum and IOM thank the following individuals for their participation in the review process:

**Roy M. Anderson,** Imperial College London, London, United Kingdom
**Ruth L. Berkelman,** Emory University, Atlanta, Georgia
**David L. Heymann,** World Health Organization, Geneva, Switzerland
**David Naylor,** University of Toronto, Toronto, Ontario
**Jeffrey L. Platt,** Mayo Clinic, Rochester, Minnesota
**Mary Wilson,** Harvard University, Boston, Massachusetts

The review of this report was overseen by **Enriqueta C. Bond, President, Burroughs Wellcome Fund, Research Triangle Park, North Carolina**. Appointed by the National Research Council she was responsible for making certain that an independent examination of this report was carried out in accordance with institutional procedures and that all review comments were carefully considered. Responsibility for the final content of this report rests entirely with the editors and the institution.

# Preface

The Forum on Emerging Infections was created in 1996 in response to a request from the Centers for Disease Control and Prevention and the National Institutes of Health. The goal of the Forum is to provide structured opportunities for representatives from academia, industry, professional and interest groups, and government[1] to examine and discuss scientific and policy issues that are of shared interest and that are specifically related to research and prevention, detection, and management of infectious diseases. In accomplishing this task, the Forum provides the opportunity to foster the exchange of information and ideas, identify areas in need of greater attention, clarify policy issues by enhancing knowledge and identifying points of agreement, and inform decision makers about science and policy issues. The Forum seeks to illuminate issues rather than resolve them directly; hence, it does not provide advice or recommendations on any specific policy initiative pending before any agency or organization. Its strengths are the diversity of its membership and the contributions of individual members expressed throughout the activities of the Forum. In September 2003 the Forum changed its name to the Forum on Microbial Threats.

## ABOUT THE WORKSHOP

The global response to the recent severe acute respiratory syndrome (SARS) epidemic has demonstrated strengths and weaknesses in national and interna-

---

[1]Representatives of federal agencies serve in an ex officio capacity. An ex officio member of a group is one who is a member automatically by virtue of holding a particular office or membership in another body.

tional capacities to address infectious disease challenges. The story of the emergence, spread, and control of SARS illustrates the considerable economic, political, and psychological effects—in addition to the impact on public health—of an unanticipated epidemic in a highly connected and interdependent world. At the same time, the rapid response to SARS reflects significant achievements in science, technology, and international collaboration.

The future is likely to bring far greater challenges. Will SARS reemerge, and with greater virulence? Can we contain a more widely disseminated epidemic? Will we have preventive or therapeutic countermeasures? Can the necessary global cooperation and resources for containment be sustained? If not SARS, are we prepared for the next emerging infection? Are our public health and research investments (human, technical, and financial) flexible enough to respond to the ever-changing profile of microbial threats?

These and other questions were explored during a September 30 and October 1 workshop of the Forum on Microbial Threats. The goals of the workshop were to:

1. Discuss the origin, emergence, and spread of SARS and the ensuing global response to the epidemic.

2. Evaluate measures employed to contain and control SARS, as well as its clinical management.

3. Examine evidence of the economic impact of this and future epidemics.

4. Look at the political repercussions of the international effort to address the threat posed by SARS.

5. Explore the future of research and technological development related to SARS.

6. Consider preparations for the next infectious disease outbreak.

The issues pertaining to these goals were addressed through invited presentations and subsequent discussions, which highlighted ongoing programs and actions taken, and also identified the most vital needs in these areas.

## ORGANIZATION OF WORKSHOP SUMMARY

This workshop summary was prepared for the Forum membership in the name of the editors, with the assistance of staff and consultants, as a collection of individually authored papers. The sections of this summary that are not specifically attributed to an individual reflect the views of the editors exclusively—they do not reflect the views of the Institute of Medicine (IOM) or of the organizations that sponsor the Forum on Microbial Threats. The contents of the unattributed sections are based on the presentations and discussions that took place during the workshop.

The SARS workshop functioned as a venue for dialogue among representatives from many sectors about their beliefs on subjects that may merit further attention. The reader should be aware that the material presented here reflects the views and opinions of those participating in the workshop and not the deliberations of a formally constituted IOM study committee. Moreover, these proceedings summarize only what participants stated in the workshop and are not intended to be an exhaustive exploration of the subject matter.

This summary is organized as a topic-by-topic description of the presentations and discussions from the SARS workshop. The purpose is to present lessons from relevant experience, delineate a range of pivotal issues and their respective problems, and put forth some potential responses as described by the workshop participants. The Summary and Assessment chapter discusses the core messages that emerged from the speakers' presentations and the ensuing discussions. Chapters 1 through 5 begin with overviews provided by the editors, followed by papers that reflect the contents of invited speaker presentations. The papers in Chapter 1 describe the emergence and detection of the SARS coronavirus and the global response to the epidemic. The papers in Chapter 2 describe the economic fallout—known and projected—of the SARS epidemic and analyze political and governmental responses to it. Chapter 3 includes papers on the microbiology, ecology, and natural history of coronaviruses, the genus of viruses to which the SARS agent belongs. The articles in Chapter 4 describe the development of diagnostics, therapeutics, and other technologies to control SARS. Finally, the papers in Chapter 5 examine how SARS might reemerge and how the world could prepare for the next major outbreak of infectious disease.

## ACKNOWLEDGMENTS

The Forum on Microbial Threats and IOM wish to express their warmest appreciation to the individuals and organizations who gave valuable time to provide information and advice to the Forum through participation in the workshop (see Appendix A for the workshop agenda and Appendix F for a list of forum, speaker, and staff biographies).

The Forum is indebted to the IOM staff who contributed during the course of the workshop and the production of this workshop summary. On behalf of the Forum, we gratefully acknowledge the efforts led by Stacey Knobler, director of the Forum, and Alison Mack, technical consultant, who dedicated much effort and time to developing this workshop's agenda, and for their thoughtful and insightful approach and skill in translating the workshop proceedings and discussion into this workshop summary. Particular recognition is given to Katherine Oberholtzer whose tireless research efforts and technical editing were essential to the framing of the workshop and its report. Considerable thanks is expressed to Laura Sivitz for her thoughtful guidance in preparing the report for review and her editing of the report. We also express our gratitude to Karl Galle who contributed greatly to the final editing and organization of the chapter overviews and technical papers. Initial drafts of the report benefited greatly from technical reviews by James Hughes, Michael Osterholm, and David Relman. We would also like to thank the following IOM staff and consultants for their valuable contributions to this activity: Patrick Kelley, Bernadette Pryde Hackley, Marcia Lewis, Amy Giamis, Joe Esparza, Harriet Banda, Dianne Stare, Marjan Najafi, Jennifer Bitticks, Bronwyn Schrecker, Porter Coggeshall, Jennifer Otten, and Sally Stanfield.

Finally, the Forum also thanks sponsors that supported this activity. Financial support for this project was provided by the U.S. Department of Health and Human Services' National Institutes of Health, Centers for Disease Control and Prevention, and Food and Drug Administration; U.S. Department of Defense; U.S. Department of State; U.S. Department of Veterans Affairs; U.S. Department of Agriculture; American Society for Microbiology; Burroughs Wellcome Fund; Pfizer; GlaxoSmithKline; and the Merck Company Foundation. The views presented in this workshop summary are those of the editors and workshop participants and are not necessarily those of the funding organizations.

Adel Mahmoud, *Chair*
Stanley Lemon, *Vice-Chair*
Forum on Microbial Threats

# Contents

## APPENDIXES

# Summary and Assessment[1]

The emergence of a novel human coronavirus in late 2002 alarmed populations across the globe, elicited a massive public health response, gave rise to a multinational research network, gripped the news media, wreaked political havoc in China, and struck a blow to the tourism and travel industries of several countries. By the time this coronavirus, labeled SCoV, apparently receded from human hosts in July 2003, nearly 10 percent of more than 8,000 individuals who fit the probable case definition had died of the disease now known as severe acute respiratory syndrome (SARS) (World Health Organization [WHO], 2003a). Analyses of this epidemic could lead to improvements in the global community's preparedness for and response to future global outbreaks of infectious disease.[2]

For these reasons, the Institute of Medicine's (IOM's) Forum on Microbial Threats convened the workshop *Learning from SARS: Preparing for the Next*

---

[1]The speed with which the SARS epidemic spread last year was matched by a similar swiftness in the rate at which the understanding of the disease and its effects evolved among scientists, public health officials, and other members of the global health community. For this reason, individual papers within this volume are likely to reflect different stages and perspectives from among the many attempts that have been made to assess the course of the epidemic at different times and places. In some cases, analyses of public health responses or variations in empirical data (such as the number of suspected SARS cases or SARS-related deaths) may reflect the fluid nature of these circumstances. For the most current updates on SARS and recommendations for clinicians and public health officials, readers are referred to the relevant websites of the WHO (http://www.who.int/csr/sars/en/) and the CDC (http://www.cdc.gov/ncidod/sars/).

[2]This report entered final production before the January 5, 2004, confirmation of the first SARS case since July 2003—explaining the references throughout the report to the uncertainty about the reemergence of the disease.

*Disease Outbreak* on September 30 and October 1, 2003. Participants discussed the emergence, detection, spread, and containment of SARS; political responses to the epidemic; its economic consequences; basic research on coronaviruses; preparations for a possible reemergence of SCoV; and lessons learned from the SARS epidemic that could shape responses to future microbial threats.

This workshop summary does not contain consensus recommendations, nor does it represent a consensus opinion of the IOM Forum on Microbial Threats. Rather, it presents the individual perspectives and research of people who made presentations at the IOM workshop on SARS or who participated in workshop discussions.

While the workshop attempted to explore a range of issues that emerged from the SARS outbreak, it is important to recognize that neither the discussions nor this report provide an exhaustive survey of the body of knowledge about SARS. Some important issues not addressed through workshop discussions include analyses of modes of transmission in indoor environments, especially airplanes; consideration of major technological breakthroughs or new fields of inquiry that would significantly advance our ability to prevent and treat infectious diseases; and comparative analyses of actions and outcomes related to the public health responses of different countries.

It should also be noted that considerable effort was made to engage the participation of more Chinese colleagues in the presentations and discussion of the workshop. The short time during which the workshop was organized made it very difficult for Chinese counterparts to obtain the necessary travel visas. Contributions from Chinese participants were important to the workshop as were additional phone and email consultations to the development of this report.

The following text summarizes what transpired during the workshop and assesses how the world's experience with SARS could potentially guide preparations by the public health community, researchers, and policy makers for future outbreaks of infectious disease.

## OVERVIEW OF THE SARS EPIDEMIC

SARS is unremarkable in certain ways among infectious diseases. For example, the transmission rate of SCoV pales in comparison with those of other known microbial threats, such as influenza, but appears to be similar to that of smallpox. Despite nationwide vaccination campaigns against influenza in the United States, an average of 36,000 U.S. residents die annually from influenza infections—nearly 50 times more people than the number killed by SARS worldwide (Centers for Disease Control and Prevention, 2002).

Yet the quality, speed, and effectiveness of the public health response to SARS brilliantly outshone past responses to international outbreaks of infectious disease, validating a decade's worth of progress in global public health networking. **Thus, in several respects, the SARS epidemic reflected fundamental** improvements in how the world responds to an outbreak of infectious disease; and at the same time, highlights the continuing need for investments in a robust response system that is prepared for the next emerging disease—whether naturally occurring or intentionally introduced.

The World Health Organization (WHO) deserves credit for initiating and coordinating much of this response through its Global Outbreak Alert and Response Network (GOARN), as do the partner organizations comprising 115 national health services, academic institutions, technical institutions, and individuals. In the future, this public health network—originally developed to manage outbreaks of influenza and other infectious diseases—ideally will encompass more partners and have the capacity to handle outbreaks of greater magnitude than SARS. Nevertheless, it is clear that multinational, collaborative, and coordinated surveillance, research, and containment measures greatly limited the spread of SCoV.

Despite the low transmission rate of SCoV and the relatively low number of SARS deaths compared to other infectious diseases, SARS had a remarkably powerful and negative psychological impact on many populations worldwide. The relatively high case fatality rate, the identification of superspreaders, the newness of the disease, the speed of its global spread, and public uncertainty about the ability to control its spread may have contributed to the public's alarm. This alarm, in turn, may have led to behavior that exacerbated the economic blows to the travel and tourism industries of the countries with the highest number of SARS cases.

In addition, the SARS epidemic starkly outlined the benefits and dangers of the impact of globalization on infectious disease. The ease and frequency of international travel facilitated the swift spread of SCoV infections to 5 countries within 24 hours and to more than 30 countries on 6 continents within 6 months (WHO, 2003a). Likewise, the increased migration of workers from rural to urban areas within their home country or into different countries (and continents) has increased the risk that new and previously unrecognized viruses will become established in worldwide human populations.

Yet at the same time, worldwide telecommunications networks facilitated collaborative research among 11 geographically distinct laboratories, helping them to identify this new infectious agent in just 1 month. The news media, individuals, and public health organizations disseminated information about SARS almost in real time, influencing behavior that helped limit the spread of the virus. It was also suggested that this information ultimately created heightened awareness and pressure within the Chinese government and public to take action against the SARS and to engage with the global efforts of research, prevention, and containment.

A complex set of factors underlies the emergence and spread of microbial threats. The extraordinary capacity of microbes to change and adapt, the disruption of human and microbial environments, and the activities that expose humans

**November 2002:** First case of SARS occurs in Guangdong Province, China.

| | |
|---|---|
| November | January |
| 2002 | 2004 |

to new microbes all play a role. The convergence of these and other factors lead to the emergence of infectious diseases, as illustrated in Figure S-1.

## Emergence of SARS

Such a convergence likely occurred during late 2002 in southern China, where merchants and farmers took small wild mammals from their native environments to local markets and sold both slaughtered and live animals for human consumption. Some of these mammals most likely carried a coronavirus resembling SCoV (Guan et al., 2003). The likelihood of human exposure to the virus is quite high when the crowded and relatively unsanitary conditions of these markets are considered. As a result, SARS emerged in the southern Chinese province of Guangdong in late 2002. The index case, retrospectively identified on November 16, occurred in the city of Foshan; by mid-December, SARS had appeared in two additional cities in the province.

An expert team from the provincial government and the national Ministry of Health went to the city of Zhongshan to investigate one of these outbreaks. The team concluded on January 21, 2003, that the infection was atypical pneumonia probably caused by a viral agent. The team recommended measures for the prevention and treatment of infection and suggested that a case reporting system be established to monitor the disease. The investigative team's findings were reported to every hospital in the province. Unfortunately, the reporting of these findings coincided with the Chinese New Year holiday. This compounded the challenge for early intervention against the disease in two ways: the report did not receive significant attention from health officials on leave; and the opportunities for disease spread were greatly enhanced by the travel that often accompanies the celebration of the New Year.[3] Additionally, as we discuss later in this chapter, the medical community's understanding of the true etiology of SARS was delayed significantly by a February announcement from a senior scientist at the Chinese Center for Disease Control that he suspected the infectious agent was *Chlamydia*—a commonly understood bacterial agent that would not have warranted heightened concern or investigation.

---

[3]Workshop presentation, Yi Guan, University of Hong Kong, September 30, 2003.

**January 21, 2003:** Guangdong provincial investigators report on "atypical" pneumonia.
**January 31, 2003:** First super-spreading SARS patient.

| November 2002 | January 2004 |

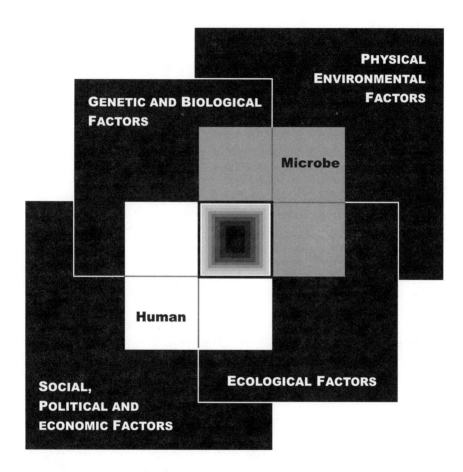

**FIGURE S-1** The Convergence Model. This diagram illustrates how four factors that influence the interaction between humans and microbes may converge in such a way that an infectious disease emerges (central box). The interior of the central box is black, representing the unknown influences on emergence, and the lightening to white at the edges of this box represents the known influences.
SOURCE: IOM (2003).

February 11, 2003: Chinese Ministry of health reports to WHO on respiratory disease in Guangdong.

---

| November | January |
| 2002 | 2004 |

On January 31, the first hyperinfective, or superspreading, case of SARS occurred in the city of Guangzhou. The patient was transferred among three hospitals and infected an estimated 200 people, many of them hospital workers.

As these events unfolded, the international public health community began to receive news of the outbreak through e-mails, Internet chat rooms, and local media outlets, whose reports were widely disseminated through electronic reporting systems such as the Global Public Health Intelligence Network (GPHIN) and Pro-MED mail (Eysenbach, 2003). Based on this information, WHO queried the Chinese government on February 10 and received a response the following day describing an outbreak of an acute respiratory syndrome involving 305 cases and five deaths in Guangdong Province (WHO, 2003b).

Some of the most severe SARS symptoms were suffered by residents of the Amoy Gardens apartment towers in Hong Kong during an outbreak in late March that sickened more than 300 people (WHO, 2003c). Rather than its usual route of transmission by respiratory droplets, the virus is thought to have spread via aerosolized fecal matter through the internal sewer system of the apartment complex (WHO, 2003f). Consequently, on March 31, Hong Kong's health authorities issued an unprecedented quarantine order to halt the spread of SARS on the island, which required some residents of the housing complex to remain in their apartments until midnight of April 9 (10 days later) (WHO, 2003c).

### Spread of the SARS Coronavirus Beyond China

Epidemiological investigations revealed that the spread of SCoV outside China began on February 21, 2003, when 12 people staying in the Metropole Hotel in Hong Kong contracted SCoV from an infected, symptomatic physician from Zhongshan University (see Figure S-2). These 12 people subsequently carried the infection with them to Singapore, Vietnam, Canada, Ireland, and the United States—initiating chains of infection in all of these countries except for Ireland. According to WHO estimates, most of the more than 8,000 probable cases of SARS worldwide originated with this superspreader (WHO, 2003a).

*Vietnam*

Dr. Carlo Urbani, a WHO infectious disease specialist based in Vietnam, reported concerns about a patient in the Hanoi French Hospital with a high

**February 18, 2003**: Senior microbiologist at Chinese Center for Disease Control announces he suspects the disease is *Chlamydia*.

| November 2002 | January 2004 |

fever and atypical pneumonia to WHO's Western Pacific office on February 28 (WHO, 2003c). Responding to Dr. Urbani's alert and other reports of atypical pneumonia in Vietnam and Hong Kong, WHO sent GOARN teams to Hong Kong and Hanoi to join the investigative and containment efforts already underway. The early detection of SARS in Vietnam, prompt sharing of that information with the international community, and aggressive containment efforts by the Vietnamese government, in partnership with a GOARN team, enabled

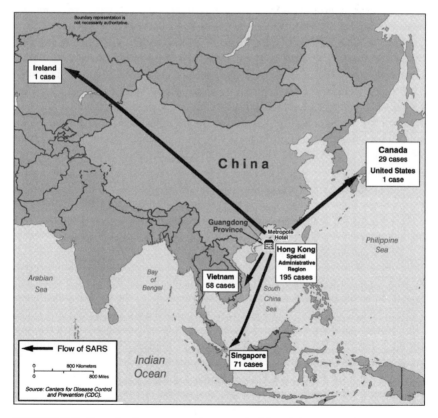

**FIGURE S-2** Portrait of a superspreader: spread of SARS from the Metropole Hotel in Hong Kong as of March 28, 2003.

the Vietnamese to eradicate SARS by the end of April. This was accomplished before SARS was contained in either Canada or Singapore, despite Vietnam's comparatively limited health care resources and lower education levels among its population. (Tragically, Dr. Urbani himself died of SARS.) It was suggested by workshop participants that containment of the disease in Vietnam was, in fact, aided by the absence of more sophisticated medical devices and facilities—such as mechanical ventilation by intubation, bronchoscopy, aerosolized medications, and large hospital facilities that exposed large numbers of individuals to undiagnosed SARS patients awaiting care—which have been identified as factors that promoted SCoV transmission considerably in Singapore and Toronto (Lee et al., 2003).

On March 12, WHO issued a global alert describing outbreaks of the yet-unnamed respiratory disease in Hong Kong and Vietnam and instituted worldwide surveillance (WHO, 2003d). A second alert on March 15 named the condition, listed its symptoms, and advised travelers to have a high level of suspicion of SARS and report to a health worker if they had SARS symptoms and had visited an area where SARS was known to be occurring. Two further alerts provided recommendations for airports to screen passengers and for travelers to avoid areas where SARS had been detected, respectively (WHO, 2003e).

*Canada*

Canada's experience with SARS illustrates the importance of identifying and isolating every infected individual in stemming the spread of the disease. There, the index patient returned to Toronto from Hong Kong on February 23, developed a febrile illness that was diagnosed as pneumonia, then died at home on March 5. Her son, who cared for her, subsequently became ill and on March 7 was admitted to a hospital, where he infected many patients and members of the staff. He died there on March 13, one day after WHO issued its first global alert. In this, the first phase of the Toronto epidemic, unrecognized patients who shared rooms with the son went on to infect scores of other patients, family members, and hospital workers. This scenario was repeated in several area hospitals, as well as others around the globe, even after increased infection control measures were undertaken.

Realizing that SARS was not contained within a single hospital, Ontario declared a provincial emergency on March 26 that halted the transfer of patients among hospitals, instituted infection control measures and created SARS units within hospitals, minimized visitor access to hospitals, and established a process

**February 28, 2003:** Atypical pneumonia reported in Hanoi, Vietnam.

| | |
|---|---|
| November | January |
| 2002 | 2004 |

to screen all persons entering hospitals for symptoms of SARS. Because the spread of SARS in Toronto was largely restricted to the hospital setting, these precautions were effective in controlling the outbreak. When a second phase of SARS occurred in mid-May, after emergency measures were relaxed, it was quickly brought under control with little spread outside the affected hospital (See D. Low in Chapter 1). A similar lapse in infection control in a Taiwan hospital ignited an outbreak in mid-April (WHO, 2003g). Health authorities responded quickly by increasing surveillance, redoubling infection control measures, and launching a mass education campaign credited with reducing the time between symptom onset and patient isolation.

### Singapore

Rapid contact tracing by health authorities in Singapore, where scores of SARS cases had been reported, linked that country's index case to the Metropole Hotel by April 4. Singaporean authorities imposed strict containment measures, including contact tracing and 10-day quarantine for all contacts of known SARS patients, as well as screening for fever among incoming and outgoing passengers at all airports and seaports. One indication of the effectiveness of these measures is the fact that 80 percent of Singapore's SARS patients did not infect anyone else (WHO, 2003h; Singapore Government, 2003).

On September 8, an isolated case of SARS was reported in Singapore, and subsequently confirmed by the U.S. Centers for Disease Control and Prevention (CDC) (WHO, 2003l). The patient, a 27-year-old microbiology postdoctoral student, had no history of travel to SARS-affected areas or contact with SARS patients. Rather, he apparently become infected through a laboratory accident stemming from the contamination of samples containing West Nile virus, the subject of the patient's research, with the SCoV, which was also being studied in the same biosafety level 3 facility.

## THE IMPACT OF THE SARS EPIDEMIC

As the SARS coronavirus spread around the globe, so did its political, sociological, and economic repercussions. Workshop participants described the official reaction to the outbreak in China, examined the political and public health implications of how China acknowledged and confronted the full dimensions of the epidemic on national and international levels, and assessed the immediate and long-term economic

**March 7, 2003:** Son of Toronto index patient enters Scarborough Grace Hospital, initiating outbreak.

| | |
|---|---|
| November | January |
| 2002 | 2004 |

impact of SARS. Central to these discussions was the recognition of the extreme pressure SARS exerted on both international and local health care systems and the frightening prospect of future outbreaks of greater contagion or virulence.

The multinational effort to contain SARS placed unprecedented demands on affected and unaffected countries to accurately identify and report cases in a timely manner, to cooperate with GOARN expert teams of scientists and medical personnel coordinated by WHO, and to sacrifice immediate economic interests (e.g., travel, trade, tourism). Without international legal obligation to report SARS, most countries did so fully. Yet this extraordinary alliance would have failed without the full cooperation of China, the epicenter of the epidemic.

## Politics, Tradition, and the Chinese Response to SARS

Workshop participants asserted that China's problems in dealing with the SARS epidemic were fundamentally rooted in organizational obstacles. Problems cited during the workshop included impediments to the flow of information through the governmental hierarchy, a lack of coordination among fragmented governmental departments, and a political system in which the value of handling problems internally overrides any recognized value of external assistance. Importantly, workshop participants noted that these systemic failings are not exclusive to China and impede the response to public health and other social problems in a large number of countries around the world.

Uniquely, the Chinese tradition of respect for senior scientists in positions of authority may have substantially influenced the behavior of the Chinese Center for Disease Control and of other Chinese scientists who were researching the epidemic (Enserink, 2003). A highly respected Chinese scientist reportedly claimed that *Chlamydia* infection caused SARS, based on an examination of only two specimens. This may have led the Chinese Center for Disease Control and other Chinese clinicians and scientists to maintain that *Chlamydia* was the SARS agent, despite other evidence inside China indicating that the agent was viral. Consequently, virologists in a Beijing laboratory refrained from announcing their discovery in early March of the SARS coronavirus, a decision that set back by weeks research on the disease and a more significant public health response in China (Enserink, 2003).

The SARS epidemic also exposed weaknesses in China's public health infrastructure, including inadequate state funding, lack of effective surveillance systems, and severe shortages in facilities and medical staff prepared for an epidemic infec-

**March 10, 2003:** WHO teams arrive in Hong Kong and Hanoi.
**March 12, 2003:** First WHO global alert issued on yet-unnamed disease.

| November | January |
|---|---|
| 2002 | 2004 |

tious disease outbreak. As a forewarning, a workshop participant observed that these same weaknesses are often cited by medical and public health experts when assessing the state of preparedness for infectious disease outbreaks in the United States.[4] These statements corresponded with other participants who suggested that, in the case of SARS, the United States was perhaps more lucky than it was prepared.

In response to the deficiencies highlighted by SARS, the Chinese government established a case reporting structure, strengthened its emergency response system, dismissed key officials who mismanaged the crisis during its initial months, and provided funding for the prevention and control of SARS. Chinese workshop participants also credited the SARS experience for increasing the recognition and understanding of government officials and the public about the importance of infectious disease control and prevention in general.[5]

## Economic Impact

While the most immediate and dramatic economic effects of SARS occurred in Asia, every market in today's global economy was at some point impacted directly or indirectly by the epidemic. Several agencies and experts have attempted to estimate the cost of SARS based on near-term expenditures and losses in key sectors such as medical expenses, travel and related services, consumer confidence, and investment. One model estimated that the short-term global cost of lost economic activity due to SARS was approximately $80 billion.[6] Participants agreed, however, that the true economic consequences of SARS remain to be determined, particularly given the possibility of its return.

An economic model presented at the workshop estimated the impact of SARS on several countries—and in aggregate, on the world. It considered two different scenarios: a short-term shock coincident with a one-time epidemic, and long-term effects typical of recurring outbreaks. The model was not intended to

---

[4]See IOM, 2003; General Accounting Office, 2001; National Intelligence Council, 2000.

[5]During the development of the this report, a Chinese author commented that the recent commitment by the highest level of Chinese government officials to the prevention and treatment of AIDS, after years of little public recognition of the disease or its victims, might in large part be credited to the new awareness by all Chinese of the threats posed by unchecked infectious diseases.

[6]Workshop presentation by Warwick McKibbin, Australia National University, September 30, 2003.

**March 15, 2003:** Second WHO global alert names SARS; first travel advisory declared.

| November<br>2002 | January<br>2004 |

calculate precise monetary effects, but rather to reveal the magnitude of the impact on countries and regions, scaled to their individual economies (see Lee and McKibbin in Chapter 2).

According to this model, the short-term SARS shock disproportionately affected Hong Kong due to its economic dependence on services (e.g., travel, tourism). Significant short-term losses also accrued in China as a result of a sharp decrease in foreign investment, a trend that could be crippling if perpetuated over several years. In the long term, the expectation of continued outbreaks of infectious disease emanating from China could engulf that entire region of Asia in a permanent "disease transmission shock."

Paradoxically, workshop participants discussed the global cost of SARS associated with lost economic activity—now estimated to have been around $40 billion, and possibly as high as $54 billion if investors remain cautious about the possibility of future outbreaks—as a potential cost of neglecting to invest in public health infrastructure. Several participants warned of a vicious spiral to be avoided: an economic downturn resulting from SARS or another pandemic which squeezes funding for public health, further weakening the world's ability to prevent or contain subsequent outbreaks. The message here: an ounce of prevention is worth a pound of cure. It was suggested by several participants that further analyses comparing the anticipated costs associated with strengthening both global and national public health systems of surveillance and response with the anticipated costs of another epidemic SARS (or other disease) outbreak might reveal important results to persuade decisionmakers to make priority investments in relevant public health and research areas.

## Impact on Global and Local Public Health Systems

Like many of the emergent diseases of the last decade, the challenge of SARS has cast a glaring spotlight on the need for greater investments in public health infrastructure. The outbreak placed a huge burden on international health systems that were already straining to address AIDS, tuberculosis, malaria, and a host of other conditions. With GOARN, WHO had an established structure to coordinate international resources and personnel and thereby muster surge capacity to address such outbreaks. That network was severely tested by SARS, but the successful containment of SARS through national actions supported by international collaboration confirms the value of this approach in addressing future epidemics (see Abdullah et al. in Chapter 1).

**March 17, 2003:** WHO establishes laboratory network to seek cause of SARS.

| | |
|---|---|
| November 2002 | January 2004 |

A key factor underlying the influence of SARS on public health, political, and economic systems was the infection of large numbers of health care workers. Nowhere was the impact of SARS felt more keenly than in the local health care systems of affected areas, where frontline caregivers all too frequently ended up as intensive care patients in need of extended hospital stays or as fatalities. This assault on the well-being of many health care personnel, coupled with the exhausting demands put on those who remained healthy, led Toronto health officials to send out a call to infectious disease professionals in the United States and Europe to come to Canada to bolster their capacity to fight the disease. Additionally, a workshop participant alleged that in Toronto, the closing of outpatient clinics in response to SARS may have caused greater morbidity and mortality than the disease itself. However, other participants argued that without a vaccine or cure for SARS, the isolation of patients and their contacts—including their caregivers—represented the most effective method of containing the epidemic.

## THE PUBLIC HEALTH RESPONSE TO SARS

### The Global Response

As noted earlier, the WHO response to SARS was spearheaded by GOARN. To extend its capacity for surveillance, reporting, and containment, WHO enlisted the support of public health services from the United States, United Kingdom, Germany, France, and other nations. GOARN recruited more than 60 teams of medical experts to assist with infection control in SARS-affected areas, which included 84 personnel from the U.S. CDC. Ultimately, more than 800 CDC employees were involved in the response to SARS.

Through GOARN, WHO also established a virtual network of 11 leading infectious disease laboratories in 9 countries. Connected by a secure website and daily teleconferences, the laboratories collaborated to identify the causative agent of SARS and to develop a diagnostic test; similar groups were also created to pool clinical knowledge and compare epidemiological data on SARS. By April 16, exactly 1 month after the laboratory network was established, its researchers had conclusively identified SCoV as the causative agent.

When evidence revealed that persons infected with SCoV continued to travel—placing adjacent passengers on airplanes at risk of infection—WHO advised airlines to screen departing passengers (WHO, 2003n). Further WHO advisories to avoid all but essential travel to certain high-risk areas were the

**March 20, 2003:** United States reports first cases of SARS.
**March 26, 2003:** Ontario declares provincial emergency.
                              ⊥ ⊥

November                                                                  January
2002                                                                         2004

most restrictive in the history of the organization (WHO, 2003c). The U.S. CDC and Health Canada also issued advisories that warned against travel to SARS-affected countries.

## Chinese Cooperation

Members of a GOARN mission to China in late March warned that country's health authorities that if SARS was not brought under control in China, there would be no chance of controlling the global threat of SARS. Within days, the GOARN team announced that Chinese authorities had agreed to join the GOARN collaborative effort to contain the outbreak and prevent further international spread (WHO, 2003i).

At a March 28 meeting with the Chinese Minister of Health, WHO officials determined that the atypical pneumonia in Guangdong was SARS and that the first cases had appeared in mid-November 2002 (WHO, 2003c). Data provided by the Chinese Center for Disease Control suggested an association between exotic food animals and SARS, indicating the possibility of a zoonosis. More than a third of the earliest SARS cases—those that emerged in China before February 2003—occurred among workers who handled, butchered, or sold wild animals in Guangdong's markets, or who prepared and served them as food. Viruses closely resembling SCoV were eventually isolated from several animal species sold in such markets; however, a natural reservoir for SCoV has yet to be found (Guan et al., 2003).

Although Chinese officials acknowledged that SARS had emerged in their country, they continued to downplay the extent and severity of the outbreak. This led the WHO team in Beijing to take the unusual measure of publicly expressing "strong concern over inadequate reporting" of SARS cases on April 16 (WHO, 2003c).

On April 20, national government leaders declared a "nationwide war on SARS" and removed the mayor of Beijing and the Minister of Health from their posts reportedly for failing to satisfactorily address the epidemic (WHO, 2003c). Thereafter, China increased both its disease control efforts and its cooperation with the international community in the effort to contain SARS. Both the Chinese government and the public took considerable action to halt the epidemic. A workshop participant described how large numbers of government offices, schools, and universities were shut down. Quarantines to prevent public gatherings and travel from cities were imposed to prevent the spread of the disease to

**March 27, 2003:** WHO instructs airlines to screen passengers in SARS-affected areas.

---

| November 2002 | January 2004 |
|---|---|

---

the rural interior of the country, where it was feared that medical resources would be unable to contain or treat the disease. In late June, after more than 5,000 cases had been reported, the disease was contained in China. By this time, Beijing had reported 348 deaths and Hong Kong, 298—the two greatest death tolls due to SARS for any city or region at that time (WHO, 2003c).

When WHO declared on July 5 that all chains of SARS transmission had been broken, the disease was thought to have spread to more than 30 countries, only 8 of which—Canada, China, Hong Kong, the Philippines, Singapore, Taiwan, the United States, and Vietnam—reported more than 10 probable cases.

## Assessing the Use of Public Health Tools

The experience of the SARS outbreak and the history of its control hold clues to the origin and spread of the disease—knowledge that will help to prevent or curtail its resurgence. In assessing the public health response to SARS at both the global and local levels, workshop participants focused on the roles of surveillance and containment in limiting the spread of SARS and anticipated the use of these tools against future microbial threats.

## Surveillance

Broad international networks of individuals and organizations within and across disciplines were responsible in large part for the successful surveillance of the SARS epidemic. Electronic communication networks such as the Global Public Health Information Network (GPHIN) and ProMED mail reported the early outbreaks. ProMED uses electronic communications to provide up-to-date news on disease outbreaks and is open to all Internet users. GPHIN, established by Health Canada in collaboration with WHO, is an Internet-based application that continuously scans global electronic media (news wires, websites) for information on global public health risks, including infectious disease outbreaks. Although these systems ultimately proved to be critical tools for effective surveillance, workshop participants questioned the ability of the existing system to rapidly identify novel emerging threats, which induce symptoms and behaviors characteristic of other infectious diseases that may not initially promote concern or further investigation. Additionally, the sensitivity of the system was considered inadequate because of its inability to correlate disparate data from multiple

**March 28, 2003:** Chinese officials share details of first SARS cases.
**March 30, 2003:** Amoy Gardens, Hong Kong, outbreak announced.

| November | January |
| --- | --- |
| 2002 | 2004 |

surveillance networks that, only when taken as a whole, might surpass a threshold that signals an alarm to public health professionals. Retrospective analyses of the reports on several surveillance networks revealed multiple reports of atypical pneumonia in China between November 2002 and January 2003. However, the lack of collaborative data analysis between multiple reporting systems and the initial absence of clustering allowed the virus to spread unchecked. GOARN identified and verified subsequent outbreaks with the help of the media, nongovernmental organizations, agencies of the United Nations, and public health teams from many countries in addition to those where the outbreaks occurred. GOARN communicated new information to authorities and the public through the WHO website, satellite broadcasts, and news conferences.

The SARS epidemic became a front-page event for the worldwide news media. Daily updates posted on the WHO website for travelers and the public sought to counter rumors with reliable information. The U.S. CDC, which spearheaded the U.S. response to SARS, provided information through its website, satellite broadcasts, and a public response hotline for clinicians and the public.

The vast Emerging Infections Network created by the Asian Pacific Economic Community (APEC) also conducted surveillance for SARS. In addition, it provided an arena for discussions relevant to both biomedical research and disease control, and it monitored the economic impact of SARS in its member countries, which comprise 2.5 billion people and conduct nearly half of the world's trade (see Kimball et al. in Chapter 5).

### Containment

While many aspects of the public health response to SARS benefited from such technological developments as global broadband telecommunications, the containment of the epidemic ultimately depended on the venerable strategies of identifying and isolating persons who fit the case definition and tracing and quarantining their contacts. In countries such as Vietnam and Singapore, where these measures were imposed soon after the identification of index cases, the chain of infection was broken quickly. By contrast, China's delayed response to the epidemic rendered contact tracing impossible and resulted in the need for broader quarantines.

The U.S. strategy to prevent an outbreak within its borders focused on the early detection of symptom onset and rapid implementation of infection control

**March 31, 2003:** Hong Kong health authorities issue quarantine order requiring some residents of the Amoy Gardens apartment complex to remain in their homes until April 9.

| November 2002 | | January 2004 |
|---|---|---|

and isolation. Only in high-risk settings such as health care facilities or airline flights carrying passengers exposed to SARS-infected individuals did CDC suggest the use of quarantine (by definition, the isolation of asymptomatic individuals believed to have been exposed to a contagion). In the absence of an outbreak, the agency directed its efforts toward informing the traveling public about high-risk areas, issuing travel advisories, distributing millions of health alert notices in seven languages at airports and U.S.–Canada border crossings, and responding to symptomatic incoming passengers. However, several other countries quarantined travelers arriving from SARS-affected areas.

The relative effectiveness of various strategies applied to SARS containment—the use of standardized case definitions and laboratory testing to identify the infected, the isolation of ill persons, and the quarantine of contacts—remains to be determined. Based on the present understanding that asymptomatic infected individuals transmit SARS at a low rate, if at all (WHO, 2003j), and that transmission occurs primarily through contact with ill individuals, workshop participants suggested that quarantine of contacts was the least effective of these strategies. However, they also recognized that quarantine could facilitate the containment of a SARS-like disease by reducing the number of contacts by infected individuals during the delay between the onset of symptoms and diagnosis. This would be particularly effective when, as in the case of SARS, symptoms are nondescript and difficult to distinguish from those of other illnesses. It was also emphasized that quarantine should not be viewed as an impermeable *cordon sanitaire* confining those at risk for illness with the known ill, but as a scalable, self-protective measure that can be adapted to local conditions.

Less problematic than quarantine, the isolation of infected individuals clearly played a central role in containing SARS. Although isolating SARS patients within hospitals could be viewed as increasing the risk of infection for health care workers and other hospital staff, evidence from Toronto indicates that hospital personnel can be protected through strict infection-control practices, such as washing hands, wearing masks and gloves, and requiring patients to wear masks. The most effective type of mask remains to be determined, however.

Finally, even if it were known which of the various strategies used to contain SARS were most effective, it is far from certain whether they would continue to be effective should SARS return. For example, although it appears that quarantine helped control SARS in China and Toronto, it did so largely because of the limited contagiousness of the virus. The likelihood that SCoV

**April 2, 2003:** WHO declares travel advisory for Hong Kong and Guangdong Province.
**April 4, 2003:** Role of Metropole Hotel in global epidemic identified.

| November | January |
|---|---|
| 2002 | 2004 |

could become more easily transmissible cannot be determined without a better understanding of its biology, ecology, and natural history—knowledge that will be essential to mounting a rational response should SARS recur (see Cetron et al. in Chapter 1).

### Evaluating SARS Containment Measures

**To plan rationally for the containment of a future SARS outbreak, it will be important to know the relative effectiveness of the various measures taken to contain the recent epidemic.** In the absence of such information, the strategy for containing SARS should emphasize overall preparedness at the local level in every community and hospital, participants agreed.

Participants discussed techniques and equipment to protect frontline caregivers of SARS patients in the hospital and at home. Simple habits such as frequent handwashing with soap and water are very important to prevent the transmission of any infectious agent. Other measures include wearing a mask that covers the nose and mouth, protective eyewear, gloves, gowns, or a containment suit. Participants noted that masks are effective only if they fit snugly and are not removed when the wearer coughs.

During the discussion of masks, participants debated the relative protectiveness of standard surgical masks compared with N-95 masks (so named because 95 percent of the time, they filter out any particle equal to or greater than 0.3 microns in size). Coronaviruses are smaller than 0.3 microns, so N-95 masks would not capture them; however, because viruses may travel in clumps, N-95 masks theoretically could capture some of the agent (University of California–Berkeley, 2003). Participants discussed a case control study in five Hong Kong hospitals in which wearers of surgical masks and N-95 masks did not contract the SARS coronavirus, while a few wearers of paper masks became infected (Seto et al., 2003). A larger study to validate this finding was proposed.

One workshop presentation described a relatively inexpensive mobile technology that potentially could be used to isolate individual patients during transport to and within hospitals, to protect staff during high-risk procedures such as intubation or bronchoscopy, to decontaminate large areas such as hospital waiting rooms or airplanes, and to create air exchange systems for isolation facilities or areas within hospitals (see Schentag et al. in Chapter 4). These mobile units remove and destroy airborne viral particles and droplets; the latter are widely believed to be the vector for SCoV transmission. Importantly however, it was

**April 16, 2003:** SARS coronavirus identified; WHO accuses Chinese government of underreporting SARS cases.

| November 2002 | | January 2004 |
|---|---|---|

noted that such technologies must be thoroughly evaluated to determine their suitability for containing SARS in a variety of clinical settings before they are recommended for use.

## CORONAVIRUS RESEARCH AND SARS

The SARS coronavirus (SCoV) appears to be zoonotic and to have originated in wild mammals in southern China. A coronavirus comprises single-stranded RNA inside a lipid envelope. Coronaviruses cause a substantial fraction of human colds and a number of common respiratory infections in other animals, including livestock and poultry (Holmes, 2003). Since its emergence, several veterinary and biomedical scientists have been called on to share their considerable knowledge of coronaviruses with a vast new audience and to join the research response to the epidemic. This experience—and the high value evident in available knowledge and understanding of coronavirus biology and molecular biology, gained at a time when coronaviruses were not recognized to be the causative agent of any severe infectious disease—attests to the value of basic research.

Based on their genetic sequences, the 14 previously known coronaviruses have been divided into three major groups. While SCoV has been linked with Group II coronaviruses, whose members include human and bovine respiratory viruses and the mouse hepatitis virus, there is still some debate over whether its genetic features might be sufficiently distinct to warrant classification within a separate, fourth class of coronaviruses.

Although coronaviruses generally cause disease in a single species, it has been demonstrated that some coronaviruses can cross species barriers. Moreover, RNA viruses are more likely to be zoonotic than DNA viruses. These findings lend credence to the hypothesis that SCoV is a zoonosis. Viruses resembling human SCoV reportedly have been detected in wild mammals of southern China that were brought to marketplaces where they were sold as exotic food. Immunological and genetic tests of these SCoV-like viruses suggest that human SCoV may be an animal virus transmitted to humans in the recent past (Guan et al., 2003).

### Understanding the Biology and Epidemiology of SARS

As one would expect of a newly characterized disease, much knowledge about the microbiology, pathogenesis, natural history, and epidemiology of SARS

**April 20, 2003:** Mayor of Beijing and Chinese Minister of Health fired.

| | |
|---|---|
| November | January |
| 2002 | 2004 |

---

**BOX S-1**
**Scientific Unknowns About SARS**

- What is the natural animal host of SCoV?
- How was the virus transmitted to humans, and under what circumstances might transmission across species recur?
- What is the potential for back-and-forth transmissions between humans and animals?
- Is there a persistent animal reservoir?
- Is the virus still present in human populations?
- Will the transmission of SCoV prove to be seasonal, as for influenza?
- What is the potential geographic range of SCoV?
- What role do cofactors play in mediating the severity of SARS symptoms?
- What explains the low rate of illness among children?
- What causes superspreading events?
- How important are routes of transmission other than infectious respiratory droplets? Under what circumstances do alternative modes of transmission occur?
- How does pathogenesis unfold at the cellular level, and especially in nonrespiratory tissues?

SOURCES: Breiman presentation; Denison presentation (see Chapters 1 and 3 respectively); WHO, 2003j.

---

remains to be discovered. For example, scientists have not yet identified the animal source of the infectious agent and have not determined whether a persistent animal reservoir of the infectious agent exists. It is also unclear whether SARS, like influenza, is a seasonal disease that would have receded on its own. Along the same lines, it remains to be seen whether SARS will reemerge on a seasonal basis, and if so, how virulent future manifestations of SCoV will be. These and other unanswered scientific questions, listed in Box S-1, were a prominent theme of workshop presentations and discussions. Answers to these questions would certainly advance the world's ability to predict and prepare for a resurgence of SARS.[7]

---

[7]The recent reemergence of human SARS infections in 2004 would indicate both an animal reservoir and a seasonality to disease emergence, but further investigation will be required for conclusive evidence.

**April 23, 2003:** WHO declares travel advisory for Beijing, Shanxi Province, and Toronto.

November
2002

January
2004

Considerable effort already has been applied to finding the animal source of SCoV. For example, viral isolates from suspected animal sources were genetically characterized and compared with samples of SCoV (see Guan et al. in Chapter 3). However, recalling previous investigations of outbreaks of Legionnaire's disease, Schistosomiasis, and *E. coli* 0157, workshop participants noted the crucial role played by epidemiological "detective work" in developing hypotheses that led ultimately to the source of transmission (Zhong et al., 2003).[8] **To this end, it was suggested at the workshop that a case control study of the first 50 to 100 SARS patients be conducted using epidemiological data collected in Guangdong Province. Such an endeavor may provide direction to further laboratory surveys of animal viruses to reveal the source of SCoV and, perhaps, its animal reservoir.[9]**

SARS researchers benefit from the wealth of literature on coronaviruses in general. Presentations by two coronavirus experts at the workshop summarized the current understanding of coronavirus biology and pathogenesis and suggested promising directions for research on SARS and other emerging zoonoses (see Saif and Denison in Chapter 3).

The pathogeneses of animal coronaviruses conform to a basic model of either intestinal (enteric) or respiratory infection. Enteric coronaviruses can cause fatal infections in young, seronegative animals. Respiratory coronavirus infections in adult animals have shown increased severity in the presence of several factors, including high exposure doses, respiratory coinfections, stress related to shipping or commingling with animals from different farms, and treatment with corticosteroids. **It is unknown whether SCoV is a respiratory virus or a pneumoenteric virus. This knowledge gap will stymie efforts to develop a vaccine or drug against SCoV.**

Studies of coronavirus replication reveal several mechanisms that account for the repeated, persistent infections typical of coronaviral disease. High rates of mutation and RNA-RNA recombination produce viruses that are extremely adaptable and capable of acquiring or regaining virulence. The relatively large coronavirus genome tolerates deletions, mutations, and substitutions and can recover from deleterious mutations. **Molecular biological studies have also identified**

---

[8]Workshop presentation by Robert Breiman, Centre for Health and Population Research, Dhaka, Bangladesh, October 1, 2003.

[9]Workshop presentation by Yi Guan, University of Hong Kong, September 30, 2003.

**April 28, 2003:** SARS contained in Vietnam.
**April 30, 2003:** WHO lifts Toronto travel advisory.

| November | January |
|---|---|
| 2002 | 2004 |

several potential targets for antiviral drug discovery, including viral binding and uncoating, replication, protein expression and processing, assembly, and release. Cellular functions on which the virus depends, such as cholesterol synthesis, membrane trafficking, and autophagy, also present opportunities for antiviral design (see Matthews et al. in Chapter 4).

The tendency of coronaviruses to undergo mutation and recombination represents a significant challenge for vaccine development. To date, no vaccine has been produced that can provide highly effective, long-term protection against respiratory coronavirus infections. Genetic approaches represent the best hope of overcoming this propensity for mutability, according to workshop presenters.[10] For example, it might be possible to find ways to limit RNA-RNA homologous recombination, or to identify areas in the genome that are more or less prone to survive mutation. Promising approaches to these challenges include the use of reverse molecular genetics to make specific mutations in the virus genome and test their functional effects.

Workshop presenters emphasized that appropriate animal models are needed immediately to advance the development of a SARS vaccine. Participants also noted that studies in existing animal models of coronavirus infection could play a role in the development of antiviral therapies against SARS. Ultimately, a range of natural and transspecies disease models will be critical to understanding the pathogenesis of this and other emerging zoonoses. **Coordinated, multidisciplinary research drawing on expertise in veterinary sciences, medicine, molecular biology, and virology will be needed to meet these goals. However, the coronavirus experts who presented at the workshop lamented that there is little encouragement or support for such critical cross-disciplinary research at present.**

## BUILDING DEFENSES AGAINST A REEMERGENCE OF SARS

### Anticipating the Reemergence

Considering the likelihood of a return of SARS under a variety of circumstances is an important first step in planning for a broad range of contingencies

---

[10]Workshop presentation by Alan Shaw, Merck Vaccine Co., October 1, 2003.

**May 3, 2003:** Taiwan outbreak grows to 100 cases; WHO sends team.
**May 8, 2003:** WHO declares travel advisory for Tianjin, Inner Mongolia, and Taipei.

| November | January |
|---|---|
| 2002 | 2004 |

and challenges. A trio of plausible scenarios was presented at the workshop (see Monaghan in Chapter 5). The first *scenario* entailed a resurgence of SARS in China, followed by limited spread to other countries in the region. Heightened surveillance and rapid response could quickly contain such an outbreak, but might also cause SARS to be viewed less as a threat and more as a public nuisance; this attitude could lead to a decline in vigilance, raising the risk of a future epidemic.

In the second scenario, SARS spreads to poor countries in Asia and Africa, where inadequate health systems, preexisting health problems, high population density, and weak government leadership result in high infection rates and mortality. Such an epidemic would prove difficult to contain and create a humanitarian emergency that would place costly demands on international policy makers and institutions as well as developed countries compelled to respond for reasons that were both humane and self-protective.

The final, scenario depicts the resurgence of SARS in key trading centers of Asia and Canada, followed by transmission to the United States, Brazil, India, Japan, and Europe.

And even if this epidemic produced fewer cases of SARS than in 2003, it would be likely to cause major disruptions in trade and investment flows.

In considering further preparations for the reemergence of SARS, workshop participants discussed the development of surveillance and containment strategies in case SARS reappears during the winter of 2004; ongoing efforts to develop diagnostic tools for SARS and other infectious diseases; and long-term prospects for the discovery and development of antiviral drugs and vaccines against this newly emergent disease.

## Continued Surveillance for SARS

For a number of reasons, workshop participants agreed that continued vigilance in light of SARS is warranted for a number of reasons. First, it is very likely that an animal reservoir for the virus exists in China. Second, the continued sale of live, small wild mammals in marketplaces and the preparation of these animals as food perpetuates a hypothesized route of SCoV transmission to humans. Third, the possibility that SARS, like influenza, is a seasonal disease means it could reappear during the winter of 2004. Finally, initial low-level transmission of the virus could elude clinical recognition and reporting of the disease.

**May 21, 2003:** WHO declares travel advisory for all of Taiwan.
**May 22, 2003:** Second wave of SARS begins in Toronto.

| November | January |
|---|---|
| 2002 | 2004 |

It was suggested that in the absence of inexpensive, accurate, and widely available SARS diagnostics, syndromic surveillance—particularly in populations at high risk for reemergence—might be important for spotting nascent outbreaks. This methodological strategy, which involves monitoring groups of signs and symptoms associated with disease activity—unusual spikes in the purchase of commonly available health remedies, for example, or surges in particular symptoms reported among routinely collected information from clinical sources—has shown some promise in the early detection of disease outbreaks in the United States (Institute of Medicine, 2003). However, because SARS symptoms are variable and difficult to distinguish from those of influenza and seasonal human coronavirus infections that emerge in the same populations, it is not clear that such methods would be capable at present of distinguishing the emergence of novel infections such as SARS without careful consideration of the utility, quantity, and specificity of the surveillance data to be collected. Until a specific diagnostic test becomes available, there will continue to be a substantial risk of both missed cases and false alarms, and syndromic surveillance methods should be evaluated as possible complements to rather than replacements for maintaining and strengthening traditional clinical reporting systems.

## Development of SARS Diagnostics

A rapid, specific, reliable, and inexpensive clinical diagnostic test for SARS would be a valuable tool for improving surveillance and limiting the transmission of SCoV. First, however, scientists must determine which tissues contain the highest concentrations of virus during the presymptomatic stage of infection. It was also noted that in confirmed cases of SARS, the virus appears to be located deep in the respiratory tract, making specimens difficult to collect.

### Available Diagnostics

Absent a clinical diagnostic test, suspected cases of SARS must be confirmed in the laboratory using reverse-transcription polymerase chain reaction (RT-PCR) or much slower methods involving serology or viral culture, isolation, and identification by electron microscopy (Yam et al., 2003).

According to WHO, the laboratory case definition of SARS requires one of the following:

**May 23, 2003:** SARS linked to masked palm civet and raccoon-dog; Hong Kong and Guangdong travel advisories lifted.

| November | January |
|---|---|
| 2002 | 2004 |

• A positive RT-PCR finding in two or more clinical specimens, sequential samples, or assays using separate RNA extracts from the same sample.
• Seroconversion or a fourfold increase in titer between the acute and convalescent phases of infection as determined by immunoassay.
• Isolation of the virus with RT-PCR validation.

Recent incidents have highlighted the critical need for both specificity and sensitivity of laboratory diagnostic procedures. To address these issues, WHO and the CDC continue to work to standardize test protocols, reagents, and controls and to establish procedures for evaluation and quality control throughout the global network of diagnostic laboratories that may handle suspected SARS cases (WHO, 2003m).

Workshop participants considered several platforms that could potentially be adapted for the rapid, clinical diagnosis of early, asymptomatic SCoV infection. For example, workshop participants considered the use of RT-PCR for detecting SCoV nucleic acids. A recent evaluation of two RT-PCR protocols found them to be highly specific for the SARS coronavirus; however, these protocols were insufficiently sensitive to detect the virus reliably in respiratory specimens. Testing two specimens from the same patient increased the probability of an accurate diagnosis (see Yam et al. in Chapter 4).

A different platform discussed at the workshop purportedly can identify the family, and possibly the genus, of known or novel infectious agents (see Sampath and Ecker in Chapter 4; Hogg, 2003). Unlike many RT-PCR techniques, which target nucleic acid sequences unique to a specific organism, this test amplifies strategically chosen, highly conserved sequences from the broadest possible grouping of organisms. The molecular weight of the amplimers is measured by electrospray ionization mass spectrometry. Then the relative amounts of each base (i.e., the percentage of adenine, cytocine, thiamine, and guanine) are deduced. The base-pair composition of the selected genetic sequence serves as a signature to identify and distinguish organisms in a sample.

Originally designed for the environmental surveillance of biowarfare agents, such technology could potentially diagnose SARS directly from a tissue sample, obviating the need for time-consuming viral culture. According to workshop presenters, their method can distinguish between SCoV and other coronaviruses and perhaps even between genetic variants of SCoV. However, it is important to note that the test's sensitivity has yet to be evaluated using samples of human SARS-infected tissue.

**May 31, 2003:** SARS contained in Singapore.

| | |
|---|---|
| November | January |
| 2002 | 2004 |

## Antiviral Drugs and Vaccines

As noted earlier, until basic research on the pathogenesis of SARS elucidates whether the infection is respiratory or pneumoenteric, it is unclear which tissues a therapeutic agent should target. That being said, preparing for a reemergence of SARS might include the strategic development of a vaccine and an antiviral drug.

Theoretically, an ideal vaccine would contain an epidemic more effectively than an ideal antiviral drug if a large segment of the population were vaccinated. Yet mathematical models of influenza described at the workshop indicate that an epidemic could be contained effectively by providing an antiviral prophylaxis to close contacts of index cases. Therefore, the parallel development of both a vaccine and a drug for SARS may be an effective course of action.

The perceived urgency of developing SARS therapeutics has led several pharmaceutical and biotechnology companies to pursue the development of countermeasures for SARS. Two advantages these companies enjoy are the panoply of veterinary vaccines against coronaviruses and the ease with which SCoV can be grown in culture.

Previous antiviral discovery efforts by researchers from Pfizer Inc., of New York, focused on the human rhinovirus 3C protease, a functional, genetic, and structural analog to a key SCoV protease named "3C-like" (3CL). This work has proved advantageous in searching for 3CL protease inhibitors. Together with scientists at the National Institute for Allergy and Infectious Diseases and the U.S. Army Medical Research Institute of Infectious Diseases, who had developed an assay to test candidate compounds for their ability to prevent death in SARS-infected monkey kidney cells, Pfizer tested existing compounds that had shown activity against the rhinovirus protease. An X-ray crystallographic atomic-level resolution model of 3C protease of human rhinovirus 14 served as the basis for structural models of the 3CL protease binding site. This structural information enabled the scientists to identify additional compounds that demonstrated significant antiviral activity. The group is currently evaluating the solubility, metabolic stability, and other physicochemical properties of some of these inhibitors in hopes of finding promising compounds for clinical development. Pfizer researchers are also employing structure-based design and combinatorial chemistry as an alternative, complementary strategy to discovering 3CL protease inhibitors (see Matthews et al. in Chapter 4).

Despite the research described earlier in this chapter and the wealth of literature on coronaviruses, it will take more time before a compound designed to

**June 13, 2003:** SARS contained in China, except Beijing.

|                                                    |                    |
|----------------------------------------------------|--------------------|
| November                                           | January            |
| 2002                                               | 2004               |

defeat SCoV reaches clinical trials. SARS vaccine development programs require biosafety level 3 conditions, which make research efforts slower and more expensive than other targets of less contagious microbes. For this reason and others, such as the genetically unstable nature of the virus and the current lack of an appropriate animal model, a vaccine for SARS could well postdate a return of the disease, perhaps by several years, even if such a product were steered through a streamlined development process. If SARS fails to reappear within the next few years, however, it is unlikely that either antiviral or vaccine development will continue, given the cost of these efforts.[11]

The Food and Drug Administration's (FDA's) Center for Biologics Evaluation and Research (CBER) conducts research to facilitate the development of needed biological products, including antiviral drugs and vaccines. Several functions handled by CBER during the SARS epidemic would pertain to future microbial threats. These include ensuring the availability of virus isolates for vaccine stock, recognizing research needs and contingencies in areas such as vaccine testing, and conducting public workshops on needed technologies, such as diagnostics.[12]

## LESSONS FROM SARS FOR FUTURE OUTBREAKS

Recognizing that it would be impossible to address the vast array of potential microbial threats individually, public health policy makers are formulating general strategies to evaluate and respond to outbreaks of all kinds. At the international level, revisions to the International Health Regulations—rules concerning infectious disease that legally bind WHO member nations—have been underway since 1995, and are expected to be completed in 2005. **Workshop participants concurred that efforts to address microbial threats should encompass and be enriched by existing strategies for defense against bioterrorism. As one participant noted, authorities do not know until well into an outbreak if it is a naturally occurring or manmade threat—in either case a robust and prepared system will be able to respond rapidly and effectively to contain disease spread.**

---

[11]Workshop presentation by Alan Shaw, Ph.D., Merck Vaccine Co., October 1, 2003.

[12]Workshop presentation by Kathryn Carbone, Ph.D., CBER, Food and Drug Administration, October 1, 2003.

**June 23, 2003:** SARS contained in Beijing.

|                                                              |              |
| ------------------------------------------------------------ | ------------ |
| November                                                     | January      |
| 2002                                                         | 2004         |

The importance of collaboration was a common theme among workshop discussions on research. It was discussed in the context of scientists around the globe who identified the causal agent of SARS, of veterinary and biomedical research communities studying zoonotic pathogens, and of private sector companies working in conjunction with government agencies and academia to develop antiviral drugs and vaccines.

Workshop participants considered what could be learned from the experience of SARS and how that knowledge could improve the public health community's response to future outbreaks of infectious disease. The principal topics discussed include:

- the early detection of outbreaks,
- effective communication to the public in the event of an outbreak,
- the promotion of research and development,
- strategies for containment, and
- multinational collaboration in implementing such strategies.

## Importance of Early Detection

The central response to SARS—surveillance and containment, when instituted promptly, rapidly, and effectively—applies to almost any microbial threat. It is clear that the initial delays in not only detecting the novel SCoV, but also alerting national and global health officials to the disease outbreak significantly increased the spread of SARS and its impact on affected countries. However, soon after the global outbreak alerts were issued, the timely recognition of the emergence of SARS in other countries proved to be an important factor in breaking all chains of transmission. The surveillance networks such as GOARN and GPHIN, supported by personnel and laboratories from 115 other partnerships, made this success ultimately possible. Along with these vital resources, workshop participants identified additional surveillance strategies for microbial threats; these include hospital-based surveillance systems capable of recognizing both known and novel diseases, and occupational clustering, with particular attention paid to illness in health care workers. Behavior-based surveillance could identify such phenomena as drug sales, or even such phenomena as the rapid rise in vinegar sales that occurred in response to SARS in Guangdong in January 2003

**July 2, 2003:** SARS contained in Toronto.

| | |
|---|---|
| November | January |
| 2002 | 2004 |

(vinegar is commonly used to combat respiratory illness in traditional Chinese medicine).

Drawing on the SARS experience, a recent WHO global consultation focused on strengthening national capacities for surveillance, response, and control of communicable diseases. After SARS, it was noted, "countries increasingly look at the integration of disease surveillance activities as an effective, efficient and sustainable approach to improving national capacities." Among recommendations issuing from this consultation was the admonition that "member states should review existing legal frameworks to further support strengthening of surveillance including participation of the private sectors and non-governmental organizations" (WHO, 2003k). Several workshop participants observed that more nationally and globally coordinated systems of information-sharing and data analyses among surveillance networks might dramatically improve the world's ability to contain microbial threats.

While discussing the critical role of laboratories for effective surveillance, concerns about laboratory safety were raised. Accidents in a Singapore clinical laboratory (described earlier in this chapter) and a Taiwan research laboratory have been responsible for SARS infections in workers (Center for Disease Control Taiwan, 2003). These incidents highlight the importance of hospital surveillance procedures and appropriate clinical management and infection control measures in preventing an outbreak. They should also raise the awareness of the research community, particularly given the many laboratories now conducting research on SARS, to the risks inherent in handling all communicable agents and the need for strict adherence to well established laboratory procedures.

Overall, workshop participants observed that surveillance must be backed up with action and reinforced by sufficient laboratory capacity, well-trained personnel, and a legal framework consistent with objectives of transparency, global cooperation, and sensitivity to the balance between public protection and the interests of individual countries and persons. Workshop discussants emphasized that investments made toward this end should capitalize on the existing networks and need not be prohibitively extensive or expensive.

### Strategies for Containing Future Threats

An estimated 75 percent of emerging human pathogens and 61 percent of all human pathogens are zoonotic (Taylor et al., 2001). Therefore, many predictions

**July 5, 2003:** SARS contained in Taiwan; WHO declares containment of worldwide epidemic.

| | |
|---|---|
| November | January |
| 2002 | 2004 |

about the nature of future novel pathogens anticipate the emergence of zoonoses. Thus, workshop participants considered the strategies for containing known zoonoses—in particular, influenza—as potential models for the containment of SARS and unidentified zoonotic diseases of the future.

*Lessons Learned from Influenza*

The same trends that ushered SARS into the human population have been apparent during a century of influenza outbreaks. The exponential increase in avian influenza virus infections among humans over the past decade has been associated with a sharp rise in the size and density of chicken and pig farm populations, their proximity to human settlements, and movement of animals through market channels, which in turn parallels the world's rapidly expanding and mobile population. As with SARS, animal markets provide the breeding ground for recent outbreaks of influenza; laboratory sources also appear to have sparked at least one epidemic. Fortunately, most of the recent influenza outbreaks did not feature the transmission of the virus to humans. However, experts agree that it is only a matter of time until a highly virulent and contagious flu, such as the strain that caused over 20 million and perhaps as many as 40 million deaths during the 1918 influenza epidemic, confronts the world (see Webby and Webster in Chapter 5).[13]

Vaccines and antiviral therapies play a significant role in containing epidemics of influenza. It is advantageous that the timing of annual outbreaks of influenza and the strain or strains of the virus can, to some extent, be anticipated. **However, strategic actions recommended against influenza that could also inform efforts to better prepare for other viral disease outbreaks have yet to be implemented. These strategies include:[14]**

---

[13]Shortly before the publication of this report in January 2004, the highly pathogenic H5N1 avian influenza virus was implicated in a human outbreak of the disease in Vietnam and Thailand. Sixteen of the 20 individuals so far infected have died. Thousands of birds in eight countries, including Vietnam, The Republic of Korea, Thailand, China, and Japan are suspected to be infected with the virus. See http://www.who.int/en/disease outbreaks for more information.

[14]Workshop presentation, Robert Webster, St. Jude's Children's Research Hospital, October 1, 2003.

**September 8, 2003:** Isolated case of SARS occurs in Singapore due to laboratory accident.

| November | January |
|---|---|
| 2002 | 2004 |

- stockpiling of broad-spectrum antiviral drugs,
- advanced development of pandemic strain vaccines,
- the establishment of surge capacity for rapid vaccine production, and
- the development of models to determine the most effective means of delivering therapies during an outbreak.

It is evident from the experience of the late 2003 influenza season that our supply and effectiveness of antiviral drugs, capabilities to accurately predict the best viral strain for annual vaccine production, and mechanisms for surge capacity production remain inadequate (Treanor, 2004; WHO, 2003o). Recognition of these vulnerabilities lead numerous workshop participants to call for greater scientific and financial investments to strengthen our defenses against these certain future threats.

*Quarantine*

Some emerging infections of the future, like SARS, may be truly novel threats for which the world—including its pharmacopoeia—is inadequately prepared. Lacking other forms of effective interventions, the implementation of quarantine or isolation strategies may prove valuable in such instances. Workshop participants discussed several ways that modeling tools might be used to improve and tailor such measures. Models based on detailed observations from previous epidemics can be used to predict demands on hospital capacity during a hypothetical epidemic and to guide the timing and nature of quarantine measures. Models that can estimate the length and severity of an unfolding epidemic will likely increase public acceptance of quarantine by permitting people to form realistic expectations of their sacrifice and its benefit to the community (see Amirfar et al. in Chapter 5).

**Evidence indicates that a modern approach to quarantine encompassing a range of options designed to reduce the frequency of social contact can significantly reduce the spread of infectious disease.** Such options include short-term, voluntary home curfew; suspension or cancellation of public activities (such as events, mass transit, or access to public buildings); and "snow day" or sheltering-in-place measures. These measures could be employed individually or in concert. In addition to or in place of these strategies, a program of contact surveillance—the monitoring of asymptomatic persons exposed to an infectious disease—could be undertaken. Modern quarantine and contact surveillance preserve individual liberties and require far less labor and other community re-

**December 5, 2003:** Taiwanese researcher contracts SARS during experiment.

| November | January |
|---|---|
| 2002 | 2004 |

sources than would be required to enforce a mandatory quarantine. Voluntary and other forms of scalable quarantine nevertheless reduce productivity and may result in public perceptions that stigmatize groups of individuals and promote irrational behavior. For example, there is evidence that consumers began to avoid Asian restaurants in the United States and other nonaffected countries during the SARS epidemic even though neither quarantine nor public health messages suggested such action. **For any quarantine to be effective, workshop participants noted, a number of needs must be met, including:**

- **education to build public trust in health authorities,**
- **compensation and job security for quarantined workers, and**
- **incentives to health care workers to maintain their morale in the face of increased risk and to pay greater attention to infection control practices.**

In the more difficult case of mandatory quarantine, enforcement requires careful planning and a clear understanding of public health law; this is particularly true in the United States, where quarantine is likely to necessitate the coordination of federal, state, and local jurisdictions and legal authorities. For example, if an infectious disease has the potential to spread across state boundaries but has not yet done so, an action by CDC to limit transmission would require the cooperation of appropriate state and local authorities. The presidential executive order adding SARS to a list of other diseases subject to federal quarantine actions eliminated such jurisdictional uncertainties (Executive Order 13295: Revised List of Quarantinable Communicable Diseases, 2003). Additional legal considerations include planning for due process—proper notice, legal representation, court-reviewed decisions, and remote communications to permit a quarantined person to be heard in court—and for practical contingencies, such as the need for law enforcement officials to serve notice of quarantine (see Matthews in Chapter 5).

Workshop participants also discussed the need to develop strategies by which hospitals—and entire communities, in the event of quarantine—can determine when precautions against infection can be scaled back. Some experts have argued that containment measures should be swiftly imposed in response to a perceived infectious disease threat (as occurred when SARS appeared in Vietnam) and reduced only after surveillance determines the absence of a threat. Clearly, the consequences of false alarms in this case must be weighed against the risks of

**December 7-10, 2003:** Infected researcher attends conference in Singapore.

| November 2002 | January 2004 |
| --- | --- |

inaction in the early stages of an epidemic, as demonstrated by China's experience with SARS.

## Informing the Public

Although no presentations exclusively addressed the subject of public communication, this topic was identified as important and was widely discussed by workshop participants. Social cohesion and compliance with quarantine in Toronto were attributed in part to a combination of clear communication and practical guidance by public health authorities. The media's sustained and intensive focus on the epidemic, heavy traffic on informational SARS websites operated by WHO and CDC, and a great volume of calls to CDC's SARS hotline reflect the public's hunger for news and information during the public health emergency.

Official travel and health advisories, though deemed necessary, were also linked to consumer avoidance of international travel, international events, and even Asian restaurants. It was suggested that such adverse effects could be mediated in the future by accompanying advisories with educational messages designed to help the public develop a realistic perception of the risks for infection and appropriate responses. **Research designed to identify why societies respond dramatically and irrationally to certain types of public health threats might help communicators to develop messages that positively influence the public's behavior during medical emergencies.**

The media's powerful role in the response to SARS was characterized in both positive and negative terms: as a cause of stigma and discrimination due to sensationalized reporting on the epidemic; as a demystifier of quarantine and other public health measures through exhaustive coverage; and, as a persuasive contributor to China's decision to cooperate with international efforts to control SARS. The Internet, recognized as a key source of early leads to the outbreak of SARS, was also viewed with concern for its potential to propagate false rumors. It is important to guard against such threats in the event of public health emergencies. Likewise, **it will be critical to make use of the media to inform and educate the public on how best to protect themselves and their communities in the event of future outbreaks**

**December 17, 2003:** Singapore authorities quarantine 70 individuals.

|  |  |
|---|---|
| November | January |
| 2002 | 2004 |

## Surge Capacity

*Health Care Personnel*

Workshop participants remarked that the strained capacity of the U.S. and global public health infrastructure—attributed to insufficient funding, labor short-ages, and a lack of facilities—impedes preparations for SARS and other threats to public health. As described earlier, even some of the highly developed health care systems of Toronto struggled to cope with inadequate numbers of health care personnel (particularly because of the inevitable toll that moderately to highly contagious diseases take on health care personnel) and were ultimately unable to sustain normal levels of care for both SARS and non-SARS patients.

**In moving forward, workshop participants suggested that up-to-date information and skills needed for containing epidemic-prone diseases must be better integrated into the training of** *all* **health care professionals**, not only those specializing in infectious diseases or infection control. In citing Toronto's call to health care personnel in other regions and countries, a participant recom-mended **the expansion and establishment of formal networks to rapidly iden-tify, transport, and enlist experienced health care personnel in the event of future outbreaks. Such contingencies would be designed for local, regional, national, and international responses and, in particular, would facilitate the mobilization of human and technical resources that are known to have pre-viously tackled certain disease outbreaks.** The question was asked, if SARS is to reemerge how will we harness the skills and new knowledge of the thousands of individuals involved with finally containing the disease? While some partici-pants lauded the efforts of GOARN and the CDC in this regard, they questioned if that was enough.

*Health Care Facilities*

The inability to effectively establish isolation areas and procedures within hospitals and other health care facilities contributed to the spread of SARS in several countries. Inadequate facilities not only promoted the spread of the dis-ease, but also forced the suspension of other vital health care procedures. As previously described, one workshop participant suspected that more patients died during the SARS outbreak in Toronto as a result of the inability to access appro-priate care for conditions other than SARS rather than from SARS itself.

**January 5, 2004:** China and WHO confirm SARS case in Guangdong Province.

| November 2002 | January 2004 |
|---|---|

As such, participants called for **preparedness planning that established procedures for rapid identification and use of facilities designated not only for treatment of suspected and confirmed cases of an epidemic disease, but also facilities that could be isolated for the conduct of other critical procedures such as emergency surgeries, trauma care, and organ transplantation.** In this regard, several participants credited the rapid construction of "SARS hospitals" in China as a key element in ultimately containing the disease.

### Supporting the Research Response

Years of investment in basic research on coronaviruses, largely in the veterinary research fields, helped the scientific community to identify the SARS coronavirus within months of its emergence. Consequently, **numerous participants noted that the potential for future outbreaks not only justifies present-day investments in basic research on viruses and microbes, but also argues for greater attention to and investment in research efforts that integrate the direct contributions of zoonotic infectious disease research with biomedical research efforts.** As noted earlier (see Box S-1), a number of basic scientific questions about the biology and epidemiology of SARS need to be answered in order to develop diagnostics and therapeutics for the disease, as well as to construct and implement targeted surveillance strategies. Apart from research that is specific to the SARS coronavirus, however, workshop participants discussed a number of broader areas of basic research that might be pursued in order to counter the threat that would arise from either a recurrence of SARS or the emergence of other new infections.

First, now that the more urgent pace of responding to an ongoing epidemic has subsided, researchers should be encouraged to thoroughly and methodically take stock of data that was accumulated over the course of fighting this epidemic. Workshop participants suggested that the public health community should not be complacent about the eventual success that was had in containing last year's SARS outbreak; **there remains a need to understand exactly what strategies were most effective, what strategies were less successful or even counterproductive, and what steps would be most essential for combating the emergence of a new and possibly more virulent or more infectious pathogen.** As part of this retrospective evaluation, for example, extant patient and hospital records should be assembled, compared, and analyzed in order to provide as exact an assessment as possible of the effectiveness of each of the many control measures that were adopted, as well as the points of greatest weakness that allowed the virus to spread. Some of the lessons to be learned will be specific to the profile of SARS, but many of them will also be readily applicable to other new infections in the crucial early stages of an epidemic when less is known about the biology of the disease than about its manner and rate of spread. On the next occasion when scientists and public health officials are confronted by a novel threat, it is important that they have a battery of well-researched studies to fall back on concerning measures that have previously been shown to be effective and feasible in controlling even a disease entity that has not yet been well characterized.

Secondly, this evaluative process should expand beyond those areas encompassed by clinical medicine and emergency care. The SARS epidemic illustrated how rapidly the impacts of a new disease can reverberate through the political and economic structures of successive countries and regions, and the decisions that were made in response to the epidemic ultimately reached into the highest levels of government and international bodies. Just as with the measures that were taken within individual hospitals and clinical settings, **the comparative effectiveness of the broader quarantine measures, travel advisories, communications with the general public, and other legal and public health directives that were issued should be gauged relative to their costs and difficulties. Any possible improvements in the measures that were adopted in the case of SARS—or recommendations for flexible options or combinations of options that might be applied in the face of different types of pathogens—may need to be examined within a broad and multidisciplinary discussion framework.**

Finally, basic research needs to be conducted into not only the measures that were most effective in containing the last epidemic but also those steps that would best facilitate research on understanding the next one. The uncertainty and confusion that are likely to be present in an epidemic's early stages may at least be ameliorated if scientists, public health officials, and governmental bodies understand and are well prepared to collect the types of data that have been shown to be most crucial in assessing the nature and magnitude of a novel threat. **A number of workshop participants commented on the need to look into better standards for data capture and coordination during the course of an epidemic, as well as the need to have better models on hand for evaluating the effects of possible intervention strategies as early as possible.** Likewise, while carefully controlled therapeutic trials are often impractical (or at best extremely difficult) during the first stages of a disease outbreak, some workshop participants lamented the fact that relatively little progress was made toward developing a standard treatment algorithm for SARS patients during last year's epidemic, and there remains significant controversy over the effectiveness of certain treatments that were applied. **It was suggested that in the case of any future epidemics, better pooling of data from scattered clinical treatment** centers could at least initiate the process of assessing the efficacy of different treatment strategies and provide groundwork for more reliable clinical advisories until the time and means are available for more thorough studies.

*Engaging the Private Sector*

Several presentations and considerable discussion concentrated on mechanisms that could potentially engage the private sector—specifically, pharmaceutical and biotechnology companies—in the research and development of products targeted at the greatest threats to public health, including infectious diseases.

For pharmaceutical researchers, streamlining the development process is crucial to productive engagement in strategic research. Means of streamlining this process include the clear identification of patient and physician needs, access to detailed biological studies of the pathogen of interest, and technologies such as computational and combinatorial chemistry that speed target selection and lead generation. Workshop presenters described the need for technology to improve predictions of the safety of drug candidates so unsafe compounds could be weeded out at an early and less expensive stage of the development process.

## Promotion of International Cooperation and Collaboration

If SARS never returns, the 2003 epidemic will nonetheless be remembered as a watershed event in the history of public health because of the degree of multinational cooperation to contain the disease. As the world becomes more conscious of microbial threats to health, countries are increasingly compelled to report infectious outbreaks and join international efforts to contain them. Recognizing that such transparency often comes at a price to a nation's economy, particularly in developing countries, workshop participants attempted to identify incentives to encourage nations and individuals to act for the common good.

Some participants offered specific ideas for incentives, including cooperative grants to support disease-monitoring efforts by academic researchers in developing countries and high-profile awards from bodies such as the Institute of Medicine or World Health Organization to countries or individuals who make important sacrifices for the health of world.

Networking can also play a vital role in local and regional preparedness for infectious disease threats. Tabletop exercises, in which detailed outbreak scenarios are presented to officials who develop a response based on the tools and resources at their disposal, encourage preparedness and provide a forum for building collaborations among the many individuals and sectors essential to an effective, coordinated response. From such exercises, the real-time compilation of epidemiological, clinical, and laboratory data that could be made available to the international community through WHO could also stimulate cooperation and collaboration. When implemented via the Internet or other communication networks, these exercises can be used to develop systems of communication, as well as working relationships, in advance of an outbreak or other emergency. Some countries are increasingly cognizant of the fact that the health of the global public affects the individual security of all nations, especially those that are most enmeshed in global networks of trade, tourism, and investment. Nevertheless, many governments continue to allocate inadequate resources to their health care systems and lack the political will to improve the quality of their public health systems and the integration of those systems nationally and internationally. This observation highlights an additional lesson offered by SARS, one that echoes what we have learned from HIV/AIDS, influenza, Ebola, malaria, and a host of other infectious diseases: the desperate state of public health infrastructure in much of the world, and especially in those countries where microbial threats are likeliest to emerge and take hold. If such lessons are to be heeded, global strategies to enhance the prevention and control capabilities of all nations will be important as the world prepares for future outbreaks of infectious disease.

Adel A.F. Mahmoud, M.D., Ph.D.          Stanley M. Lemon, M.D.
*Chair,* Forum on Microbial Threats     *Vice-Chair,* Forum on Microbial Threats

## REFERENCES

Center for Disease Control Taiwan. A report on the laboratory-acquired SARS in Taiwan. [Online] Available: http://www.cdc.gov.tw/sarsen/ [accessed January 19, 2004].

Centers for Disease Control and Prevention. Public health and aging: influenza vaccination coverage among adults aged ≥50 years and pneumococcal vaccination coverage among adults aged ≥65 years—United States, 2002. *MMWR* 52(41):987-92.

Enserink M. 2003. SARS in China. China's missed chance. *Science* 301(5631):294-6.

Eysenbach G. 2003. SARS and population health technology. *Journal of Medical Internet Research* 5(2):e14.

General Accounting Office. 2001. *Challenges in Improving Infectious Disease Surveillance Systems.* GAO-01-722. Washington, DC: GAO.

Guan Y, Zheng BJ, He YQ, Liu XL, Zhuang ZX, Cheung CLLSW, Li PH, Zhang LJ, Guan YJ, Butt KM, Wong KLCKW, Lim W, Shortridge KF, et al. 2003. Isolation and characterization of viruses related to the SARS coronavirus from animals in southern China. *Science* 302(5643):276-8.

Hogg C. 2003. Test for early detection of SARS. *BBC News.*

Holmes KV. 2003. SARS coronavirus: a new challenge for prevention and therapy. *Journal of Clinical Investigation* 111(11):1605-9.

Institute of Medicine. 2003. *Microbial Threats to Health: Emergence, Detection, and Response.* Washington, DC: The National Academies Press.

Lee N, Hui D, Wu A, Chan P, Cameron P, Joynt GM, Ahuja A, Yung MY, Leung CB, To KF, Lui SF, Szeto CC, Chung S, Sung JJ. 2003. A major outbreak of severe acute respiratory syndrome in Hong Kong. *New England Journal of Medicine* 348(20):1986-94.

National Intelligence Council. 2000. *National Intelligence Estimate: The Global Infectious Disease Threat and Its Implications for the United States.* NIE 99–17D. Washington, DC: NIC.

Seto WH, Tsang D, Yung RW, Ching TY, Ng TK, Ho M, Ho LM, Peiris JS. 2003. Effectiveness of precautions against droplets and contact in prevention of nosocomial transmission of severe acute respiratory syndrome (SARS). *Lancet* 361(9368):1519-20.

Singapore Government. 2003. Singapore government SARS website. [Online] Available: http://www.sars.gov.sg/ [accessed January 18, 2004].

Taylor LH, Latham SM, Woolhouse ME. 2001. Risk factors for human disease emergence. *Philosophical Transactions of the Royal Society of London-Series B: Biological Sciences* 356(1411):983-9.

Treanor J. 2004. Influenza vaccine—outmaneuvering antigenic shift and drift. *New England Journal of Medicine* 350(3):218-20.

University of California–Berkeley. 2003. Will a mask protect you? *UC Berkeley Wellness Letter.* [Online] Available: http://wellnessletter.com/html/wl/2003/wlFeatured0703.html.

World Health Organization (WHO). 2003a. Summary of probable SARS cases with onset of illness from November 2, 2002 to July 42, 2003. [Online] Available: http://www.who.int/csr/sars/country/table2003_09_23/en/ [accessed December 17, 2003].

WHO. 2003b. Acute respiratory syndrome in China—Update. [Online] Available: http://www.who.int/csr/don/2003_2_20/en/ [accessed December 17, 2003].

WHO. 2003c. Update 95—SARS: chronology of a serial killer. [Online] Available: http://www.who.int/csr/don/2003_07_04/en/.

WHO. 2003d. WHO issues a global alert about cases of atypical pneumonia. [Online] Available: http://www.who.int/csr/sars/archive/2003_03_12/en/.

WHO. 2003e. World Health Organization issues emergency travel advisory. [Online] Available: http://www.who.int/csr/sars/archive/2003_03_15/en/.

WHO. 2003f. Update 47—Studies of SARS virus survival, situation in China. [Online] Available: http://www.who.int/csr/sars/archive/2003_05_05/en/print.html.

WHO. 2003g. Update 96—Taiwan, China: SARS transmission interrupted in last outbreak area. [Online] Available: http://www.who.int/csr/don/2003_07_05/en/print.html.

WHO. 2003h. Update 70—Singapore removed from list of areas with local SARS transmission. [Online] Available: http://www.who.int/csr/don/2003_05_30a/en/print.html.

WHO. 2003i. Severe Acute Respiratory Syndrome (SARS)-multi-country outbreak-Update 13: China joins WHO collaborative network. [Online] Available: http://www.who.int/csr/don/2003_03_28/en/.

WHO. 2003j. WHO issues consensus document on the epidemiology of SARS. [Online] Available: http://www.who.int/csr/sars/archive/epiconsensus/en/print.html.

WHO. 2003k. Revision process of the International Health Regulations (IHR). [Online] Available: http://www.who.int/csr/ihr/revision/en/print.html.

WHO. 2003l; Severe acute respiratory syndrome (SARS) in Singapore—update 2: SARS case in Singapore linked to accidental laboratory contamination. [Online] Available: http://www.who.int/csr/don/2003_09_24/en/ [accessed January 18, 2004].

WHO. 2003m. Summary of the discussions and recommendations of the SARS laboratory workshop, October 22, 2003. [Online] Available: http://www.who.int/csr/sars/guidelines/en/SARS Lab meeting.pdf [accessed January 14, 2004].

WHO. 2003n. Update 11—WHO recommends new measures to prevent travel-related spread of SARS. [Online] Available: http://www.who.int/csr/sars/archive/2003_03_27/en/ [accessed January 20, 2004].

WHO. 2003o. Avian influenza ("bird flu") and the significance of its transmission to humans. [Online] Available: http://www.who.int/csr/don/2004_01_15/en/ [accessed January 26 2003].

Yam WC, Chan KH, Poon LLM, Guan Y, Yuen KY, Seto WH, Peiris JSM. 2003. Evaluation of reverse transcription-PCR assays for rapid diagnosis of severe acute respiratory syndrome associated with a novel coronavirus. *Journal of Clinical Microbiology* 41(10):4521-4.

Zhong NS, Zheng BJ, Li YM, Poon, Xie ZH, Chan KH, Li PH, Tan SY, Chang Q, Xie JP, Liu XQ, Xu J, Li DX, Yuen KY, Peiris, Guan Y. 2003. Epidemiology and cause of severe acute respiratory syndrome (SARS) in Guangdong, People's Republic of China, in February 2003. *Lancet* 362(9393):1353-8.

# 1

# SARS: Emergence, Detection, and Response

## OVERVIEW

The story of the emergence, spread, and control of severe acute respiratory syndrome (SARS) is the latest, most vivid episode of a microbial threat in our highly connected world. The SARS epidemic of 2002–2003 not only demonstrated the ease with which a local outbreak can rapidly transform into a worldwide epidemic, but also how news of such a threat can travel faster than a microbe. Notably, the experience demonstrated how effectively the global public health community can collaborate to contain a novel microbial threat.

SARS emerged in November 2002 in the southern Chinese province of Guangdong and has been linked with the handling and preparing of exotic mammals for human consumption. The virus ultimately spread to 30 countries and administrative regions within 6 months. Key points in the chronology of the epidemic are included in the Summary and Assessment.

This chapter begins with a description of the World Health Organization's (WHO) coordination of a massive and multinational public health response to SARS. While the authors emphasize that the actions of individual nations ultimately contained the epidemic, they describe the many ways that WHO supported governments through its Global Outbreak Alert and Response Network (GOARN) and its country offices. These efforts served to highlight the important brokering role that can be played by the WHO in catalyzing and galvanizing the capacity of its member states in response to global public health challenges. This is followed by a discussion of the contributions made by the U.S. Centers for Disease Control and Prevention (CDC) in responding to and helping contain the SARS outbreak in the U.S. and overseas. In both of these papers, the authors describe not just the actions taken by the WHO and the CDC during the recent epidemic but also the lessons that were learned and the preparations being made to handle any future challenges that may arise from SARS or other emerging diseases.

The chapter continues with a broad overview of what is known and hypothesized about the emergence of SCoV, the natural history of the epidemic, the evolution of the virus, and the clinical profile of SARS. The authors suggest studies to answer some of the many remaining questions about this new disease.

Given the likelihood of an animal reservoir for the virus in China that could reinfect the human population, continued vigilance for SARS is warranted. This chapter explores the value of modern quarantine in curtailing the spread of infectious disease in general and SARS in particular. Risks for the reintroduction of SARS include the possibility of initial low-level transmission that eludes surveillance and a laboratory-acquired infection, as occurred in Singapore in September 2003 and in Taiwan in December 2003.

During the epidemic, hospitals in Hong Kong, Singapore, Vietnam, and Canada struggled to contain SARS within their walls. For example, in the first phase of the Toronto epidemic, which began on February 23, unrecognized SARS patients infected scores of other patients, family members, and hospital workers. Even after increased infection control measures were undertaken, this scenario was replayed in several area hospitals, as well as others around the globe. A sobering analysis of mistakes made in the communication and practice of hospital and community hygiene during the epidemic concludes the chapter.

## THE WHO RESPONSE TO SARS AND PREPARATIONS FOR THE FUTURE

*J.S. Mackenzie, P. Drury, A. Ellis,*[1] *T. Grein, K.C. Leitmeyer,*
*S. Mardel, A. Merianos, B. Olowokure, C. Roth, R. Slattery, G. Thomson,*
*D. Werker, and M. Ryan*
Global Alert and Response, Department of Communicable Disease
Surveillance and Response

Severe acute respiratory syndrome (SARS) is the first severe and readily transmissible new disease to emerge in the 21st century. Initially recognized as a global threat in mid-March 2003, SARS was successfully contained in less than 4 months, largely because of an unprecedented level of international collaboration and cooperation. The international response to SARS was coordinated by the World Health Organization (WHO) with the assistance of the Global Outbreak

---

[1]Strategy for Development and Monitoring Zoonoses, Foodborne Diseases and Kinetoplastidae, Department of Communicable Diseases Control, Prevention and Eradication, World Health Organization, Geneva, Switzerland.

Alert and Response Network (GOARN) and its constituent partners made up of 115 national health services, academic institutions, technical institutions, and individuals. The SARS outbreak has also shown how, in a closely interconnected and interdependent world, a new and poorly understood infectious disease can have an adverse affect not only on public health, but also on economic growth, trade, tourism, business and industrial performance, and political and social stability.

The chronology of the outbreak has been published on the WHO website (WHO, 2003a). The first recorded case occurred in mid-November in the city of Foshan, Guangdong Province, China. The Chinese Ministry of Health officially reported to WHO in mid-February that there had been 300 cases and 5 deaths in an outbreak of "acute respiratory syndrome" in which symptoms were clinically consistent with atypical pneumonia, and that the outbreak was coming under control. To complicate the issue, however, there were also cases of avian influenza, influenza A (H5N1), with three deaths among members of a Hong Kong family who had traveled to Fujian Province. WHO activated its global influenza laboratory network and called for heightened global surveillance on February 19, 2003; GOARN partners were alerted on February 20.

The SARS virus was carried out of southern China on February 21, when a 64-year-old medical doctor who had treated patients in Guangzhou and was himself suffering from respiratory symptoms checked into a room on the ninth floor of the Metropole Hotel in Hong Kong. Through mechanisms that are not yet fully understood, he transmitted the SARS virus to at least 16 other guests, all linked to the ninth floor. Those guests carried the disease to Toronto, Singapore, and Hanoi, or they entered hospitals in Hong Kong. The medical doctor fell severely ill the following day, was hospitalized immediately, and died on March 4. A global outbreak was thus seeded from a single person on a single day on a single floor of a Hong Kong hotel.

A businessman, infected in the Metropole Hotel, traveled to Hanoi, fell ill, and was hospitalized on February 26. He was attended by a WHO official, Dr. Carlo Urbani, following concerns raised by hospital staff. Alarmed at the unusual disease and concerned that it could be an avian influenza, Dr. Urbani contacted the WHO Western Pacific Regional Office (WPRO) on February 28.

On March 10, the Ministry of Health in China asked WHO to provide technical and laboratory support to clarify the cause of the Guangdong outbreak of atypical pneumonia. On March 12, WHO alerted the world to the appearance of a severe respiratory illness of undetermined cause that was rapidly spreading among hospital staff in Vietnam and Hong Kong. Three days later, on March 15, it became clear that the new disease was carried along major airline routes to reach new areas, and WHO issued a further global alert, giving the new disease its name: severe acute respiratory syndrome, or SARS.

## The WHO Response

As the outbreak of SARS moved into the spotlight of intense global concern, an unprecedented multifaceted, multilateral, and multidisciplinary response was coordinated jointly by WHO Headquarters, Switzerland, and by WHO WPRO, the Philippines. The management of the global SARS response involved intense daily coordination in the areas of etiology and laboratory diagnosis, surveillance and epidemiology, clinical issues, animal sources, and field operations.

WHO Regional Offices, working through a worldwide network of Country Offices and intercountry networks, were the main channels for support to affected countries. While the six WHO Regional Offices were fully engaged in the global coordination of the SARS response, the Western Pacific Regional Office—covering the area where the vast majority of cases were occurring—bore the brunt of the response, deploying a total of 116 additional experts as short-term consultants during the outbreak. At WHO Headquarters, 75 people worked on the SARS outbreak response, with additional surge capacity provided by partners in the GOARN.

The GOARN is a global technical partnership, coordinated by WHO, to provide rapid multidisciplinary support for outbreak response to affected populations (WHO, 2000; 2001). The GOARN provided critical operational capacity for the initial response to SARS. Responding to requests for assistance from several countries, WHO and its GOARN partners mobilized field teams to support outbreak response in China, Hong Kong, Singapore, Taiwan, and Vietnam. Throughout the outbreak, WHO continued to work with GOARN partners to ensure ongoing support to health authorities, and GOARN teams continued in the field until the chains of transmission were conclusively broken.

Through GOARN, WHO coordinated development of a number of networks that proved pivotal in developing tools and standards for containment of the epidemic. The networks met regularly by teleconference, usually on a daily basis, to share information and data in real time. They were also assisted by dedicated, secure websites on which network participants were able to share preliminary information. The networks brought frontline workers and international experts together, and demonstrated the international collaboration and cooperation that was characteristic of the response to the SARS outbreak. A virtual network of clinicians was set up to exchange experiences, thoughts, and findings about SARS in an attempt to better understand and treat the disease effectively. The clinical network linked infection control issues closely with every aspect of case management, from clinical diagnosis and investigation to therapy. The discussions also allowed the rapid evaluation of the infection control risks of a number of interventions and helped to indicate potential alternative approaches.

A virtual network of epidemiologists brought together public health institutions, ministries of health, and WHO Country Offices to analyze the spread of SARS and to define appropriate public health measures. Activities of the *epidemiology network* have included the preparation of a consensus document on the epidemiology of SARS (WHO, 2003b). The *laboratory network* was established to assist with identifying the etiologic agent of SARS and to develop specific and robust laboratory diagnostic tests for the agent responsible. The network comprised members of the international influenza laboratory network in those countries in which cases of SARS had been reported. Thus a total of 11 expert laboratories in nine countries were included in the network. The success of the laboratory network was quickly demonstrated by the discovery and characterization of the etiological agent, the SARS coronavirus (SCoV), and the rapid development of the first generation of diagnostic tests.

### WHO Country Offices: A Critical In-Country Presence

WHO Country Offices work as direct partners with Member States on all issues related to health, including those related to health and poverty, health and macroeconomic reforms, and the Millennium Development Goals. SARS dramatically illustrated the effects of a new disease on the broader health and development agenda.

Traditionally, the Ministry of Health is the primary working partner at the national level; however, in many countries WHO is encouraging a more inclusive definition of the nature of the health sector, leading to greater collaboration with other government institutions, United Nations agencies, nongovernmental organizations (NGOs), and the international donor community—this was particularly important in the SARS outbreak response.

During the SARS outbreak, WHO was widely recognized as a key organization to assist health authorities with national policy formulation and multisectoral coordination of preparedness activities and the SARS outbreak response. WHO provided objective and neutral policy and technical advice to strengthen the capacity of national health administrations to better manage preparedness activities and the SARS outbreak response and to build local capacity. WHO Country Offices—particularly in China and Vietnam—provided extensive technical input on policy development, guidelines and strategies, dissemination of information on key issues, and technical advice for preparedness and response activities. The WHO Country Offices in Beijing and Hanoi, supported considerably by experts from partners in GOARN and WPRO, worked with national authorities to address rapidly developing needs: strengthening disease surveillance and reporting systems; improving the classification and reporting of cases; and advising on field epidemiology, contact tracing, infection control in health care settings, rumor management, and risk communications.

Ultimately, controlling the course of SARS in China and elsewhere was the result of concerted multisectoral preparedness and outbreak response activities by national authorities. WHO's activities and advice played an important role in catalyzing and coordinating this reponse. These activities are increasingly the routine work of a WHO Country Office anywhere in the world; however, the scale of the SARS outbreak and the attendant political and media interest ensured that the scale of operations was enormous.

In addition to providing direct support through WHO to affected areas, many GOARN partners were also involved in other SARS activities, including providing bilateral assistance to affected areas and supporting other countries in the Western Pacific and Southeast Asia regions. The International Federation of Red Cross and Red Crescent Societies helped to ensure that marginalized sections of society were reached by social mobilization activities. International NGOs and United Nations organizations were also involved in addressing humanitarian aspects of the response and preparedness activities. National surveillance and response institutions provided experts for field teams and, participating in the virtual networks, were also working at their own national levels to enhance preparedness and reporting on SARS cases to WHO. Regional disease surveillance networks provided information on measures and activities to be undertaken to prevent and control outbreaks of SARS.

The initial call for global surveillance was followed by a more detailed description of the surveillance system, which had as its objectives describing the epidemiology of SARS and monitoring the magnitude and spread of the disease in order to provide advice on prevention and control. This description, including revised case definitions and reporting requirements to WHO, was distributed with tools for its implementation through the WHO network to national public health authorities. It was also published on April 4, 2003, in the *Weekly Epidemiological Record* (Anonymous, 2003). With some minor changes, this global surveillance system remained in place until July 11, 2003, a week after the last chain of human transmission was broken.

Global SARS surveillance was primarily based on the reporting mechanism established through the *Daily Country Summary of Cases of SARS*. This form requested national public health authorities to report to WHO Geneva (with a copy to the WHO country and regional office) the number of new cases and deaths since the previous report, the cumulative number of probable cases and their geographic distribution, and the areas where local chains of transmission had occurred. Case numbers and information on areas with local transmission were updated daily on the WHO website in accordance with the information received by the national public health authorities. Local transmission was defined as one or more reported probable case(s) of SARS having most likely acquired the infection locally, regardless of the setting in which this may have occurred. An area was removed from the list 20 days after the last reported locally acquired probable case died or was appropriately isolated.

By July 11, 2003, 29 countries had reported a total of 8,437 probable cases, including 813 deaths (crude case fatality ratio 8.6 percent) from November 1, 2002. Ninety-two percent ($n = 7,754$) of the reports were received from China (including Hong Kong, Macao, and Taiwan). In the final compilation of reports received from public health authorities, there were 18 areas in 6 countries that experienced local transmission of SARS, with the first reported chain transmission starting on November 16, 2002, in Guangdong Province, China (WHO, 2003c).

## The Origin of the Etiological Agent

As the SARS outbreak spread, and before the etiological agent was identified, questions were being raised as to where this new infection had originated. Early discussions between members of the first WHO Mission in China and colleagues from the Chinese Centers for Disease Control (CDC and Guangdong CDC implicated food preparers possibly connected with preparation of animals for food as being a particular risk group. As a result, on April 10 WHO formed an internal working group to address the potential that SARS could be a zoonotic disease. With the collaboration of the Food and Agriculture Organization (FAO) and the Office of International des Epizooties (OIE), an international working group on the animal reservoir of SARS was established. Animal susceptibility studies were carried out in various laboratories around the world. Subsequently, findings from Guan et al. (2003) from the University of Hong Kong indicated that masked palm civets and raccoon dogs sampled in a Shenzen market carried a virus very similar to SCoV.

In mid-July, WHO received permission to organize a mission to China to review animal studies conducted by Chinese scientists and recommend further research on the role of animals in the transmission of SCoV. The mission was carried out as a joint endeavor among the government of China, FAO, and WHO from August 10 to 22, 2003. A comprehensive report of the mission and recommendations were provided to the government of China for review. Important collaborations were established between members of the mission and Chinese scientists. Collaborative projects are ongoing and focus on developing a screening test for animals, animal susceptibility studies, and further testing of animals from markets. As part of enhanced SARS surveillance in China, wild animal handlers are considered a high-risk group. Protocols have been developed to prompt an appropriate epidemiological investigation should this group begin presenting at hospitals with symptoms of SARS.

## Preparations for the Future

### Reemergence

Will SARS return? This is difficult to answer without recourse to a crystal ball. If SARS is to return, it has to reemerge from one of three sources: (1) from undetected transmission cycles in areas with little or no health care facilities; (2) from an animal source; or (3) from a laboratory accident. With respect to the first possible source, it is difficult to believe that there have been continued, undetected transmission cycles. However, as SCoV is believed to have spread into the human population from a wild animal source, this has to remain a possibility, but whether it will occur this year or sometime in the future remains unknown. Preliminary results would indicate that SCoV, or a related virus, occurs in a number of wildlife species. However, the ability of the virus to cross the species barrier to cause disease in humans, and then to become adapted to transmit between humans, may be a relatively rare event. Of greater immediate concern is the threat posed by stocks of SCoV and clinical specimens potentially containing SCoV, which are kept in many laboratories globally, as well as the paucity of safer biosafety level 3 (BSL3) facilities in many parts of south and eastern Asia.

*Surveillance and Laboratory Safety*

WHO has been very active in preparing for the possible return of SARS. Of particular importance has been the preparation of an epidemiological and surveillance document, *Alert, Verification and Public Health Management of SARS in the Post-Outbreak Period,* which was posted on the WHO website on August 14 (WHO, 2003d); a workshop concerned with laboratory preparedness and planning to ensure rapid, sensitive, and specific early diagnosis of SCoV infections, and aspects of biosafety in the laboratory (WHO, 2003e); clinical trial preparedness; a meeting to determine SARS research priorities; training courses on SARS diagnosis and epidemiology; a meeting to discuss the development of SCoV vaccines (WHO, 2003f); and a series of capacity-building developments and assistance to countries within the Western Pacific Region as well as a continuing dialogue with and assistance to China.

Health authorities in nodal areas, where cases had occurred previously, and in areas of potential re-emergence (WHO, 2003d) have maintained heightened SARS surveillance established during the outbreak period, and continue doing so for the foreseeable future. WHO will also continue to identify and verify rumors about SARS through its usual, well-established mechanisms.

Laboratory preparedness has been a major concern as the northern hemisphere has approached the winter season with the prospects of increased influenza activity and other respiratory diseases, potentially leading to a significant increase in requests for diagnostic tests for SCoV. This could lead to an unsustainable surge in the work of clinical diagnostic laboratories, and the strong possibility of false-positive test results. Thus a number of recommendations were made at a SARS laboratory workshop held in Geneva in October 2003, all of which have been introduced or are in the process of being introduced (WHO, 2003e). The major outcomes have been the establishment of an International SARS Reference and Verification Laboratory Network to provide a diagnostic service to those countries and areas that do not have the necessary diagnostic facilities and to verify any laboratory-diagnosed case of SCoV infection reported in the interepidemic period; the development of a panel of positive control sera; and the formulation of strong recommendations about laboratory safety. Indeed, biosafety has become a major issue since the occurrence of the laboratory-acquired cases in Singapore and Taiwan (WHO, 2003f), and a major biosafety document is nearing completion with respect to the containment level and conditions under which work is undertaken with live SCoV. This document will support and extend the earlier document posted on the WHO website (WHO, 2003g). Finally, the workshop attendees considered the algorithms under which laboratory diagnosis should be undertaken, and these have been incorporated into the algorithms developed in the epidemiological document *Alert, Verification and Public Health Management of SARS in the Post-Outbreak Period.*

### Diagnostics and Therapeutic Countermeasures

Insufficient evidence is available to evaluate the effectiveness of specific treatment measures, including antivirals, steroids, traditional Chinese medicine, and the appropriate type of mechanical ventilation. Therefore, generic protocols urgently need to be developed for SARS and other future disease outbreaks. The WHO SARS Clinical team hosted a workshop to plan future clinical trials for SARS with the following objectives: (1) to review treatment experiences in different countries during the last outbreak; (2) to share existing plans for future clinical trials and identify candidate therapies; (3) to agree on basic trial design, including a hierarchy of outcome parameters and agreed standards of care; and (4) to assist in preparedness for clinical trials at relatively short notice.

A SARS Research Advisory Committee was established to determine the major gaps in our knowledge of the origin, ecology, epidemiology, clinical diagnosis and treatment, and social and economic impacts of SARS, and to discuss research needs required to fill these gaps for effective public health management of SARS, including preparedness and response to future outbreaks. The committee was asked to prioritize the research issues with the aim that the prioritized list of issues could be widely circulated to international and national funding bodies as a consensus blueprint of international research objectives aimed at achieving a better understanding of the virus, its origins, and pathogenesis, so that public health management could be improved if SCoV returns. A report on the meeting is available on the WHO website (WHO, 2003h), and the full recommendations will be placed on the website in early 2004.

Training courses on laboratory diagnosis of SCoV were held in the fall in collaboration with WHO Regional Offices in Europe and Africa, and a further "train-the-trainer" course is being planned in association with the WHO Regional Office for the Americas (AMRO/PAHO) in 2004.

WHO has also held a meeting to discuss possible SCoV vaccines, and a number of recommendations were made to facilitate and accelerate SARS vaccine development and evaluation (WHO, 2003i).

In the Western Pacific Region, a number of activities have been started that are aimed at improving preparedness for the possible reemergence of SCoV, including updating existing guidelines for surveillance and response activities in the interoutbreak period, updating an assessment protocol for national preparedness, and developing a WPRO SARS risk assessment and preparedness framework (WHO Western Pacific Regional Office, 2003). Other priorities have been to strengthen infection control and establish a regional laboratory network. The objectives of the latter are to ensure proper laboratory diagnosis by providing coordination, technical support, and communication among country and regional reference laboratories.

### Concluding Comments

WHO's vision for global health security is a world on alert and ready to respond rapidly—both locally and globally—to epidemic-prone and emerging disease threats, whether they are natural or intentional in origin, minimizing their impact on the health and economy of the world's populations.

Defense against the threat posed by epidemics such as SARS requires a collaborative, multifaceted response. National and international public health systems represent a major pillar of action for rapid and effective containment.

Through unprecedented collaboration the world community has demonstrated that it is possible to contain a serious infectious threat to the world population. Pivotal to addressing future threats is the need for a global coordinating mechanism that allows the worldwide community to be alerted and to respond to health events of international concern as rapidly, appropriately, and effectively as possible. The World Health Assembly recognized the role played by WHO, its staff, and GOARN partners during the 56th Assembly in passing a resolution, WHA56.29, in which it strongly supported the GOARN partnership and WHO's global role in surveillance and response to infectious disease threats.

Harnessing the undoubted global capacities for detection, characterization, and containment of epidemic threats will require sustained strategic investment in initiatives like GOARN. However, at the end of the day these threats can only truly be faced with the courage and personal sacrifice as made by the thousands of individuals who came together to put a genie back in the bottle.

## THE CENTERS FOR DISEASE CONTROL AND PREVENTION'S ROLE IN INTERNATIONAL COORDINATION AND COLLABORATION IN RESPONSE TO THE SARS OUTBREAK

*James W. LeDuc and Anne Pflieger*
National Center for Infectious Diseases, Centers for Disease Control and Prevention, Atlanta, Georgia

The global outbreak of an acute respiratory illness that became known as severe acute respiratory syndrome (SARS) was the first major international outbreak of the 21st century and clearly had a dramatic, worldwide effect far exceeding the morbidity and mortality that directly resulted from infection with the novel coronavirus that causes SARS. In addition to the infection and hospitalization of several thousand individuals and the nearly 900 deaths that occurred in the countries with SARS cases, the entire global economy was affected by SARS, leading to serious losses of revenue, collapse of regional tourist and travel industries, and significant decreases in the gross national product among the nations affected (Lee and McKibbin, 2003). Despite several introductions of the virus from returning infected travelers, the United States was spared from the worst of SARS, given that there was no significant secondary spread, no large hospital-based outbreaks as seen in several countries, and no fatalities.

The fact that the United States had relatively few cases belies the enormous effort put forth by public health officials in responding to the outbreak. The Centers for Disease Control and Prevention (CDC) worked closely with state and local governments, the health care delivery industry, and other federal agencies to actively alert the traveling public about the risks of SARS, to prepare the health care delivery system to recognize and treat suspected SARS patients, and to assure the public that appropriate interventions to protect them from infection were being taken. These efforts were undertaken in close collaboration with international partners in the World Health Organization (WHO) and in the countries most affected by SARS. The collaborative international response can be considered in five parts: coordination of response, collaborations in science, communications at home and abroad, capacity building and response preparedness, and challenges and lessons learned.

## Coordination of Response

More than 800 CDC staff members were organized into 13 domestic teams, with core members serving throughout most of the 7-month response period. Domestic teams each focused on one critical aspect of the response, including clinical care and infection control, epidemiology of the outbreak, diagnostics and laboratory studies, quarantine issues, information management, occupational health issues (included staff from the National Institute for Occupational Safety and Health), communications, environmental issues, and community outreach programs focused on the challenges of providing accurate information to special groups such as immigrants and the Asian community. In addition, two teams were organized to review and offer constructive criticism of the response as it unfolded and to plan for possible pandemic transmission of SARS, and two other teams engaged in international efforts to respond to the outbreak and conduct subsequent scientific studies. Each group worked closely with experts from throughout the CDC Centers and often included members from other federal agencies (e.g., Department of Defense, Department of State, and National Institutes of Health, Food and Drug Administration [FDA], and others from the Department of Health and Human Services [DHHS]) or affected countries (specifically Canada). Many of the groups held frequent telephone conference calls with their constituents and academic experts to brainstorm and discuss next steps. For example, weekly telephone conference calls with virologists from several academic centers were held to coordinate laboratory studies, share results, and design collaborative studies, which often were undertaken by these same scientists at their own facilities.

CDC staff were deployed either directly to affected countries, as was the case with Taiwan, or as part of the WHO-coordinated Global Outbreak Alert and Response Network deployments. A total of 84 staff members were dispatched on 92 deployments to 11 countries affected by the SARS outbreak (CDC, unpublished) (see Tables 1-1 and 1-2). The largest group of personnel, 30 individuals, was sent to Taiwan, where a total of 696 person-days of assistance were provided. In all, staff were deployed for a total of 1,959 days, or 7.8 work-years, as determined on the basis of the standard U.S. federal work schedule. Deployed staff contributed diverse skills and expertise to these deployments (Table 1-2). Medical officers and epidemiologists were dispatched most often, with these personnel going to Taiwan (17), China (12), Vietnam (8), Singapore (2), the Philippines (3), Hong Kong (4), Canada (4), Switzerland and Thailand (2 shared), and Cambodia and Laos (1 shared). Other critical staff included pathologists and laboratory scientists, infection control officers, industrial hygienists, information management specialists, public health administrators, and communications experts. As the outbreak continued and staff rotations were required, it soon became apparent that CDC staff alone would be insufficient to meet a sustained demand for deployment of skilled personnel. As a result, the search to identify appropriate and available personnel was expanded to include public health professionals at state and local health departments, hospitals, other public health agencies, and academic centers.

**TABLE 1-1** CDC's 2003 International SARS Response by Center, Institute, Office (CIO)

| CIO | Number (%) of Staff Deployed | Number (%) of Days Deployed |
| --- | --- | --- |
| EPO | 7   (8.3) | 197   (10) |
| NCCDPHP | 3   (3.6) | 68   (3.5) |
| NCEH | 1   (1.2) | 29   (1.5) |
| NCHSTP | 4   (4.8) | 115   (5.9) |
| NCID | 59 (70.2) | 1,345 (68.7) |
| NIOSH | 6   (7.1) | 83   (4.2) |
| NIP | 4   (4.8) | 122   (6.2) |
| Total number | 84 | 1,959 |

NOTE: EPO = Epidemiology Program Office; NCCDPHP = National Center for Chronic Disease Prevention and Health Promotion; NCEH = National Center for Environmental Health; NCID = National Center for Infectious Diseases; NIOSH = National Institute for Occupational Safety and Health; NIP = National Immunization Program.

**TABLE 1-2** CDC International SARS Response: Staff Deployed by Country and Area of Technical Expertise

| Country | Number (%) of Staff Deployed | No. (%) of Days Deployed | Med/Epi | Path/Lab | Inf Cont | Ind Hyg | Data/IT | PHA | Consult | Media |
|---|---|---|---|---|---|---|---|---|---|---|
| Taiwan | 30 (32.6) | 696 (35.5) | 17 | 1 | 5 | 4 | | 3 | | |
| China | 17 (18.5) | 498 (25.4) | 12 | 5 | | | | | | |
| Vietnam | 10 (10.9) | 226 (11.5) | 8 | 1 | 1 | | | | | |
| Singapore | 5 (5.4) | 137 (7) | 2 | 2 | | | 1 | | | |
| Philippines | 4 (4.3) | 98 (5) | 3 | | 1 | | | | | |
| Hong Kong | 6 (6.5) | 88 (4.5) | 4 | | 1 | | 1 | | | |
| Thailand | 4 (4.3) | 60 (3.1) | 2 | | | | | 2 | | |
| Canada/ Ottawa | 5 (5.4) | 57 (2.9) | 3 | | | | | | | 2 |
| Canada/ Toronto | 4 (4.3) | 46 (2.5) | 1 | | | 3 | | | | |
| Switzerland | 4 (4.3) | 33 (1.7) | | | | | | | 2 | |
| Cambodia | 1 (1.1) | 15 (0.8) | | | | | | | | |
| Laos | 2 (2.2) | 5 (0.3) | 1 | | | | | 1 | | |
| **Total:** | | | | | | | | | | |
| By deployment | 92 | | 53 | 9 | 8 | 7 | 2 | 6 | 2 | 2 |
| and **by staff** | **84** | **1,959** | 52 | 8 | 7 | 7 | 2 | 4 | 2 | 2 |

NOTES: Areas of technical expertise: Consult = scientific consultant; Data/IT = data manager/analyst or information technology specialist; Ind Hyg = industrial hygienist or environmental engineer; Inf Cont = nurse or infection control specialist; Med/Epi = physician or epidemiologist; Media = communications or media relations specialist; Path/Lab = pathologist or laboratorian; PHA = public health advisor. The difference in the total number of personnel deployed (84) versus the total number of deployments (92) reflects the redeployment of 8 staff members, whose areas of expertise are shown by the differences in the totals for 4 public health specialties.

Fortunately, the outbreak peaked before serious personnel shortages were encountered; however, it is clear that CDC must both enhance retention of the uniquely skilled staff needed to assist with such outbreak responses and identify external partners who can be recruited when needed to help meet such challenges. The outbreak also highlighted the benefit of having well-established laboratory Infections Program, which was established in 2001 in partnership with the Thailand Ministry of Health, repeatedly proved its value as skilled staff were deployed rapidly to assist affected countries within the region and to work with Thai health officials responding to the importation of SARS cases. The CDC staff assisted Thai officials with caring for Dr. Carlo Urbani, the WHO physician who acquired SARS and died early in the course of the outbreak.

## Collaborations in Science

Early in the course of the outbreak, WHO facilitated the exchange of laboratory information being generated in response to the SARS outbreak by establishing daily conference calls with representatives of the 11 leading laboratories participating in the response (WHO, 2003j). They also created a secure website where laboratory findings could be posted and shared with others, and they assisted with the acquisition and distribution of clinical material for laboratory testing (Stohr, 2003). These critical steps led to the rapid and virtually simultaneous recognition by several international laboratories of a new coronavirus (SCoV) as the likely cause of the outbreak (Ksiazek et al., 2003; Peiris et al., 2003a), and soon thereafter, the determination of the complete genomic sequence of the virus (Rota et al., 2003). The rapidity with which these results were obtained was truly historic and clearly emphasized the benefits of global data sharing and scientific collaboration. Despite widespread application of molecular techniques to determine the cause of the outbreak, it was the traditional virologic procedure of inoculation of acutely acquired patient specimens into cell cultures and laboratory animals that ultimately proved successful in isolating SCoV.

## Communications at Home and Abroad

One of the most daunting challenges faced by public health officials in responding to the SARS outbreak was meeting the need for timely, accurate, and consistent information regarding the evolving outbreak and response activities. WHO did an exceptional job in providing information through nearly daily press briefings and updates on its website, by hosting global conference calls with international partners to discuss specific issues, and by effectively using a secure website to post sensitive information, such as results of ongoing laboratory investigations. Video conferences were arranged between the Director General of WHO, the Secretary of DHHS, and the Director of CDC to provide an opportunity for direct dialogue between agency leaders and their key staff. All of these activities served to calm a nervous world by rapidly providing accurate information on the evolution of the outbreak and interventions under way and on the evolving discovery of the cause of the outbreak and development of treatment and prevention strategies.

The communications burden faced by CDC was enormous and as intense as any previous public health emergency experienced by the agency. More than 10,000 news media calls were handled, 12 SARS news releases were issued, and 21 live telebriefings and news conferences were broadcast. Thirty specialized conference calls were made to the health care provider community, and nearly 35,000 public inquires were answered by telephone. A special clinical hotline was established for physicians inquiring about SARS, and more than 2,000 such calls were answered. Over 1.9 million global participants are estimated to have seen one or more of the three SARS satellite broadcasts directed to health care workers, and more than 17 million hits were recorded on the CDC SARS websites, with 3.8 million hits occurring during the week of April 20–26 alone (Personal

**TABLE 1-3** CDC Shipments of Diagnostic Materials During the 2003 SARS Outbreak, by Recipient

| Recipient | RNA | Virus | Antigen | Total, All Materials |
|---|---|---|---|---|
| Academic centers | 32 | 13 | 1 | 46 |
| Commercial companies | 26 | 15 | 1 | 42 |
| Government agencies | 21 | 18 | 4 | 43 |
| Total, all recipients | 79 | 46 | 6 | 131 |

communications, Dan Rutz and Bill Pollard, CDC, September 26, 2003). Providing accurate, real-time information to meet these demands was one of the most challenging aspects of the entire outbreak response effort.

## Capacity Building and Response Preparedness

With recognition that SCoV was responsible for the outbreak, laboratory efforts quickly turned to establishment of diagnostic tests to identify infected patients. Several laboratories rapidly developed prototype assays to measure SCoV—specific nucleic acid sequences, viral antigen in tissues, and the serologic response to infection. CDC distributed assays to measure both SCoV genomic material by polymerase chain reaction and specific immunoglobulin response by enzyme immunoassay; recipients of these assays included state health departments, members of the Laboratory Response Network established to respond to bioterrorism threats, and several countries following their requests for assistance. CDC also reisolated SCoV under formal Good Laboratory Practices conditions, using FDA-approved certified cells provided by Aventis Pasteur and clinical material obtained from an acutely ill American traveler who had returned recently from Hong Kong. This isolate was made available to vaccine manufacturers free of charge and has now been used in the development of candidate new vaccines by several companies (WHO, 2003i). In all, CDC provided purified RNA, virus, or antigen to more than 130 academic centers, commercial firms, and government agencies (Personal communication, Betty Robertson, CDC, September 26, 2003) (see Table 1-3).

## Challenges and Lessons Learned

The SARS outbreak of 2003 gave the world a clear example of future challenges in addressing emerging infectious diseases. As demonstrated by SARS, an outbreak of infection even in seemingly remote areas of the world can pose a threat to the health and economies of countries worldwide. All nations need to have access to accurate and timely information and must be prepared to respond appropriately. The benefit of having well-established partnerships with countries was demonstrated repeatedly, especially as it became apparent that there is a serious shortage of available United States–based skilled personnel. Similarly, because specialized skill sets, such as infection control expertise, were in critically short supply, future preparedness planning should include establishing contingency plans whereby partners from outside the government can assist with outbreak response efforts as needed. The benefit of global collaboration in addressing scientific challenges was well documented; nevertheless, serious challenges were encountered in the acquisition and transport of clinical material critical to establishing the cause of the outbreak, clearly indicating the need to further facilitate technology transfer and enhance preparedness. Once the cause of the outbreak was determined, an enormous demand for validated diagnostics, training, and technical assistance emerged. Meeting this demand proved to be a major undertaking as well. Last, the long-standing political obstacle in regard to WHO's interactions with Taiwan was highlighted as the SARS outbreak exploded across the island. Initially, only CDC experts responded to Taiwan's call for assistance; however, a decision by the director general of WHO soon led to formal WHO participation in the outbreak response. Once again, we learned that infectious diseases respect neither geographic nor political boundaries.

## ROLE OF CHINA IN THE QUEST TO DEFINE AND CONTROL SARS

*Robert F. Breiman,*[1] *Meirion R. Evans,*[2] *Wolfgang Preiser,*[3] *James Maguire,*[4] *Alan Schnur,*[5] *Ailan Li,*[5] *Henk Bekedam,*[5] *and John S. MacKenzie*[6]

China holds the key to solving many questions crucial to global control of severe acute respiratory syndrome (SARS). The disease appears to have originated in Guangdong Province, and the causative agent, SARS coronavirus, is likely to have originated from an animal host, perhaps sold in public markets. Epidemiologic findings, integral to defining an animal-human linkage, may be confirmed by laboratory studies; once animal host(s) are confirmed, interventions may be needed to prevent further animal-to-human transmission. Community seroprevalence studies may help determine the basis for the decline in disease incidence in Guangdong Province after February 2002. China will also be

[1]International Centre for Diarrheal Disease Research, Bangladesh–Centre for Health and Population Research, Dhaka, Bangladesh.
[2]National Public Health Service for Wales, Cardiff, United Kingdom.
[3]Institute for Medical Virology, Frankfurt, Germany.
[4]Centers for Disease Control and Prevention, Atlanta, Georgia.
[5]World Health Organization, Beijing, China.
[6]University of Queensland, Brisbane, Australia.

able to contribute key data about how the causative agent is transmitted and how it is evolving, as well as identifying pivotal factors influencing disease outcome.

SARS is a newly emerged disease, caused by a previously unknown coronavirus. The first known cases occurred in Guangdong Province in southern China in November and December 2002. During late February 2003, a physician who was incubating SARS traveled from Guangzhou, the provincial capital, to Hong Kong, Special Administrative Region of China, and stayed at a hotel. There, the virus was transmitted from him to local residents and to travelers, who became ill and transmitted disease to others when they returned to Vietnam, Singapore, Canada, and Taiwan, Province of China (Tsang et al., 2003). SARS has now occurred in >8,450 people with >800 deaths worldwide.

The tally of SARS climbed rapidly in China through May 2003, then decelerated markedly during June. The disease has now been reported in 24 of China's 31 provinces. By June 26, 2003, a total of 5,327 SARS cases and 348 deaths had been reported from mainland China, including 2,521 cases in Beijing and 1,512 in Guangdong Province.

Since February 2003, teams of technical consultants for the World Health Organization have been working in China to provide assistance to the Ministry of Health and provincial governments on public health responses to the SARS outbreak. A team that began working in China in March reviewed considerable clinical, epidemiologic, and laboratory data with scientists and officials from a variety of settings in Guangdong Province and Beijing. The team worked closely with colleagues from the National and Guangdong Provincial Centers for Disease Control, and together were able to establish that cases occurring in Guangdong beginning in November were clinically and epidemiologically similar to subsequent cases of SARS documented elsewhere.

The team observed detailed, comprehensive data collection forms, which are completed for activities and behaviors and clinical manifestations of patients with SARS. The team was informed that serum and respiratory secretion specimens collected from many patients from Guangdong were being held under appropriate storage conditions, awaiting further laboratory testing.

While a dedicated, collaborative international effort has resulted in substantial understanding of this disease with remarkable speed, critical information is still lacking. We detail a variety of knowledge gaps that should be addressed through a set of activities to optimize prevention and control of SARS.

## Emergence of SARS-Associated Coronavirus in Humans

Available evidence suggests that SARS emerged in Guangdong Province, in southern China. How and when did it emerge? Did the causative agent evolve in an animal species and jump to humans (or perhaps first to other animal species), or did the virus evolve within humans? The genetic sequence of the virus has been obtained in several laboratories, and phylogenetic analyses have shown that it is unlike other coronaviruses of animal and human origin. Indeed, the virus has been tentatively placed in a new fourth genetic group (Marra et al., 2003; Rota et al., 2003).

Why is it so important to answer the question of how SARS emerged? Most recently recognized novel emergent viruses have been zoonotic, usually with a reservoir in wildlife (Ludwig et al., 2003; Williams et al., 2002). Thus, SARS coronavirus, if zoonotic, may provide the basis for modeling and predicting the appearance of other potential zoonotic human pathogens. More importantly, the information may be crucial for control of SARS. If this disease is to be curtailed or eliminated by strict public health measures, blocking further animal-to-human transmission is indicated. Only about half of the cases in Guangdong are attributed to contact with a SARS patient. Transmission from an unknown, but persisting animal reservoir might explain this finding; however, a nonspecific case definition (i.e., many "cases" might not actually be SARS) and limitations in contact-tracing capacity are other potential explanations.

Finding a potential animal source is, however, a daunting task. The province is famous for its "wet markets," where a bewildering variety of live fauna are offered for sale (sometimes illegally) for their medicinal properties or culinary potential. The opportunity for contact, not only with farmed animals but also with a variety of otherwise rare or uncommon wild animals, is enormous. More than one third of early cases, with dates of onset before February 1, 2003, were in food handlers (persons who handle, kill, and sell food animals, or those who prepare and serve food) (Guangdong Province Center for Disease Control and Prevention, unpub. data,).

Hypothesis-generating epidemiologic studies are indicated to focus on early cases of SARS and cases in persons without known contact with infected persons. These studies should also collect information from appropriately selected controls (i.e., matched by categories such as community and age), regarding exposures to animals of any kind in any setting (including food preparation, dietary habits, pets, and a variety of other activities and behaviors in the community).

Plausible hypotheses generated by epidemiologic studies should be briskly followed by intensive, focused, laboratory studies where relevant, including surveys of specific animal populations to identify SARS-associated coronaviruses (by culture and polymerase chain reaction [PCR]) or to measure specific antibodies. Some virologic surveys have already been conducted among prevalent animal populations, including those known to harbor other coronaviruses or other viruses transmissible to humans or wild animals, handled and sold in the markets; a variety of animals, most notably masked palm civets, have been reported to harbor SARS-associated coronavirus. However, whether these animals are transmitting virus or are recipients of virus transmission is not yet clear. Solutions will lie with identifying epidemiologic links, which should guide targeted animal studies. Molecular epidemiologic and genetic studies can then be helpful in evaluating viruses isolated from animals and from humans.

## Natural History of the Epidemic

Since the earliest known cases were in Guangdong Province, China has had more time than any other location to observe disease incidence over time. Evidence from Guangdong Provincial Centers for Disease Control suggests that the disease incidence peaked in mid-February, and declined weekly through May. What were the reasons for the decline? Introduction of stringent infection-control measures in hospital settings undoubtedly resulted in reduced incidence in healthcare settings but would not likely have accounted for reductions in community transmission. Efforts have been made to reduce the interval between onset of illness and hospitalization (minimizing the potential for community transmission). This effort likely had substantial impact in reducing disease incidence, as shown elsewhere (Riley et al., 2003).

The initial hypothesis was that the virus attenuated after multiple generations of transmission; this hypothesis now seems unlikely. We note several other considerations. Were there a limited number of susceptible people within the population to begin with? Such a concept is possible if there had been earlier spread of a less virulent coronavirus, providing some immunity to a proportion of the population. If so, whether this occurrence was unique to Guangdong will be important to determine.

Alternatively, did the population develop widespread immunity to the causative agent itself? This scenario would require a good deal of asymptomatic or mildly symptomatic disease. At this stage, no reason exists to exclude the possibility of a much wider spectrum of disease than is currently appreciated, since the spectrum of illness has not been fully evaluated.

Another possibility is that a second agent might be required, in addition to coronavirus, to produce severe illness; if this is the case, the epidemiology (like seasonality) of the second agent (perhaps a less recently emerged pathogen for which there is already fairly widespread immunity), rather than coronavirus, may actually be responsible for the decline of the incidence of SARS in Guangdong.

Extensive seroprevalence studies will be helpful for sorting through these possibilities. Analyzing stored serum samples, collected before the onset of this outbreak, could be of immense value in evaluating the possibility of preexisting immunity. Some researchers have found human metapneumoviruses (Poutanen et al., 2003) and species of *Chlamydia* in patients with SARS, but the importance of these findings is unclear. Systematic evaluation of specimens available from all cases, severe cases, and healthy controls in China regarding the presence of antibodies to coronavirus, as well as hypothesized co-infecting agents, should be done. Important clues may come from seroprevalence and other epidemiologic studies in children. As in other affected countries, children were disproportionately less affected by SARS than adults. Carefully working through the bases for reduced incidence and severity may uncover cross-protecting infectious or immunizing agents or crucial host factors for protection.

## Superspreading Events

When documenting the source of person-to-person transmission of SARS has been possible, a substantial proportion of cases have emanated from single persons, so-called superspreaders (Tsang et al., 2003). While contact tracing is undoubtedly incomplete, most infected patients have transmitted illness to few other people. Understanding the differentiating characteristics of persons who transmit, especially patients who are able to transmit to several other people, often after minimal contact, may provide important clues for public health strategies focused on preventing transmission. In addition, better defining environmental settings or circumstances that facilitate high transmission rates would be helpful. China is not unique in documenting superspreaders. The country could participate in multinational studies to define the characteristics of superspreaders and their role in the epidemiology of SARS. Of particular interest is the virus load of superspreaders, compared with those of other infected persons.

Little is known about the importance of fecal-oral transmission or about the length of time that infectious virus shedding occurs in the gastrointestinal tract. Virus shedding in feces has major implications for control strategies and for the possibility of continued carriage and shedding by clinically recovered patients. China has the opportunity to explore the role of fecal spread in the transmission of SARS.

## Evolution of the Virus

The causative agent is a coronavirus, and the entire genome of several strains has been fully sequenced by many laboratories globally (Marra et al., 2003; Rota et al., 2003; Ruan et al., 2003). Tests have been developed to detect coronavirus genetic sequences by PCR. In addition, tests to detect SARS-associated coronavirus antibodies have been developed, but the sensitivity and specificity of these tests are low, especially early in the illness when public health and clinical needs are greatest. A good test for SARS would be important not only for diagnosis and management but also for investigating the origin of the disease and for defining its epidemiology.

If the causative agent can be isolated from stored specimens from the earliest group of patients (from November 2002 to January 2003), how their genetic sequences compare with those from viruses isolated later from various parts of China and elsewhere, and from animals from Guangdong and Guanxi Provinces, would be useful to know. Mutations may be important for a number of reasons. They may affect transmissibility and virulence; they may provide (or frustrate) therapeutic targets for new drugs; and they may pose challenges for development of diagnostic tests and vaccines. Specimens from Chinese patients provide the longest observation window with which mutational tendencies can be evaluated.

An analysis of 14 full-length sequences suggests that two genetic lineages might have arisen from Guangdong. One lineage is represented by the chain of transmission associated with the physician from Guangzhou who traveled to Hong Kong, Special Administrative Region, in February. The other lineage is associated with isolates from Hong Kong, Guangzhou, and Beijing (Ruan et al., 2003). If two genetic lineages arose in Guangdong, were there two separate transmission events from an animal host to humans, or did the lineage diverge within humans? Specimens from early cases in Guangdong may be helpful in addressing this question.

## Outcomes of Infection

Epidemiologic, immunologic, and microbiologic factors associated with severe outcome are not fully defined. Clearly, though, a principal determinant for poor outcome is advancing age. As with other respiratory diseases, age-related coexisting conditions reduce the capacity to compensate to conditions associated with severe disease. Understanding other specific factors that result in poor outcome will have value for optimizing therapeutic approaches.

Clinicians disagree about the value of early treatment with ribavirin and high-dose corticosteroids,[7] and some are reticent to ventilate patients because of high risk for transmission to health-care workers associated with intubation. More data are needed to help define the most effective treatment strategy, particularly for areas with limited resources.

Extraordinary clinical expertise exists among health professionals in Guangdong Province. They have substantial experience with a variety of antivirals, antibiotics, alternative (herbal) medicines, and corticosteroids, and with using assisted ventilation in the treatment of patients with SARS (Zhong and Zeng, 2003). While randomized clinical trials have not been conducted, careful compilations of existing case series data would be helpful in evaluating the potential effectiveness of various management regimens.

The store of clinical data, accumulated from treating hundreds of SARS cases, needs to be put to good use. One priority is to investigate clinical, epidemiologic, and laboratory predictors of poor outcome. Such experience will supplement other recently published data from Hong Kong, Special Administrative Region (Donnelly et al., 2003; Lee et al., 2003; Peiris et al., 2003b; Tsang et al., 2003), and Singapore (Hsu et al., 2003).

Several questions remain unanswered. Do patients exposed to high viral doses (for which a short incubation period may be a surrogate) or to a co-infecting pathogen have poorer outcomes? What is the impact of multiple exposures to SARS-associated coronavirus, like that which occurred among health-care workers early in the epidemic? Do patients infected early in the transmission cycle perform more poorly than those infected during subsequent cycles of transmission?

---

[7][IOM editor's note: For more on the controversy over ribavirin use, see Zhaori, G., 2003, Antiviral treatment of SARS: Can we draw any conclusions? *Canadian Medical Association Journal* 169(11): 1165-6.]

## Learning from the SARS Epidemic

Seldom have intersections between politics, economic development, and public health been more graphically demonstrated. While awaiting the development of effective prophylactic and therapeutic options, many countries have had to muster substantial political will for quick and transparent steps to declare the presence of a lethal pathogen within their borders; conduct surveillance and report the results; use contact tracing, quarantine, and border control measures when needed; and apply stringent infection control measures in health-care settings. Providing the general public with timely and candid information about the magnitude of the problem, the known risks, and how persons can protect themselves has also been necessary. These actions were necessary even when they appeared contrary to economic interests in the short run. Delaying implementation can result in major public health consequences, in addition to damage to the economy and national image.

The work outlined here involves descriptive and epidemiologic inquiry, fundamental to establishing an understanding of this new pathogen and disease. While refined and esoteric research will likely also be conducted, support must first be established for systematically addressing these basic questions and rapidly disseminating results through publication in international journals, presentations at international meetings, and public communications. In China, in contrast with many other settings globally, scientific inquiry and dissemination of results to the international community are subject to institutional interference. The SARS pandemic has shown that virulent pathogens are beholden to no political philosophy or edict. Only careful and rapid application of knowledge and reason through a variety of public health measures has been effective in minimizing the spread and severity of the SARS epidemic. More information and data generated from studies of the epidemic in China are needed immediately to save lives and to prevent fear and disease, both in China itself and elsewhere in the world.

SARS became a public health emergency for China, where investment in health services has been given low priority for many years. Maintaining control in a country so large and diverse will be a major challenge for the months, and perhaps years, to come. Each of China's mainland provinces (including municipalities with equivalent status, autonomous regions, and special administrative regions) is like a country within a country. Many are larger than most countries in Europe. Some, such as Shanghai, are wealthy and highly developed, while others such as Guangxi (bordering Guangdong and Vietnam) are poor and typical of developing countries. Given the potential for reemergence of SARS in the future, if sustained control measures are not in place in China, the possibility of controlling the global threat posed by the disease until new technology (i.e., an effective vaccine) is available may be slight. Key strategies include effective disease surveillance and reporting with early detection and isolation; hospital infection control during triage and treatment of cases; and transparent, open public communication about risk and disease magnitude.

China has recently begun to vigorously address the need for better surveillance, accurate reporting, and forthright public communication. Substantial epidemiologic, clinical, virologic, and immunologic expertise and interest are available within China to address the fundamental questions. International expertise is also available to provide guidance, feedback, and assistance when requested. Identifying the modest resources needed to implement the work should not be a barrier. Support from the government will be needed to carry out valid, transparent studies, and for permission to report the findings, regardless of the conclusions. SARS provides a jarring reminder of the preparedness that is needed to respond to emerging and existing disease threats; it highlights the need to reinvest in health in China, and strengthen public health programs, including surveillance systems and response capacity.

While disease incidence has abated in China and in other locations globally, the disease may still represent an important threat in the future. Many of the solutions to solve the multifaceted puzzle of SARS and to prevent future epidemics must come from China. Without solutions from that country, the degree of difficulty for sustained control of the problem globally is raised still higher.

## SARS: LESSONS FROM TORONTO

*Donald E. Low, M.D., FRCPC*
Toronto Medical Laboratories, Mt. Sinai Hospital, Toronto

Toronto's experience with severe acute respiratory syndrome (SARS) illustrated how quickly the disease can spread in hospitals and highlighted the dangerous phenomenon of SARS superspreaders (see Figure 1-1). Unrecognized cases in Toronto caused significant morbidity and mortality (see Tables 1-4 and 1-5). The absence of rapid tests to distinguish this new disease from pneumonia, influenza, or other common diseases bodes ill for future outbreaks. In the meantime, however, it is clear that a number of simple precautionary measures can significantly reduce hospital-based transmission of the SARS coronavirus, SCoV, during an outbreak.

During the first phase of the outbreak in Toronto, SARS chiefly affected health care workers (HCW), patients, and their visitors at four hospitals (see Table 1-6). The second phase of the outbreak occurred primarily in the workers and visitors of a single hospital ward. The following text chronicles the two phases of the SARS outbreak in Ontario and describes the preventive measures taken by hospitals and individual HCWs once the outbreak became apparent.

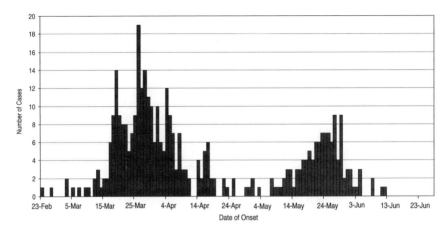

**FIGURE 1-1** SARS Toronto: Phases I and II. The two SARS outbreaks that occurred in Toronto and the age distribution of cases. The majority of cases, which occurred between the ages of 18 and 64, were among health care workers, patients, and visitors to patients in hospitals.

**TABLE 1-4** Case Distribution by Age Group

| Age Group | Phase I | | Phase II | |
|---|---|---|---|---|
| | No. | % | No. | % |
| <18 | 18 | 7 | 2 | 2 |
| 18-35 | 71 | 28 | 20 | 17 |
| 36-64 | 132 | 51 | 70 | 59 |
| >64 | 36 | 14 | 26 | 22 |
| Total | 257 | 100 | 118 | 100 |

**TABLE 1-5** Case Fatality by Age Group

| Age Group | Phase I | | Phase II | |
|---|---|---|---|---|
| | No. | % | No. | % |
| <18 | 0 | 0 | 0 | 0 |
| 18-35 | 0 | 0 | 0 | 0 |
| 36-64 | 10 | 38 | 6 | 31 |
| >64 | 16 | 62 | 11 | 69 |

## Phase I of the Toronto SARS Outbreak

The index case and her husband had vacationed in Hong Kong and had stayed at a hotel in Kowloon from February 18 to 21, 2003. The index case began to experience symptoms after her return on February 23 and died at home

**TABLE 1-6** SARS Toronto: Phases I and II

| | Phase | |
|---|---|---|
| | I | II |
| Exposure | No. (%) | No. (%) |
| 2002 | 91 (33%) | 52 (42%) |
| Hospital -worker patient/visitor | 49 (18%) | 64 (51%) |
| Other health care (clinic, EMS) | 8 (2.9%) | 2 (1.6%) |
| Household contact | 76 (28%) | 9 (7.2%) |
| "Community" | 16 (5.9%) | — |
| Travel | 12 (4.4%) | — |
| Under investigation | 21 (7.7%) | — |

on March 5. During her illness, family members, including her son (case A), provided care at home. Case A became ill on February 27 and presented to the index hospital on March 7 (Varia et al., 2003).

Nosocomial transmission in the hospital began when case A presented to the emergency department on March 7 with severe respiratory symptoms. He was placed in a general observation area of the emergency department and received nebulized salbutamol. During this time, SARS was transmitted to two other patients in the emergency department (cases B and C). Case B, who had presented with rapid atrial fibrillation, was in the bed adjacent to case A, about 1.5 meters away and separated by a curtain, and was discharged home after 9 hours in the emergency department. Case C, who had presented with shortness of breath secondary to a pleural effusion, was three beds (about 5 meters) away from case A and was transferred to a hospital ward and later discharged home on March 10. The three patients were cared for by the same nurse.

Case A was transferred briefly to a medical unit, then to the intensive care unit (ICU) 18 hours after his presentation to the emergency department. Three hours later, he was placed in airborne isolation because tuberculosis was included in his differential diagnosis. Contact and droplet precautions were implemented on March 10 by ICU staff caring for case A, and the patient remained in isolation until his death, on March 13. Case A's family visited him in the ICU on March 8, 9, and 10. During this time, some family members were febrile, and two were experiencing respiratory symptoms. Chest radiographs were taken of the family members on March 9 and again on March 11. Four members had abnormal radiographs and were instructed to wear masks at all times, wash their hands upon entering and leaving the ICU, and limit their visits to the ICU.

On March 12, the WHO alerted the global community to a severe respiratory syndrome that was spreading among HCWs in Hanoi, Vietnam, and Hong Kong. The alert was forwarded to infectious disease and emergency department physicians in Toronto. The following day, case A died and it became clear that several other family members had worsening illness. The clinicians involved and the local public health unit suspected the family's illnesses might be linked to cases of atypical pneumonia reported in Hong Kong. Four family members were admitted to three different hospitals on March 13, and another family member was admitted to hospital on March 14. All were managed using airborne, droplet, and contact precautions. No further transmission from these cases occurred after admission to hospital.

Case B became febrile on March 10, 3 days after exposure to case A in the emergency department and discharge home. Respiratory symptoms evolved over the next 5 days. He was brought to the index hospital on March 16 by two Emergency Medical Services paramedics, who did not immediately use contact and droplet precautions. After 9 hours in the emergency department, where airborne, contact and droplet precautions were used, case B was transferred to an isolation room in the ICU. His wife became ill on March 16. She was in the emergency department with case B on March 16 (no precautions used) and visited him in the ICU on March 21 (precautions used); he died later that day. The infection also spread to three other members of case B's family. SARS developed in a number of people who were in contact with case B and his wife on March 16, including the 2 paramedics who brought him to the hospital, a firefighter, 5 emergency department staff, 1 other hospital staff, 2 patients in the emergency department, 1 housekeeper who worked in the emergency department while case B was there, and 7 visitors who were also in the emergency department at the same time as case B (symptom onset March 19 to 26). The 16 hospital staff, visitors, and patients transmitted the infection to 8 household members and 8 other family contacts. In the ICU, intubation for mechanical ventilation of case B was performed by a physician wearing a surgical mask, gown and gloves. He subsequently acquired SARS and transmitted the infection to a member of his family. Three ICU nurses who were present at the intubation and who used droplet and contact precautions had onset of early symptoms between March 18 and 20. One transmitted the infection to a household member.

Case C became ill on March 13 with symptoms of a myocardial infarction and was brought to the index hospital by paramedics. It was unknown that he had been in contact with case A on March 7, and thus it was not recognized that he had SARS. As a result, he was not isolated, and other precautions were not used. He was admitted to the coronary care unit (CCU) for 3 days and then transferred to another hospital for renal dialysis. He remained in the other hospital until his death, on March 29. Subsequent transmission of SARS occurred within that hospital (Dwosh et al., 2003). Case C's wife became ill on March 26. At the index hospital, case C transmitted SARS to 1 patient in the emergency department, 3 emergency department staff, 1 housekeeper who worked in the emergency department while case C was there, 1 physician, 2 hospital technologists, 2 CCU, patients, and 7 CCU staff. One of the paramedics who transported case C to the index hospital also became ill. Further transmission then occurred from ill staff at the index hospital to 6 of their family members, 1 patient, 1 medical clinic staff, and 1 other nurse in the emergency department.

On March 23, 2003, officials recognized that the number of available negative pressure rooms in Toronto was being exhausted. In a 4-hour period on the
afternoon of March 23, staff at West Park Hospital, a chronic care facility in the
city, recommissioned 25 beds in an unused building formerly used to house patients with tuberculosis. Despite the efforts of West Park physicians and nurses,
and assistance from staff at the Scarborough Grace and Mount Sinai Hospitals,
qualified staff could be found to care for only 14 patients.

Faced with increasing transmission, the Ontario government designated
SARS as a reportable, communicable, and virulent disease under the *Health Protection and Promotion Act* on March 25, 2003. This move gave public health
officials the authority to track infected people, and issue orders preventing them
from engaging in activities that might transmit the new disease. Provincial public
health activated its emergency operations center.

By the evening of March 26, 2003, the West Park unit and all available negative pressure rooms in Toronto hospitals were full; however, 10 ill Scarborough
Hospital staff needing admissions were waiting in the emergency department,
and others who were ill were waiting at home to be seen. Overnight, with the
declaration of a provincial emergency, the Ontario government required all hospitals to create units to care for SARS patients.

By March 25, 2003, Health Canada was reporting 19 cases of SARS in
Canada—18 in Ontario and the single case in Vancouver. But 48 patients with a
presumptive diagnosis of SARS had in fact been admitted to hospital by the end
of that day. Many more individuals were starting to feel symptoms, and would
subsequently be identified as SARS patients. Epidemic curves later showed that
this period was the peak of the outbreak. On March 19, nine Canadians developed
"probable" SARS, the highest single-day total. Taking "suspect" and "probable"
cases together, the peak was March 26, and the 3 days, March 25 to 27 are the
highest 3-day period in the outbreak.

The Ontario government declared SARS a provincial emergency on March
26, 2003. Under the Emergency Management Act, the government has the power
to direct and control local governments and facilities to ensure that necessary
services are provided.

All hospitals in the Greater Toronto Area (GTA) and Simcoe County were
ordered to activate their "Code Orange" emergency plans by the government.
"Code Orange" meant that the involved hospitals suspended nonessential services. They were also required to limit visitors, create isolation units for potential
SARS patients, and implement protective clothing for exposed staff (i.e., gowns,
masks, and goggles). Four days later, provincial officials extended access restrictions to all Ontario hospitals.

On May 14, 2003, WHO removed Toronto from the list of areas with recent
local transmission. This was widely understood to mean that the outbreak had
come to an end. Consistent with the notion that the disease was contained, the
government of Ontario lifted the emergency on May 17. Directives continued to

reinforce the need for enhanced infection control practices in health care settings. Code Orange status for hospitals was revoked.

It appeared that the total number of cases had reached a plateau—140 probable and 178 suspect infections. Twenty-four Canadians had died, all in Ontario.

## Phase II of the Toronto SARS Outbreak

During early and mid-May, as recommended by provincial SARS-control directives, all hospitals discontinued SARS expanded precautions (i.e., routine contact precautions with use of an N95 or equivalent respirator) for non-SARS patients without respiratory symptoms in all hospital areas other than the emergency department and the ICUs. In addition, staff no longer were required to wear masks or respirators routinely throughout the hospital or to maintain distance from one another while eating.

On May 20, five patients in a rehabilitation hospital in Toronto were reported with febrile illness. One of these five patients was determined to have been hospitalized in the orthopedic ward of North York General (NYG) Hospital during April 22 to 28, and a second was found on May 22 to have SARS-associated SCoV by nucleic acid amplification test. On investigation, a second patient was determined to have been hospitalized in the orthopedic ward of NYG hospital during April 22 to 28. After the identification of these cases, an investigation of pneumonia cases at NYG hospital identified eight cases of previously unrecognized SARS among patients.

The first patient linked to the second phase of the Ontario outbreak was a man aged 96 years who was admitted to NYG hospital on March 22 with a fractured pelvis. On April 2, he was transferred to the orthopedic ward, where he had fever and an infiltrate on chest radiograph. Although he appeared initially to respond to antimicrobial therapy, on April 19, he again had respiratory symptoms, fever, and diarrhea. He had no apparent contact with a patient or an HCW with SARS, and aspiration pneumonia and *Clostridium difficile*—associated diarrhea appeared to be probable explanations for his symptoms. In the subsequent outbreak investigation, other patients in close proximity to this patient and several visitors and HCWs linked to these patients were determined to have SARS. At least one visitor became ill before the onset of illness of a hospitalized family member, and another visitor was determined to have SARS although his hospitalized wife did not.

On May 23, NYG hospital was closed to all new admissions other than patients with newly identified SARS. Soon after, new provincial directives were issued, requiring an increased level of infection-control precautions in hospitals located in several greater Toronto regions. HCWs at NYG hospital were placed under a 10-day work quarantine and instructed to avoid public places outside work, avoid close contact with friends and family, and wear a mask whenever public contact was unavoidable. As of June 9, of 79 new cases of SARS that resulted from exposure at NYH hospital, 78 appear to have resulted from exposures that occurred before May 23.

## Transmission

The SCoV has been isolated in sputum, nasal secretions, serum, feces, and bronchial washings (Drosten et al., 2003; Peiris et al., 2003b). Evidence suggests that SCoV is transmitted via contact and/or droplets (Peiris et al., 2003a; Poutanen et al., 2003) and that the use of any mask (surgical or N95) significantly decreases the risk of infection (Seto et al., 2003). However, there are cases that defy explanation based on these modes of transmission suggesting that alternative modes of transmission may also occur (Varia et al., 2003). SCoV remains viable in feces for days and the outbreak at the Amoy Gardens apartments highlights the possibility of an oral-fecal or fecal-droplet mode of transmission (WHO, 2003m,n).

A number of cases occurred in HCWs wearing protective equipment following exposure to high risk aerosol- and droplet-generating procedures such as airway manipulation, administration of aerosolized medications, noninvasive positive pressure ventilation, and bronchoscopy or intubation (Lee et al., 2003; Ofner et al., 2003). When intubation is necessary, measures should be taken to reduce unnecessary exposure to health care workers, including reducing the number of health care workers present and adequately sedating or paralyzing the patient to reduce cough. Updated interim infection control precautions for patients who have SARS are under development and will be available from CDC at http://www.cdc.gov/ncidod/sars/index.htm.

Currently, epidemiological evidence suggests that transmission does not occur prior to the onset of symptoms or after symptom resolution. Despite this, shedding of SCoV in stool has been documented by reverse-transcription polymerase chain reaction (RT-PCR) for up to 64 days following the resolution of symptoms (Ren et al., 2003). A small group of patients appear to be highly infectious and have been referred to as superspreaders (CDC, 2003a). Such superspreaders appear to have played an important role early in the epidemic but the reason for their enhanced infectivity remains unclear. Possible explanations for their enhanced infectivity include the lack of early implementation of infection control precautions, higher load of SCoV, or larger amounts of respiratory secretions.

## Clinical Disease

*Case Definition*

The Centers for Diseases Control and Prevention in Atlanta (CDC) has classified SARS into suspect and probable with further classification based on laboratory findings (CDC, 2003b). The World Health Organization has a similar case classification (WHO, 2003d). Although these classifications have proven epide-miologically useful, they have a low sensitivity for diagnosis in patients early in disease (sensitivity, 26 percent; specificity, 96 percent) (Rainer et al., 2003), un-derscoring the importance of a rapid, accurate diagnostic test.

*Presentation*

The typical incubation period of SARS ranges from 2 to 10 days but may rarely be as long as 16 days (Booth et al., 2003; Lee et al., 2003). The prodrome includes influenza-like symptoms such as fever, myalgias, headache, and diarrhea (Booth et al., 2003; Lee et al., 2003). Fever can vary from low to high grade, and can occasionally be absent on presentation, particularly in older patients. The respiratory phase, consisting of an early and late stage, starts 2-7 days after the prodrome and can be associated with watery diarrhea (Booth et al., 2003; Lee et al., 2003; Peiris et al., 2003b). The early stage includes a dry nonproductive cough and mild dyspnea. Patients may only have prodromal or early respiratory symp-toms at the time of presentation making the diagnosis of SARS difficult. Chest radiographic and laboratory findings may help in making an early diagnosis. Early chest radiographs often show subtle peripheral pulmonary infiltrates, that can be more readily detected as consolidation or ground-glass appearance using high-resolution computed tomographic (CT) lung scans (Wong et al., 2003a, b). Atypi-cal presentations of the disease have been described also complicating the diag-nosis (Fisher et al., 2003; Wu and Sung, 2003). Interestingly, the disease has been rare in children and if present appears to be milder (Hon et al., 2003; Li et al., 2003).

*Natural History*

SARS is characterized by a spectrum of disease. Asymptomatic cases have been described but only in small number (Gold et al., 2003). Another infrequent subset of cases includes those who have a febrile illness without a respiratory component. More frequent is a mild variant of the disease that includes mild respiratory symptoms with fever. Within this category is a cough variant with persistent intractable cough. The classic moderate-severe variant is characterized by a more serious later respiratory phase with dyspnea on exertion or at rest, and hypoxia. This later respiratory phase often occurs 8 to 12 days after the onset of symptoms (Booth et al., 2003; Lee et al., 2003; Peiris et al., 2003b). In 10-20 percent of hospitalized patients, persistent or progressive hypoxia results in intu-bation and mechanical ventilation (Booth et al., 2003; Fowler et al., 2003; Lew et al., 2003). Among patients developing respiratory failure, intubation was required at a median of 8 days following symptom onset. Subtle but progressive declines in oxygen saturation are often indicative of impeding respiratory failure and should trigger more intensive monitoring and preparation for intubation under controlled circumstances. In total, the respiratory phase lasts approximately 1 week. The recovery phase begins approximately 14 to 18 days from the onset of symptoms with resolution of the lymphopenia and thrombocytosis.

## Clinical Outcome

The case fatality rate during recent outbreaks was 9.6 percent ranging from 0 to 40 percent (WHO, 2003o). Advanced age is the most important risk factor for death with patients older than 60 years having a case fatality rate of 45 percent (Booth et al., 2003; Peiris et al., 2003b). Other risk factors for death include diabetes mellitus and hepatitis B virus infection (Booth et al., 2003; Fowler et al., 2003; Lee et al., 2003; Lew et al., 2003; Peiris et al., 2003b). Little data exist regarding the long-term morbidity of SARS although preliminary studies suggest that the psychological impact of the disease is considerable (Maunder et al., 2003; Styra et al., 2003).

## Conclusion

The experience with SARS in Toronto indicates that this disease is entirely driven by exposure to infected individuals. Transmission occurred primarily within health care settings or in circumstances where close contacts occurred. The infectious agent was spread by respiratory droplets in the great majority of cases, and some patients were more infectious than others. Ultimately, the strict adherence to precautions—and practice implementing them—was critical to the containment of SARS in Toronto and the restoration of safe conditions for hospital staff and patients.

## ISOLATION AND QUARANTINE: CONTAINMENT STRATEGIES FOR SARS 2003

*Martin Cetron, M.D., Susan Maloney, M.D., M.H.Sc., Ram Koppaka, M.D., and Patricia Simone, M.D.*
National Center for Infectious Diseases, Centers for Disease Control and Prevention

Quarantine is an ancient tool used to prevent the spread of disease. The Bible describes the sequestering of persons with leprosy, and the practice was used widely in 14th-century Europe to control the spread of bubonic and pneumonic plague. To prevent disease transmission, ships were required to stay in harbor for 40 days before disembarkation (thus the term quarantine, which derives from the Latin *quadragina* or the Italian *quaranta*, meaning 40).

Quarantine has been used for centuries, but because it was often implemented in a way that equated disease with crime, the practice has negative connotations.

Persons under quarantine were often detained without regard to their essential needs. Those who were exposed but not yet ill were not always separated from the ill, allowing disease to spread within the detained group. Populations targeted for quarantine, such as foreigners, were stigmatized. In some cases, the power of quarantine was abused; for example, at the end of the 19th century, the steerage passengers on arriving ships were frequently quarantined while the first- and second-class passengers were allowed to disembark without being examined for illness.

Despite its history, quarantine—when properly applied and practiced according to modern public health principles—can be a highly effective tool in preventing the spread of contagious disease. It may play an especially important role when vaccination or prophylactic treatment is not possible, as was the case with severe acute respiratory syndrome (SARS). Even when direct medical countermeasures are available (e.g., smallpox and pneumonic plague), reducing mobility in the at-risk population may enable the most rapid and efficient delivery of postexposure vaccination and chemoprophylaxis.

## Isolation and Quarantine

Before discussing the role of quarantine as a component of community response and containment for SARS, it is necessary to distinguish, from a public health perspective, between the related practices of isolation and quarantine. Both are usually imposed by health officials on a voluntary basis; however, federal, state, and local officials have the authority to impose mandatory quarantine and isolation when necessary to protect the public's health.

**Isolation** refers to the separation and restricted movement of *ill* persons who have a contagious disease in order to prevent its transmission to others. It typically occurs in a hospital setting, but can be done at home or in a special facility. Usually individuals are isolated, but the practice may be applied in larger groups.

**Quarantine** refers to the restriction of movement or separation of *well* persons who have been exposed to a contagious disease, before it is known whether they will become ill. Quarantine usually takes place in the home and may be applied at the individual level or to a group or community of exposed persons.

Contact surveillance, in the context of quarantine, is the process of monitoring persons who have been exposed to a contagious disease for signs and symptoms of that disease. Surveillance may be done *passively*, for example, by informing contacts to seek medical attention if signs or symptoms occur. Contact surveillance can also be performed *actively*, for example, by having health workers telephone contacts daily to inquire about signs and symptoms or even having health workers directly assess contacts for fever or other symptoms. All quarantined persons should be monitored for development of signs and symptoms of disease to ensure appropriate isolation, management, and/or treatment. For persons without a known contact but believed to be at increased risk for disease or exposure, enhanced surveillance and education can be used for risk assessment monitoring. During the SARS epidemic, this approach was used effectively with airline passengers arriving in the United States from areas of high transmission during the SARS epidemic.

### Principles of Modern Quarantine

Quarantine as it is now practiced is a public health tool and a collective action for the common good. Today's quarantines are more likely to involve a few people exposed to contagion in a small area, such as on an airplane or at a public gathering, and only rarely are applied to entire cities or communities. The main goal of modern quarantine is to reduce transmission by increasing the "social distance" between persons; that is, reducing the number of people with whom each person comes into contact (see Figure 1-2).

If quarantine is to be used, the basic needs of those infected and exposed must be met. The following key principles of modern quarantine ensure that it strikes the appropriate balance between individual liberties and the public good:

- Quarantine is used when persons are exposed to a disease that is highly dangerous and contagious.
- Exposed well persons are separated from those who are ill.
- Care and essential services are provided to all people under quarantine.
- The "due process" rights of those restricted to quarantine are protected.

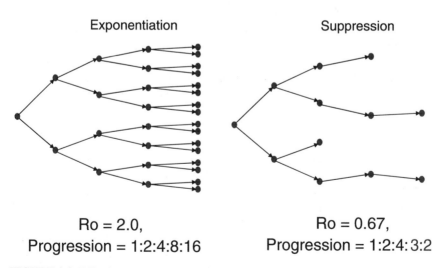

Exponentiation

Ro = 2.0,
Progression = 1:2:4:8:16

Suppression

Ro = 0.67,
Progression = 1:2:4:3:2

**FIGURE 1-2** Effectiveness of vaccination and quarantine to contain a smallpox outbreak after the release of bioengineered, aerosolized smallpox in an airplane carrying 500 people.

- Quarantine lasts no longer than is necessary to ensure that quarantined persons do not become ill. Its maximum duration would be one incubation period from the last known exposure, but it could be shortened if an effective vaccination or prophylactic treatment is available and can be delivered in a timely fashion.
- Quarantine is used in conjunction with other interventions, including—
  - Disease surveillance and monitoring for symptoms in persons quarantined.
  - Rapid diagnosis and timely referral to care for those who become ill.
  - The provision of preventive interventions, including vaccination or prophylactic antibiotics.

Quarantine encompasses a range of strategies that can be used to detain, isolate, or conditionally release individuals or populations infected or exposed to contagious diseases, and should be tailored to particular circumstances. Quarantine activities can range from only passive or active symptom monitoring or short-term voluntary home curfew, all the way to cancellation of public gatherings, closing public transportation, or, under extreme circumstances, to a *cordon sanitaire:* a barrier erected around a geographic area, with strict enforcement prohibiting movement in or out. In a "snow day" or "sheltering in place" scenario, schools may be closed, work sites may be closed or access to them restricted, large public gatherings may be cancelled, and public transportation may be halted or restricted. People who become ill under these conditions would need specific instructions for seeking evaluation and care; they would only expose others in their households—or perhaps no one at all, if precautions are taken as soon as symptoms develop. The fact that most people understand the concept of sheltering at home during inclement weather, regarding home in these circumstances as the safest and most sensible place to be, increases the likelihood that similar conditions of quarantine will be accepted. "Snow day" measures can be implemented instantaneously, and most essential services can be met without inordinate additional resources, especially if the quarantine lasts only a few days.

Another important feature of quarantine is that it need not be absolute to be effective. Even a partial or "leaky" quarantine, such as occurs with voluntary compliance, can reduce the transmission of disease. Voluntary measures, which rely on the public's cooperation, reduce or remove the need for legal enforcement and leverage the public's instinct to remain safely sheltered. In contrast, compulsory confinement may precipitate the instinct to "escape." If an effective vaccine is available, partial quarantine can be an effective supplement to vaccination, further reducing transmission of disease. For example, Figure 1-3 shows a model illustrating various outcomes of a hypothetical scenario of 500 people, all of whom are vaccinated against smallpox, exposed to an intentional aerosol release of that contagion on an airplane. In the model,

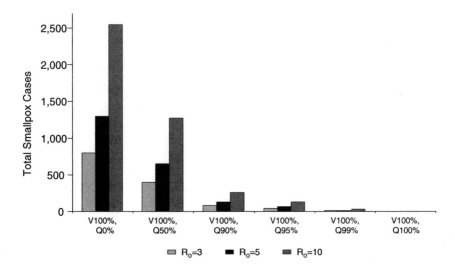

**FIGURE 1-3** Impact of varying $R_o$ and percent quarantined on total smallpox cases. Even with 100 percent vaccination against smallpox, quarantine effectively reduces the spread of disease in the community. This effect remains significant even at lower reproductive rates, and differs little between 90 and 100 percent quarantine.

all 500 people are offered postexposure smallpox vaccine; the model assumes that the vaccine is 95 percent effective. Even under these unlikely and theoretical circumstances, the addition of even partial (50 percent to 90 percent) quarantine to vaccination can have a profound effect on reducing the number of eventual cases in the community. This trend remains significant even at low rates of transmission ("reproductive rates").

In order to implement modern quarantine effectively, there must be a clear understanding of the roles of public health staff at federal, state, and local levels, and each group should know their legal authorities. Effective implementation also requires identifying appropriate partners, including transportation authorities and law enforcement officials, and engaging them in coordinated planning. Finally, quarantine can be most successful if the public has advance knowledge of the disease threat and understands the role of quarantine in containing an epidemic. People who are actually quarantined need to believe that their sacrifice is justified and that they will be supported during the period of quarantine.

### Quarantine and the Response to SARS

Containment strategies employed during the recent SARS epidemic included case and contact management, infection control in hospitals and other facilities, community-wide temperature screening, mask use, isolation and quarantine, and

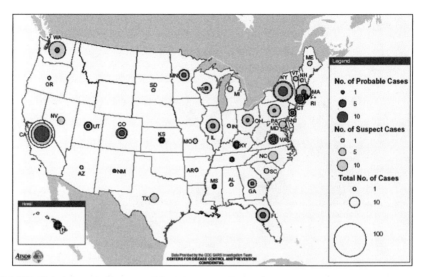

**FIGURE 1-4** Reported cases of SARS, United States, May 19, 2003.

the monitoring of travelers and response at national borders. Various combinations of these strategies were applied in different places, depending on factors such as the magnitude and scope of the local outbreak, the availability of resources to support containment, and the level of public cooperation and trust. In the United States, where only eight laboratory-confirmed cases of SARS and no community transmission occurred (see Figure 1-4), the principal strategies of containment were education of high-risk populations (e.g., international travelers and health-care workers); early detection of suspected and probable cases; and rapid implementation of isolation and other infection control tools. Additional measures such as quarantine were used in other countries where SARS presented a greater threat.

*Case and Contact Management*

In the United States, most people with suspected or probable SARS were isolated at home; hospital isolation was reserved for those who required such care or had no suitable home environment. (e.g., homeless, out-of-town visitors). Isolation was continued while symptoms persisted and for 10 days thereafter. In some other countries, most persons with suspected or probable SARS were isolated in the hospital. For contact management, the U.S. Centers for Disease Control and Prevention (CDC) recommended quarantine only for health-care workers who had a high-risk exposure to a SARS patient. In several states, however, local health officials "furloughed" health-care workers who were exposed to high-risk probable cases. In general, CDC recommended only passive surveillance. Persons who were exposed to suspected or probable SARS, as well as travelers returning from areas with SARS transmission, were asked to monitor their health for 10 days and seek medical attention immediately if fever or respiratory symptoms developed. Active surveillance was reserved for probably and lab-confirmed cases and their high risk close contacts; this was usually conducted by members of the local or state health departments.

In some countries other than the United States (e.g., China, Taiwan [ROC],[8] Singapore, and Canada), home quarantine was used for most close contacts of people with suspected or probable SARS. Designated quarantine facilities were used in some situations for homeless persons, travelers, and people who did not wish to be quarantined at home. In some situations, as a result of staffing shortages and relatively high exposure rates in hospitals, exposed health-care workers and ambulance personnel were placed on "work quarantine," which entailed working during their regular shifts, using comprehensive infection control precautions and personal protective equipment, and staying either at home or in a building near the hospital when off duty. Most persons in home quarantine were asked to monitor their temperature regularly, once or twice a day; health workers called them twice a day to get a report on temperature and symptoms. Other health-care workers had their temperature checked twice a day or more at work. In Singapore, video cameras linked to telephones were occasionally used to monitor patients.

Authorities used a variety of methods to enforce quarantine during the SARS epidemic. In select places, quarantine orders were given to all persons placed in quarantine, while in the majority, only those who demonstrated noncompliance were given orders. Under some orders, noncompliant individuals were isolated in guarded rooms; others were confined at home wearing security ankle bracelets; yet others received fines or even jail sentences. However, these instances of compulsory enforced quarantine orders were clearly the exception rather than the norm during the SARS epidemic.

*Community Containment*

In the United States, community containment strategies consisted mainly of coordinating the SARS response activities through emergency operations centers and providing information and education to the public, health workers, and others. This strategy included publishing guidelines and fact sheets on websites, holding press conferences, making presentations to a variety of audiences, and meeting with groups and communities who were experiencing stigmatization.

---

[8]ROC stands for Republic of China.

On some occasions, such as occurred in mainland China, Hong Kong (SAR), Taiwan (ROC), and Singapore, large-scale quarantine was imposed on travelers arriving from other SARS areas, work and school contacts of suspected cases, and, in a few instances, entire apartment complexes where high attack rates of SARS were occurring.

In addition to imposing large-scale quarantine in some cases, many areas with high transmission (e.g., Hong Kong, Singapore, Taiwan, Toronto, and mainland China) used strategies such as mandated fever screening before entry to schools, work, and other public buildings; requiring masks in certain settings; and implementing populationwide temperature monitoring and disinfection campaigns. Community mobilization programs were also developed to educate the public about SARS and what to do to prevent and control it; for example, a populationwide body temperature monitoring campaign and a SARS hotline to promote early detection of fever as a warning sign for SARS. Taiwan and mainland China also undertook a series of community disinfection campaigns in which streets, buildings, and vehicles were sprayed with bleach and bleach was distributed free throughout the community.

Several important lessons can be gained from the experience of countries where large-scale quarantine measures were imposed in response to SARS. First, when the public was given clear messages about the need for quarantine, it was well accepted—far better, in fact, than many public health officials would have anticipated. Indeed, voluntary quarantine was effective in the overwhelming majority of cases. Yet, despite the widespread acceptance of and cooperation with quarantine, it represented a great sacrifice for many people through consequences such as loss of income, concerns for the health of their families, feelings of isolation, and stigma. Finally, large-scale quarantine was found to be complicated and resource intensive to implement, creating enormous logistic, economic, ethical, and psychological challenges for public health authorities. Recent data evaluating the efficacy of quarantine in Taiwan and Beijing, China, during the SARS epidemic suggest that efficiency could be improved by focusing quarantine activities on persons with known or suspected contact with SARS cases. In order to prepare for future epidemics, enhanced systems and personnel will need to be established to deliver essential services to persons in quarantine, to monitor their health and refer them to necessary medical care, and to offer mental health and other support services.

## Border and Travel Response

Several strategies for border and travel response were used in the United States, including issuing travel advisories and alerts, distributing health alert notices at ports of entry, and meeting planes and responding to reports of ill passengers. Additional strategies used in other countries (e.g., Canada, China, and Singapore) included predeparture screening of temperature, SARS symptoms,

**TABLE 1-7** Travel Alerts and Advisories for SARS, March–July 2003

| Region | Advisory Started | Advisory Stopped | Alert Started | Alert Stopped |
|---|---|---|---|---|
| Mainland China | 3/13/03 | 6/17/03 | 6/17/03 | 7/3/03 |
| Beijing, China | 6/17/03 | 6/25/03 | 6/25/03 | 7/11/03 |
| Taiwan | 6/25/03 | 6/25/03 | 6/25/03 | 7/15/03 |
| Hong Kong | 5/1/03 | 6/25/03 | 6/25/03 | 7/1/03 |
| Hanoi, Vietnam | 3/13/03 | 4/29/03 | 4/29/03 | 5/15/03 |
| Toronto | Never had an advisory | Never had an advisory | 4/23/03 restarted: 5/23/03 | 5/20/03 restopped: 7/8/03 |
| Singapore | 3/13/03 | 5/4/03 | 5/4/03 | 6/4/03 |

and recent exposures to SARS patients; postarrival disembarkation screening with questions about travel and exposure to SARS, maintaining "stop lists" of people with suspected SARS and their contacts at airports to prevent such individuals from traveling, isolation of ill travelers with suspected or probable SARS, and quarantine of healthy travelers returning from other areas with high SARS transmission.

In the United States, CDC issued a series of travel alerts and advisories related to SARS (see Table 1-7). A *travel alert* describes a health situation in a particular area and gives recommendations about appropriate precautions, while a *travel advisory* goes a step further and recommends postponement of nonessential travel to an affected area. During the SARS epidemic, CDC staff met nearly 12,000 flights and distributed more than 2.7 million health alert notices to passengers arriving directly and indirectly from affected areas. The notices instructed travelers to monitor their health for fever and respiratory symptoms for 10 days and immediately seek medical attention (with advance notice to the health-care facility) if the symptoms occurred. Health alert notices (HANs) were also distributed at 13 U.S.–Canada land crossings, as well as in the predeparture area at the Toronto airport. If an ill passenger was reported on a flight arriving in the United States, it was met by members of the CDC quarantine staff. They evaluated the affected passenger for possible SARS, provided referral to a health-care provider, collected locating information from other passengers, and coordinated with federal, state, and local public health authorities.

## Preparedness Planning

Preparations for a resurgence of SARS (or indeed an outbreak of any contagious disease) should be made at all levels of government. Plans must encompass general logistics and planning for case and contact management, including quarantine. A framework for the community containment of SARS (see Figure 1-5) lists several criteria for establishing movement restrictions and a range of options for containment that could be applied in response. In deciding whether and how

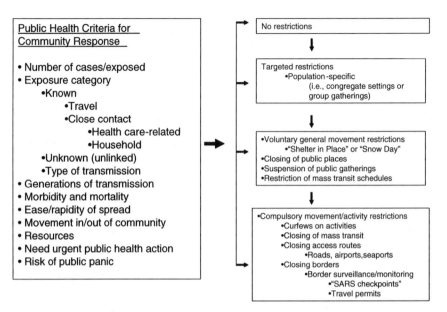

**FIGURE 1-5** Range of available responses to SARS at the national, state, and community levels.

to restrict movement during an epidemic, community officials would consider factors such as:

- the number of suspected, probable, and confirmed cases;
- whether cases have well-defined exposure risks;
- how many potential new exposures each case has been in contact with;
- what type of transmission is predominant (e.g., airborne, droplet, fomite);
- how many generations of transmission have occurred; and
- the morbidity and case-fatality rate of the epidemic.

Decision makers would also need to consider the baseline amount of movement in the community, the impact of curtailing movement on critical infrastructure, the resources available to support containment, and the public's reaction to the epidemic.

### Planning for Community Containment

In some circumstances, containment of SARS or other microbial threats at the community level could be accomplished without restricting movement, with the focus instead on educating the public through such means as press releases and travel alerts and advisories (as was done in the United States in 2003). In other situations, targeted restrictions, including quarantine of close contacts and restriction of some group gatherings, would be appropriate. A more restrictive option would include general voluntary movement restrictions, including measures such as fever screening at entrances of public places, "snow-day" or "shelter-in-place" quarantines, closing public places, canceling public gatherings, and restricting mass transit. Rarely, in the most extreme circumstances, compulsory movement restrictions, including the closing of airports and borders, would be warranted.

Advance planning is necessary to enable officials to assess risk, make decisions, and implement necessary measures as effectively as possible in the event of a disease outbreak. Jurisdictions should establish an emergency operations center structure and a legal preparedness plan, and forge connections among essential partners such as law enforcement officials, first responders, health-care facilities, educators, the media, and the legal community. Provisions must be made to monitor and assess factors such as those above to determine response level for both implementing and scaling back interventions and movement restrictions. Educational message strategies should be developed to disseminate information to government decision makers, health-care providers and first responders, and the public; it will be especially important to address the possibility that some people may experience stigmatization as a result of containment. A draft of the CDC SARS Preparedness Plan entitled, "Public Health Guidance for Community-Level Preparedness and Response to Severe Acute Respiratory Syndrome (SARS) is posted at http://www.cdc.gov/ncidod/sars/updatedguidance.htm. Appendices D and E specifically address Community Containment and Border Strategies, respectively. A SARS preparedness checklist (available at http://www.astho.org) also provides guidance for public health officials in developing such plans.

To plan for case and contact management, jurisdictions should secure necessary protocols for clinical evaluation and monitoring, contact tracing and monitoring, and reporting of disease. Standards, tools, and supplies must be established for home and nonhospital isolation facilities. A telecommunications plan should be developed to provide for case and contact monitoring and fever triage, as well as to provide information to decision makers, health-care workers, and the public. Provisions must be made to ensure that all isolated and quarantined individuals receive food, medicine, and mental health and other supporting services, including transportation to medical facilities. Jurisdictions should also identify and develop assessment procedures for appropriate nonhospital residential facilities. These sites could be used for quarantining contacts or persons for whom "home isolation" is indicated, but who do not have an appropriate "home" environment.

To prepare for the implementation of community containment measures, jurisdictions must establish legal authorities and procedures to implement all levels

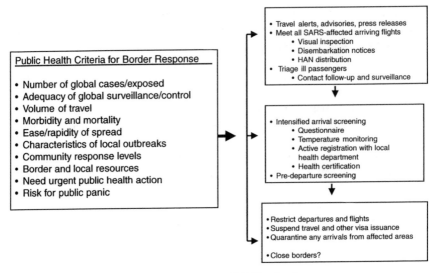

**FIGURE 1-6** Range of available responses to SARS at borders.

of movement restrictions. Essential personnel for the implementation of quarantine and other movement restrictions will include law enforcement officials, first responders and other deployable government services workers, and key personnel from the transportation, business, and education sectors. Training programs and deployment drills should be developed for these partners, as well as for public health personnel.

*Preparing to Respond and Secure National Borders*

Similar criteria to those used to determine community-level containment policy must be considered when determining appropriate responses to SARS at national borders (see Figure 1-6). In addition to considering circumstances in their area, officials contemplating movement across national borders must also monitor events in adjacent areas and, given the frequency of global travel, throughout the world. A limited border response could resemble that mounted by the United States in 2003 (i.e., issuing travel advisories and alerts; meeting flights from SARS areas to triage arriving ill passengers; and monitoring contacts for symptoms of illness). More intensive arrival screening could include questionnaires on symptoms and exposure to SARS, temperature screening, or even requiring health certification or registration with the local health department. In some circumstances, predeparture screening also would be appropriate. A further step would be to quarantine arriving passengers from affected areas, and under the most extreme circumstances, restriction of inbound and outbound travel may be necessary.

## Conclusion

Modern quarantine represents a wide range of scalable interventions to separate or restrict movement (e.g. detain, isolate, or conditionally release) of individuals or populations infected by or exposed to highly dangerous contagions. These strategies can be an important part of the public health toolbox for suppressing transmission and stopping epidemics such as SARS. However, the ethical implementation of modern quarantine can be resource and labor intensive. Quarantine is most effective when it is tailored to specific circumstances and used in conjunction with other containment measures; people affected by quarantine must be ensured appropriate support services. The effectiveness of quarantine is further improved by comprehensive preparedness planning. Effective communication and public trust are quintessential components; consequently, the public must receive clear messages about the role and importance of quarantine as a means of containing certain infectious disease in advance of, as well as during, the epidemic.

If a future epidemic affects the United States as SARS did other countries in 2003, it may be necessary to recommend quarantine, among other containment measures, in this country. Thus, it is essential that planning for the effective implementation of quarantine and other containment measures be undertaken at every level of government, and well in advance of the need. Strategic and operative plans should be exercised at all levels to expose and rectify gaps and pitfalls in nonurgent settings to ensure our readiness in an emergency.

## Acknowledgments

The authors thank Alison Mack, Katherine Oberholtzer, Alexandra Levitt, and Ava Navin for technical assistance in the preparation and review of the manuscript.

## IMPACTS OF SARS ON HEALTH CARE SYSTEMS AND STRATEGIES FOR COMBATING FUTURE OUTBREAKS OF EMERGING INFECTIOUS DISEASES

*Abu Saleh M. Abdullah,*[9] *Brian Tomlinson,*[10]
*G. Neil Thomas,*[9] *and Clive S. Cockram*[10]

Severe acute respiratory syndrome (SARS), resulting from a novel coronavirus, originated in November 2002 in, Guangdong Province, China. By February 2003 it had spread to Hong Kong and subsequently to 32 countries or regions on most continents, infecting about 8,098 patients and resulting in 774 deaths

[9]Department of Community Medicine, The University of Hong Kong.
[10]Department of Medicine and Therapeutics, Chinese University of Hong Kong, Hong Kong.

(WHO, 2003k). The overall case fatality ratio is approximately 15 percent (WHO, 2003b). The nonspecific disease presentation, coupled with a long incubation period and the initial absence of a reliable diagnostic test, limited the understanding of the magnitude of the outbreak. The outbreak has identified a number of deficiencies in hospital and community infection control systems in Hong Kong. The lessons learned should be applied on a worldwide basis to help prevent the spread of other new infections that may emerge (Abdullah et al., 2003). In this chapter we outline our experience with medical and public health issues that have arisen in dealing with the outbreak of SARS in Hong Kong and suggest appropriate strategies for combating future infections.

## The SARS Epidemic in Hong Kong

The first case of SARS to be identified in Hong Kong was a physician, who had been treating patients in Guangzhou. He traveled to Hong Kong on February 21, 2003. He rapidly became ill and was hospitalized, and he died soon after. This doctor apparently was able to warn his medical attendants of the highly infectious nature of his illness based on his own experience. Precautions were taken to prevent the spread of infection, so there were few cases of transmission within the hospital from this case (Tsang et al., 2003).

In contrast, the index case at the Prince of Wales Hospital who was the source of the first large hospital-based outbreak was not known to be highly infectious (Lee et al., 2003; Tomlinson and Cockram, 2003). This patient was admitted before the discovery of the SARS coronavirus and any international recognition of the disease. The clinical picture was that of "typical" community-acquired pneumonia with no suspicious circumstances. This patient was thus treated using standard protocols established for previous cases in Hong Kong—in an eight-bed cubicle of an open general medical ward. Heightened infection control precautions were not instituted.

During the epidemic, cases who were admitted to hospitals who did not show symptoms suggestive of SARS may not have been treated with strict isolation precautions, and this resulted in larger hospital outbreaks in areas such as Hong Kong and Toronto (Simmerman et al., 2003). In Hong Kong, this first received attention when 11 health care workers from the same ward of a hospital went on sick leave simultaneously in early March 2003. At that point different hypotheses were tested and different control measures were instituted to combat the disease. However, the prolonged epidemic affected a total of 1,755 individuals over a period of 3 months in Hong Kong. The last case was confirmed on June 11, 2003.

## Learning from the Experience

A few important lessons were learned over the course of the SARS outbreak. Cardiopulmonary resuscitation and endotracheal intubation were identified as procedures causing very high risk to medical personnel. During some resuscitation procedures and difficult intubations, cases were reported of health care workers becoming infected despite the use of what was believed to be appropriate protective equipment. The use of nebulizers received particular attention in relation to the index patient at the Prince of Wales Hospital in Hong Kong (Lee et al., 2003). Other procedures such as nasopharyngeal aspiration, bronchoscopy, airway suction, and noninvasive ventilation procedures such as Bi-level Positive Airway Procedure (BiPAP) were also suspected to increase the dissemination of infection. It soon became apparent that respiratory secretions were not the only source of transmission of infection. Feces and urine were recognized to be major hazards. Cleaning the patient and the bedding after fecal incontinence, often performed by health care workers less trained in infection control procedures, proved to be a high-risk duty.

Another problem found with the hospital management of SARS patients was that even after implementation of usual infection precautions for staff with gloves, gowns, and face masks, new infections in health care workers continued to occur (Lee and Sung, 2003). These may have been partly related to lapses in following standard procedures and partly because of initial lack of awareness of the mode of spread of the virus. Although it was concluded at an early stage that the infection was spread by droplets, it was not immediately recognized that the virus was so tenacious that it could survive outside the body on surfaces for long periods of time. The estimates of the time that the virus could survive on various surfaces grew longer and longer—from hours to days over the period of the outbreak—as understanding of the virus increased.

Another contributing factor to the spread of infection within hospitals in Hong Kong was probably the relative inexperience of most hospital staff with respiratory pathogens with such a degree of infectivity. In recent years the only common infective respiratory conditions encountered in Hong Kong hospitals have been tuberculosis and influenza, and these generally have been contained quite easily within hospitals without specialized isolation facilities. Lack of experience in dealing with such a novel agent as the SARS coronavirus must have contributed to the high rate of infection within hospitals. *This must be addressed by appropriate training, with repeated reinforcement and checking of infection control techniques so that hospital staff are ready for the next emerging infection.*

It is also likely that over the years a degree of complacency has developed, and that procedures that should be considered routine, such as washing hands between examining different patients, are no longer strictly implemented. Furthermore, the use of face masks in Hong Kong hospitals was previously a rarity except in operating rooms and designated high-risk areas.

Guidelines need to be developed that are based on the best available evidence. In hospital settings in Hong Kong, such guidelines were established at a relatively early stage of the outbreak (Ho, 2003), but in the general community, it was more difficult to provide clear guidelines apart from applying the principles of common hygiene. *The use of face masks outside of the hospital environment was adopted by a large percentage of the population, but guidelines for the use of this and other preventive measures were often vague and inconsistent.*

In the community setting, contact tracing and quarantining of people who had been in close contact with cases who developed SARS was rapidly introduced and was of vital importance in curtailing the spread of the disease and bringing the epidemic to an end (Riley et al., 2003). Again much experience was gained during the course of the outbreak, particularly regarding communication between different sectors of the health services, and mechanisms have been introduced to improve such communications. The initial case of the Guangzhou doctor was reported to the Hong Kong Department of Health, but contact tracing was not initially conducted at the Metropole Hotel where he stayed because there were no other reports of atypical pneumonia related to that hotel and little was understood about the nature of the condition. In retrospect such contact tracing clearly should have been attempted, although it is unlikely that it could have prevented the spread of disease to other countries. The other people who were infected at the hotel would have left Hong Kong soon afterward, at a time when they were still asymptomatic.

International travel provides a means to disseminate an infection like SARS throughout the world. Fortunately few cases seem to have actually acquired the infection during air travel. Although measures were instituted to stop people with fever from traveling by air, those who were incubating the disease and were still asymptomatic would not be identified, so perhaps stricter measures are needed to effectively reduce the risk of spread of such diseases to other countries. The ease and frequency of international travel demand effective channels be established for rapid international communication of information about infectious diseases. Rapid alerting to potential threats will help ensure that appropriate measures can be instituted and official public information can be disseminated to mitigate public alarm.

## Conclusion

Based on our current understanding about its pathogenicity and transmissibility, SARS needs to be regarded as a serious disease. Health care workers and service providers should use SARS as an example to prepare themselves with potential measures to combat any future outbreak of infectious disease. The SARS outbreak provides a timely reminder of the importance of the reorganization of health care systems with an international focus to ensure adequate surveillance mechanisms, rapid response to epidemics, effective prevention and control strategies, and maintenance of optimal infrastructure nationally and internationally (Lee and Abdullah, 2003). In advance of future disease outbreaks, countries where no SARS cases have been reported should be prepared with clear national and provincial contingency plans and mechanisms for integrating such plans into an international response (Lee and Abdullah, 2003).

# REFERENCES

Abdullah AS, Tomlinson B, Cockram CS, Thomas GN. 2003. Lessons From the severe acute respiratory syndrome outbreak in Hong Kong. *Emerging Infectious Diseases* 9(9):1042-5.

Anonymous. 2003. Global surveillance for severe acute respiratory syndrome (SARS). *Weekly Epidemiological Record* 78(14):100-19.

Booth CM, Matukas LM, Tomlinson GA, Rachlis AR, Rose DB, Dwosh HA, Walmsley SL, Mazzulli T, Avendano M, Derkach P, Ephtimios IE, Kitai I, Mederski BD, Shadowitz SB, Gold WL, Hawryluck LA, Rea E, Chenkin JS, Cescon DW, Poutanen SM, Detsky AS. 2003. Clinical features and short-term outcomes of 144 patients with SARS in the greater Toronto area. *JAMA* 289(21):2801-9.

CDC. 2003a. Severe acute respiratory syndrome—Singapore, 2003. *MMWR* 52(18):405-11.

CDC. 2003b. Updated interim surveillance case definition for severe acute respiratory syndrome (SARS)—United States, April 29, 2003. *MMWR* 52(17):391-3.

Donnelly CA, Ghani AC, Leung GM, Hedley AJ, Fraser C, Riley S, Abu-Raddad LJ, Ho LM, Thach TQ, Chau P, Chan KP, Lam TH, Tse LY, Tsang T, Liu SH, Kong JH, Lau EM, Ferguson NM, Anderson RM. 2003. Epidemiological determinants of spread of causal agent of severe acute respiratory syndrome in Hong Kong. [Erratum Appears in *Lancet*. May 24, 2003. 361(9371): 1832]. *Lancet* 361(9371):1761-6.

Drosten C, Gunther S, Preiser W, van der Werf S, Brodt HR, Becker S, Rabenau H, Panning M, Kolesnikova L, Fouchier RA, Berger A, Burguiere AM, Cinatl J, Eickmann M, Escriou N, Grywna K, Kramme S, Manuguerra JC, Muller S, Rickerts V, Sturmer M, Vieth S, Klenk HD, Osterhaus AD, Schmitz H, Doerr HW. 2003. Identification of a novel coronavirus in patients with severe acute respiratory syndrome. *New England Journal of Medicine* 348(20):1967-76.

Dwosh HA, Hong HH, Austgarden D, Herman S, Schabas R. 2003. Identification and containment of an outbreak of SARS in a community hospital. *Canadian Medical Association Journal* 168(11):1415-20.

Fisher DA, Lim TK, Lim YT, Singh KS, Tambyah PA. 2003. Atypical presentations of SARS. *Lancet* 361(9370):1740.

Fowler RA, Lapinsky SE, Hallett D, Detsky AS, Sibbald WJ, Slutsky AS, Stewart TE. 2003. Critically ill patients with severe acute respiratory syndrome. *JAMA* 290(3):367-73.

Gold WL, Mederski B, Rose D, Simor A, Minnema B, Mahoney J, Petric M, MacArthur M, Willey BM, Chua R, Pong-Porter S, Rzayev Y, Tamlin P, Henry B, Green K, Low DE, Mazzulli T. 2003. Prevalence of asymptomatic (AS) infection by severe acute respiratory syndrome coronavirus (SARS-CoV) in exposed healthcare workers (HCW). Interscience Conference on Antimicrobial Agents and Chemotherapy Abstract: K-1315c.

Guan Y, Zheng BJ, He YQ, Liu XL, Zhuang ZX, Cheung CLLSW, Li PH, Zhang LJ, Guan YJ, Butt KM, Wong KLCKW, Lim W, Shortridge KF, Yuen KY, Peiris JSM, Poon LLM. 2003. Isolation and characterization of viruses related to the SARS coronavirus from animals in southern China. *Science* 302(5643):276-8.

Ho W, Hong Kong Hospital Authority Working Group on SARS, Central Committee of, Infection Control. 2003. Guideline on management of severe acute respiratory syndrome (SARS). *Lancet* 361(9366):1313-5.

Hon KL, Leung CW, Cheng WT, Chan PK, Chu WC, Kwan YW, Li AM, Fong NC, Ng PC, Chiu MC, Li CK, Tam JS, Fok TF. 2003. Clinical presentations and outcome of severe acute respiratory syndrome in children. *Lancet* 361(9370):1701-3.

Hsu LY, Lee CC, Green JA, Ang B, Paton NI, Lee L, Villacian JS, Lim PL, Earnest A, Leo YS. 2003. Severe acute respiratory syndrome (SARS) in Singapore: clinical features of index patient and initial contacts. *Emerging Infectious Diseases* 9(6):713-7.

Ksiazek TG, Erdman D, Goldsmith CS, Zaki SR, Peret T, Emery S, Tong S, Urbani C, Comer JA, Lim W, Rollin PE, Dowell SF, Ling AE, Humphrey CD, Shieh WJ, Guarner J, Paddock CD, Rota P, Fields B, DeRisi J, Yang JY, Cox N, Hughes JM, LeDuc JW, Bellini WJ, Anderson LJ, SARS Working Group. 2003. A novel coronavirus associated with severe acute respiratory syndrome. *New England Journal of Medicine* 348(20):1953-66.

Lee A, Abdullah AS. 2003. Severe acute respiratory syndrome: a challenge for public health practice in Hong Kong. *Journal of Epidemiology & Community Health* 57(9):655-8.

Lee JW, McKibbin WJ. 2003. *Globalization and Disease: The Case of SARS*. Australian National University Working Paper.

Lee N, Hui D, Wu A, Chan P, Cameron P, Joynt GM, Ahuja A, Yung MY, Leung CB, To KF, Lui SF, Szeto CC, Chung S, Sung JJ. 2003. A major outbreak of severe acute respiratory syndrome in Hong Kong. *New England Journal of Medicine* 348(20):1986-94.

Lee N, Sung JJ. 2003. Nosocomial Transmission of SARS. *Current Infectious Disease Reports* 5(6):473-6.

Lew TW, Kwek TK, Tai D, Earnest A, Loo S, Singh K, Kwan KM, Chan Y, Yim CF, Bek SL, Kor AC, Yap WS, Chelliah YR, Lai YC, Goh SK. 2003. Acute respiratory distress syndrome in critically ill patients with severe acute respiratory syndrome. *JAMA* 290(3):374-80.

Li G, Zhao Z, Chen L, Zhou Y. 2003. Mild severe acute respiratory syndrome. *Emerging Infectious Diseases* 9(9):1182-3.

Ludwig B, Kraus FB, Allwinn R, Doerr HW, Preiser W. 2003. Viral zoonoses—A threat under control? *Intervirology*. 46(2):71-8.

Marra MA, Jones SJ, Astell CR, Holt RA, Brooks-Wilson A, Butterfield YS, Khattra J, Asano JK, Barber SA, Chan SY, Cloutier A, Coughlin SM, Freeman D, Girn N, Griffith OL, Leach SR, Mayo M, McDonald H, Montgomery SB, Pandoh PK, Petrescu AS, Robertson AG, Schein JE, Siddiqui A, Smailus DE, Stott JM, Yang GS, Plummer F, Andonov A, Artsob H, Bastien N, Bernard K, Booth TF, Bowness D, Czub M, Drebot M, Fernando L, Flick R, Garbutt M, Gray M, Grolla A, Jones S, Feldmann H, Meyers A, Kabani A, Li Y, Normand S, Stroher U, Tipples GA, Tyler S, Vogrig R, Ward D, Watson B, Brunham RC, Krajden M, Petric M, Skowronski DM, Upton C, Roper RL. 2003. The genome sequence of the Sars-associated coronavirus. *Science* 300(5624):1399-404.

Maunder R, Hunter J, Vincent L, Bennett J, Peladeau N, Leszcz M, Sadavoy J, Verhaeghe LM, Steinberg R, Mazzulli T. 2003. The immediate psychological and occupational impact of the 2003 SARS outbreak in a teaching hospital. *Canadian Medical Association Journal* 168(10):1245-51.

Ofner M, Lem M, Sarwal S, Vearncombe M, Simor A. 2003. Cluster of severe acute respiratory syndrome cases among protected health care workers-Toronto, April 2003. *Canada Communicable Disease Report* 29(11):93-7.

Peiris JS, Lai ST, Poon LL, Guan Y, Yam LY, Lim W, Nicholls J, Yee WK, Yan WW, Cheung MT, Cheng VC, Chan KH, Tsang DN, Yung RW, Ng TK, Yuen KY, SARS study group. 2003a. Coronavirus as a possible cause of severe acute respiratory syndrome. *Lancet* 361(9366):1319-25.

Peiris JS, Chu CM, Cheng VC, Chan KS, Hung IF, Poon LL, Law KI, Tang BS, Hon TY, Chan CS, Chan KH, Ng JS, Zheng BJ, Ng WL, Lai RW, Guan Y, Yuen KY, HKU/UCH SARS Study Group. 2003b. Clinical progression and viral load in a community outbreak of coronavirus-associated SARS pneumonia: a prospective study. *Lancet* 361(9371):1767-72.

Poutanen SM, Low DE, Henry B, Finkelstein S, Rose D, Green K, Tellier R, Draker R, Adachi D, Ayers M, Chan AK, Skowronski DM, Salit I, Simor AE, Slutsky AS, Doyle PW, Krajden M, Petric M, Brunham RC, McGeer AJ, National Microbiology Laboratory Canada, Canadian Severe Acute Respiratory Syndrome Study Team. 2003. Identification of severe acute respiratory syndrome in Canada. *New England Journal of Medicine* 348(20):1995-2005.

Rainer TH, Cameron PA, Smit D, Ong KL, Hung AN, Nin DC, Ahuja AT, Si LC, Sung JJ. 2003. Evaluation of WHO criteria for identifying patients with severe acute respiratory syndrome out of hospital: prospective observational study. *British Medical Journal* 326(7403):1354-8.

Ren Y, Ding HG, Wu QF, Chen WJ, Chen D, Bao ZY, Yang L, Zhao CH, Wang J. 2003. [Detection of SARS-CoV RNA in stool samples of SARS patients by nest RT-PCR and its clinical value]. *Zhongguo Yi Xue Ke Xue Yuan Xue Bao* 25(3):368-71.

Riley S, Fraser C, Donnelly CA, Ghani AC, Abu-Raddad LJ, Hedley AJ, Leung GM, Ho LM, Lam TH, Thach TQ, Chau P, Chan KP, Lo SV, Leung PY, Tsang T, Ho W, Lee KH, Lau EM, Ferguson NM, Anderson RM. 2003. Transmission dynamics of the etiological agent of SARS in Hong Kong: impact of public health interventions. *Science* 300(5627):1961-6.

Rota PA, Oberste MS, Monroe SS, Nix WA, Campagnoli R, Icenogle JP, Penaranda S, Bankamp B, Maher K, Chen MH, Tong S, Tamin A, Lowe L, Frace M, DeRisi JL, Chen Q, Wang D, Erdman DD, Peret TC, Burns C, Ksiazek TG, Rollin PE, Sanchez A, Liffick S, Holloway B, Limor J, McCaustland K, Olsen-Rasmussen M, Fouchier R, Gunther S, Osterhaus AD, Drosten C, Pallansch MA, Anderson LJ, Bellini WJ. 2003. Characterization of a novel coronavirus associated with severe acute respiratory syndrome. *Science* 300(5624):1394-9.

Ruan YJ, Wei CL, Ee AL, Vega VB, Thoreau H, Su ST, Chia JM, Ng P, Chiu KP, Lim L, Zhang T, Peng CK, Lin EO, Lee NM, Yee SL, Ng LF, Chee RE, Stanton LW, Long PM, Liu ET. 2003. Comparative full-length genome sequence analysis of 14 SARS coronavirus isolates and common mutations associated with putative origins of infection. [Erratum Appears in *Lancet*. May 24, 2003. 361(9371):1832]. *Lancet* 361(9371):1779-85.

Seto WH, Tsang D, Yung RW, Ching TY, Ng TK, Ho M, Ho LM, Peiris JS. 2003. Effectiveness of precautions against droplets and contact in prevention of nosocomial transmission of severe acute respiratory syndrome (SARS). *Lancet* 361(9368):1519-20.

Simmerman JM, Chu D, Chang H. 2003. Implications of unrecognized severe acute respiratory syndrome. *Nurse Practitioner* 28(11):21-31.

Stohr K. 2003. A multicentre collaboration to investigate the cause of severe acute respiratory syndrome. *Lancet* 361(9370):1730-3.

Styra R, Gold W, Robinson S. 2003. Post-traumatic stress disorder and quality of life in patients diagnosed with SARS. Interscience Conference on Antimicrobial Agents and Chemotherapy Abstract: V-796a.

Tomlinson B, Cockram C. 2003. SARS: experience at Prince of Wales Hospital, Hong Kong. *Lancet* 361(9368):1486-7.

Tsang KW, Ho PL, Ooi GC, Yee WK, Wang T, Chan-Yeung M, Lam WK, Seto WH, Yam LY, Cheung TM, Wong PC, Lam B, Ip MS, Chan J, Yuen KY, Lai KN. 2003. A cluster of cases of severe acute respiratory syndrome in Hong Kong. *New England Journal of Medicine* 348(20):1977-85.

Varia M, Wilson S, Sarwal S, McGeer A, Gournis E, Galanis E, Henry B. 2003. Investigation of a nosocomial outbreak of severe acute respiratory syndrome (SARS) in Toronto, Canada. *Canadian Medical Association Journal* 169(4):285-92.

WHO Western Pacific Regional Office. *Interim Assessment Protocol for National SARS Preparedness*. 2003. Manila, Philippines: WHO.

Williams ES, Yuill T, Artois M, Fischer J, Haigh SA. 2002. Emerging infectious diseases in wildlife. *Revue Scientifique Et Technique* 21(1):139-57.

Wong KT, Antonio GE, Hui DS, Lee N, Yuen EH, Wu A, Leung CB, Rainer TH, Cameron P, Chung SS, Sung JJ, Ahuja AT. 2003. Thin-section CT of severe acute respiratory syndrome: evaluation of 73 patients exposed to or with the disease. *Radiology* 228(2):395-400.

WHO (World Health Organization). 2000. *Global Outbreak Alert and Response: Report of a WHO Meeting*. Geneva, Switzerland: WHO.

WHO. 2001. *A Framework for Global Outbreak Alert and Response*. WHO/CDS/CSR/2000/2. Geneva: WHO.

WHO. 2003a. Update 95—SARS: chronology of a serial killer. [Online] Available: http://www.who. int/csr/don/2003_07_04/en/.

WHO. 2003b. *Consensus Document on the Epidemiology of Severe Acute Respiratory Syndrome (SARS).* WHO/CDS/CSR/GAR/2003.11. Geneva: WHO.

WHO. 2003c. Summary table of areas that experienced local transmission of SARS during the outbreak period from November 1, 2002, to July 31, 2003. [Online] Available: http://www.who.int/ csr/sars/areas/areas2003_11_21/en/ [accessed January 15, 2004].

WHO. 2003d. Alert, verification and public health management of SARS in the post-outbreak period. [Online] Available: http://www.who.int/csr/sars/postoutbreak/en/ [accessed January 15, 2004].

WHO. 2003e. Summary of the Discussions and Recommendations of the SARS Laboratory Workshop, 22 October 2003. [Online] Available: http://www.who.int/csr/sars/guidelines/en/ SARSLabmeeting.pdf [accessed January 14, 2004].

WHO. 2003f. *Biosafety and SARS Incident in Singapore September 2003.* Geneva: WHO.

WHO. 2003g. WHO biosafety guidelines for handling of SARS specimens. [Online] Available: http: //www.who.int/csr/sars/biosafety2003_04_25/en/ [accessed January 14, 2004].

WHO. 2003h. WHO SARS Scientific Research Advisory Committee concludes its first meeting. [Online] Available: http://www.who.int/csr/sars/archive/research/en/ [accessed January 15, 2004].

WHO. 2003i. WHO consultation on needs and opportunities for SARS vaccine research and development [Online] Available: http://www.who.int/vaccine_research/diseases/sars/events/2003/11/en/ [accessed January 15, 2004].

WHO. 2003j. *Severe Acute Respiratory Syndrome (SARS): Status of the Outbreak and Lessons for the Immediate Future.* Geneva: WHO.

WHO. 2003k. Summary table of SARS cases by country, November 1, 2002, to August 7, 2003. [Online] Available: http://www.who.int/csr/sars/country/2003_08_15/en/ [accessed January 15, 2004].

WHO. 2003m. Update 15—Situation in Hong Kong, activities of WHO team in China. [Online] Available: http://www.who.int/csr/sars/archive/2003_03_31/en/ [accessed January 17, 2004].

WHO. 2003n. Inadequate plumbing systems likely contributed to SARS transmission. [Online] Available: http://www.who.int/mediacentre/releases/2003/pr70/en/ [accessed January 14, 2004].

WHO. 2003o. Summary of probable SARS cases with onset of illness from November 1, 2002, to July 31, 2003. [Online] Available: http://www.who.int/csr/sars/country/table2003_09_23/en/ [accessed December 17, 2003].

Wu EB, Sung JJ. 2003. Haemorrhagic-fever-like changes and normal chest radiograph in a doctor with SARS. *Lancet* 361(9368):1520-1.

Zhong NS, Zeng GQ. 2003. Our strategies for fighting severe acute respiratory syndrome (SARS). *American Journal of Respiratory & Critical Care Medicine* 168(1):7-9.

# 2

# Political Influences on the Response to SARS and Economic Impacts of the Disease

## OVERVIEW

As the severe acute respiratory syndrome (SARS) coronavirus spread around the globe, so too did its political, economic, and sociological repercussions. The ensuing multinational effort launched in response to SARS placed unprecedented demands on affected countries for timely, accurate case reporting; cooperation with expert teams coordinated by the World Health Organization (WHO); and the sacrifice of immediate economic interests, such as trade, tourism, and investment.

The first paper in this chapter presents an economic model of the past and projected costs of the SARS epidemic (see Lee and McKibbin). As one would expect, the model indicates that significant short-term economic losses in China resulted from a sharp decrease in foreign investment. Although the most immediate and dramatic economic effects of SARS occurred in Asia, nearly every major market was impacted directly or indirectly by the epidemic. Several agencies and experts have attempted to estimate the cost of SARS based on expenditures and near-term losses in key areas such as medical expenses, travel and related services, consumer confidence, and investment. The extent of the long-term economic consequences resulting from SARS will depend on whether—and how—the disease returns.

The chapter continues with two political analyses that reflect upon issues of both national and global governance impacted by the SARS epidemic. The first political analysis frames the issue in terms of the new rules of international engagement during the age of globalization, described by the author as the post-Westphalian era (see Fidler) in which nonstate actors such as multinational corporations and multilateral organizations have increasing influence on global governance.

The second article hypothesizes that the structure and operation of China's central government account for most of that country's initial resistance to international collaboration at the onset of the SARS epidemic (see Huang). The author describes considerable internal and external pressures that ultimately influenced the Chinese government to declare its "war on SARS." He identifies both improvements in the Chinese public health infrastructure and challenges the country may face if SARS reemerges.

## ESTIMATING THE GLOBAL ECONOMIC COSTS OF SARS[*]

*Jong-Wha Lee and Warwick J. McKibbin*
Korea University and The Australian National University, The Australian
National University and The Brookings Institution

While the number of patients affected by the SARS coronavirus and its broader impact on the global public health community have been surveyed in considerable detail, the consequences of the disease in other areas are less well calibrated. The purpose of this paper is to provide an assessment of the global economic costs of SARS. Our empirical estimates of the economic effects of the SARS epidemic are based on a global model called the G-Cubed (Asia-Pacific) model. Most previous studies on the economic effects of epidemics focus on the economic costs deriving from disease-associated medical costs or forgone incomes as a result of the disease-related morbidity and mortality. However, the direct consequences of the SARS epidemic in terms of medical expenditures or demographic effects seem to be rather small, particularly when compared to other major epidemics such as HIV/AIDS or malaria. A few recent studies—including Chou et al. (2003), Siu and Wong (2003), and Wen (2003)—provide some estimates on the economic effects of SARS on individual Asian regions such as mainland China, Hong Kong (SAR), and Taiwan. But these studies focus mostly

[*]This paper is adapted from an article that will appear later this year in Asian Economic Papers (MIT Press). An earlier version of the paper was originally presented to the Asian Economic Panel meeting held in Tokyo, May 11–12, 2003, and the Pacific Economic Cooperation Council (PECC) finance forum, Hua Hin, Thailand, July 8–9, 2003. We have updated that original paper to include the last known case of SARS as well as adjusting the scale of some shocks given the knowledge that the SARS epidemic lasted approximately 6 months rather than the full year originally assumed. The authors particularly thank Andrew Stoeckel for interesting discussions and many participants at the conferences, particularly Ifzal Ali, Richard Dorbnick, George Von Furstenberg, Yung Chul Park, Jeffrey Sachs, Wing Thye Woo, and Zhang Wei for helpful comments. Alison Stegman provided excellent research assistance and Kang Tan provided helpful data. See also the preliminary results and links to the model documentation at http://www.economicscenarios.com. The views expressed in the paper are those of the authors and should not be interpreted as reflecting the views of the institutions with which the authors are affiliated, including the trustees, officers, or other staff of the Brookings Institution.

on assessing the damages by SARS in affected industries such as tourism and the retail service sector.

However, just calculating the number of canceled tourist trips, declines in retail trade, and similar factors is not sufficient to get a full picture of the impact of SARS because there are linkages within economies, across sectors, and across economies in both international trade and international capital flows. The economic costs from a global disease such as SARS go beyond the direct damages incurred in the affected sectors of disease-inflicted countries. This is not just because the disease spreads quickly across countries through networks related to global travel, but also because any economic shock to one country is quickly spread to other countries through the increased trade and financial linkages associated with globalization. As the world becomes more integrated, the global cost of a communicable disease like SARS can be expected to rise. Our global model is able to capture many of the important linkages across sectors as well as countries through capital flows and the trade of goods and services, thereby providing a broader assessment of disease-associated costs.

The G-Cubed model also incorporates rational expectations and forward-looking intertemporal behavior on the part of individual agents. This feature is particularly important when we are interested in distinguishing the effects of a temporary shock from those of a persistent shock. For example, when foreign investors expect that SARS or other epidemics of unknown etiology can break out in some Asian countries not just this year but persistently for the next few years, they would demand a greater risk premium from investing in affected economies. Their forward-looking behavior would have immediate global impacts.

Needless to say, our empirical assessment is preliminary and relies on our limited knowledge about the disease and constrained methodology. For instance, there is speculation that SARS could reemerge in an even deadlier form in the next influenza season. There is also no consensus yet on the likely developments of any future epidemic and the precise mechanism by which SARS affects economic activities. Although a global model is better than simple back-of-the-envelope calculations, it is a coarse representation of a complex world. Nonetheless, even simple calculations are important inputs into the model. We saw this with the Asian Crisis of 1997, when the transmission of shocks in Asia to the rest of the world and the adjustment within economies in Asia were poorly predicted when only trade flows were considered.[1] Thus it is important to go beyond the rough estimates that currently permeate commentary on the economic consequences of SARS. Because we take into account the interdependencies among economies and the role of confidence, our costs are larger than many of the estimates that currently appear in the media.

---

[1]See McKibbin (1998) for a study of the Asia crisis that included the critical role of capital flow adjustment.

## Economic Impacts of SARS

Despite the catastrophic consequences of infectious diseases such as malaria and HIV/AIDS, the impact of epidemics has been considerably under-researched in economics.[2] Traditionally, studies have attempted to estimate the economic burden of an epidemic based on the private and nonprivate medical costs associated with the disease, such as expenditures on diagnosing and treating the disease. The costs are magnified by the need to maintain sterile environments, implement prevention measures, and conduct basic research. Such economic costs can be substantial for major epidemics such as HIV/AIDS. According to UNAIDS (the Joint United Nations Programme on HIV/AIDS), 42 million people globally are living with HIV/AIDS. The medical costs of various treatments of HIV patients, including highly active antiretroviral therapies (HAARTs), are estimated to be more than $2,000 per patient per year. In the Southern African regions, the total HIV-related health service costs, based on an assumed coverage rate of 10 percent, ranges from 0.3 to 4.3 percent of gross domestic product (GDP) (Haacker, 2002).

The costs of disease also include income forgone as a result of disease-related morbidity and mortality. Forgone income is normally estimated by the value of workdays lost due to the illness. In the case of mortality, forgone income is estimated by the capitalized value of future lifetime earnings lost to the disease-related death, based on projected incomes for different age groups and age-specific survival rates. This cost can be substantial for some epidemics. Malaria kills more than 1 million people a year, and HIV/AIDS is estimated to have claimed 3.1 million lives in 2002.

Previous researchers have also focused on long-term effects from the demographic consequences of epidemics. The first and foremost impact of epidemics is a negative shock to population and labor force. However, economic theory provides conflicting predictions regarding the economic effects of negative population shocks. A disease that kills mostly children and the elderly without affecting the economically active population aged 15 to 54 can lead to an initial increase in GDP per head. Even when the disease mostly attacks prime earners, its long-term economic consequences are not unambiguous. Standard neoclassical growth models predict that a negative shock to population growth can lead to a faster accumulation of capital and subsequently faster output growth (see Barro and Sala-I-Martin, 1995). Conversely, an exogenous, one-time reduction in labor force raises the capital-labor ratio and lowers the rate of return to capital, which subsequently leads to slower capital accumulation and thereby lower output growth.

Empirical studies also present conflicting results. Brainerd and Siegler (2002) show that the Spanish flu epidemic of 1918–1919, which killed at least 40 million

---

[2]Exceptions can be found in the Commission on Macroeconomics and Health (2002).

people worldwide and 675,000 in the United States, had a positive effect on per capita income growth across states in the United States in the 1920s. In contrast, Bloom and Mahal (1997) show no significant impact of that epidemic on acreage sown per capita in India across 13 Indian provinces.

Epidemics can have further effects on demographic structures by influencing fertility decisions of households. According to the "child-survivor hypothesis," parents desire to have a certain number of surviving children. Under this theory, risk-averse households raise fertility by even more than expected child mortality. Evidence shows that high infant and child mortality rates in African regions of intense malaria transmission are associated with a disproportionately high fertility rate and high population growth (Sachs and Malaney, 2002). Thus, the increase in fertility has a further negative impact on long-term growth.

Aside from the direct demographic consequences of an epidemic, another important mechanism by which a disease has an adverse impact on the economy's long-term growth is the destruction of human capital. Human capital, the stock of knowledge embodied in the population, is considered an important determinant of long-term growth (Barro and Sala-I-Martin, 1995). Furthermore, the decline in "health capital," as measured in general by life expectancy, has negative effects on economic growth (Bloom et al., 2001). Epidemics also adversely affect labor productivity by inhibiting the movement of labor across regions within a country as well as across countries. Restricted mobility thus inhibits labor from moving to the places where it is most productive. Researchers simulating the effect of AIDS on growth in Southern African countries find that AIDS has had significant negative effects on per capita income growth mainly through the decline in human capital (Haacker, 2002).

While previous studies have emphasized the economic cost of disease associated with private and nonprivate medical costs, this doesn't seem to be the principal issue in the case of SARS. The number of probable SARS cases is still small in comparison to other major historical epidemics. Furthermore, unlike AIDS, the duration of hospitalization of the infected patients is short, with more than 90 percent of the patients recovering in a relatively short period, thereby rendering the medical costs comparatively very low. The SARS-related demographic or human capital consequences are also currently estimated to be insignificant. The fatality rate of the SARS coronavirus is high, but, with current estimates indicating fewer than 800 deaths from SARS worldwide, the death toll is tiny compared with the 3 million who died of AIDS last year or at least 40 million people worldwide who died in the Spanish flu epidemic of 1918–1919. Therefore, forgone incomes associated with morbidity and mortality as a result of SARS appear to be insignificant. If SARS became endemic in the future, it would substantially increase private and public expenditures on health care and would have more significant impacts on demographic structure and human capital in the infected economies. However, based on information to date, this is unlikely to happen with the SARS epidemic.

Although the medical expenditures and demographic consequences associated with SARS are insignificant, SARS apparently has already caused substantial economic effects by other important channels. We summarize three mechanisms by which SARS influences the global economy.

First, fear of SARS infection leads to a substantial decline in consumer demand, especially for travel and retail sales service. The fast speed of contagion makes people avoid social interactions in affected regions. The adverse demand shock becomes more substantial in regions that have much larger service-related activities and higher population densities, such as Hong Kong or Beijing, China. The psychological shock also ripples around the world, not just to the countries of local transmission of SARS, because the world is so closely linked by international travel.

Second, the uncertain features of the disease reduce confidence in the future of the affected economies. This effect seems to be potentially very important, particularly as the shock reverberates through China, which has been a key center of foreign investment. The response by the Chinese government to the epidemic was fragmented and nontransparent. The greater exposure to an unknown disease and the less effective government responses to the disease outbreaks must have elevated concerns about China's institutional quality and future growth potential. Although it is difficult to measure directly the effects of diseases on decision making by foreign investors, the loss of foreign investors' confidence would have potentially tremendous impacts on foreign investment flows, which would in turn have significant impacts on China's economic growth. This effect is also transmitted to other countries competing with China for foreign direct investment (FDI).

Third, SARS undoubtedly increases the costs of disease prevention, especially in the most affected industries such as the travel and retail sales service industries. This cost may not be substantial, at least in global terms, as long as the disease is transmitted only by close human contact. However, the global cost could become enormous if the disease is found to be transmitted by other channels such as through international cargo.

## Simulations Using the G-Cubed (Asia Pacific) Model

Given the important linkages among affected countries in the region through capital flows and the trade of goods and services, any analysis of the implications of SARS on the global economy needs to be undertaken with a model that adequately captures these interrelationships. The G-Cubed (Asia Pacific) model, based on the theoretical structure of the G-Cubed model outlined in McKibbin and Wilcoxen (1998), is ideal for such analysis, having both a detailed country coverage of the region and rich links between countries through goods and asset markets.[3] A number of studies—summarized in McKibbin and Vines (2000)—

---

[3]Full details of the model, including a list of equations and parameters, can be found online at http://www.gcubed.com.

show that the G-Cubed model has been useful in assessing a range of issues across a number of countries since the mid-1980s.[4] A summary of the principal characteristics of the G-Cubed model is presented as an annex at the end of this paper.

We make two alternative assumptions in generating a range of possible scenarios under this model. In an earlier analysis, we assumed in the first scenario that the shock lasted for a year. To capture the fact that the shock lasted 6 months, in reality we now scale down the shocks by 50 percent to capture the shorter duration. This is called a temporary shock. The second assumption is that the shocks are the same magnitude in the first year as the temporary shock, but are more persistent in that they fade out equiproportionately over a 10-year period. This illustrates the impact of expectations of the future evolution of the disease on the estimated costs in 2003. It also gives some insight into what might happen to the region if the SARS virus is considered the beginning of a series of annual epidemics emerging from China.

### Initial Shock to China and Hong Kong

We first calculate the shocks to the economies of mainland China and Hong Kong (SAR), which were hit most heavily by the disease, and then work out some indexes summarizing how these shocks are likely to occur in other economies. There are three main shocks, based on observations of financial market analysts about the existing data emerging from China and Hong Kong:[5]

- A 200 basis-point increase in country risk premium.[6]
- A sector-specific demand shock to the retail sales sector, amounting to a 15 percent drop in demand for the exposed industries in the service sector.
- An increase in costs in the exposed activities in the service sector of 5 percent.

These shocks are then scaled to last only 6 months rather than 1 year.

We could also consider several other shocks, such as the impact on health expenditures and fiscal deficits. It is not clear how large this shock should be for the persistent shock, nor even whether the schock should have a positive or negative sign. Because SARS kills a higher proportion of vulnerable people in a very short period, it may be that the large expenditure for these people will be reduced

---

[4]These issues include Reaganomics in the 1980s, German unification in the early 1990s, fiscal consolidation in Europe in the mid-1990s, the formation of NAFTA, the Asian crisis, and the productivity boom in the United States.

[5]These are also consistent with other papers on particular countries presented at the Asian Economic Panel in May 2003.

[6]In the May version of this paper we assumed a 300 basis-point shock. We follow the updated research of Australian Treasury (2003) in adjusting this shock to 200 basis points.

as a result of SARS. There might also be a reaction by medical authorities to substantially increase investments in public health. Given the current state of information, we would be forced to speculate concerning all of these potential effects on health expenditures. We therefore explicitly ignore such fiscal impacts of SARS in this version of the paper.

*Shocks to Other Countries*

The transmission of SARS, as distinct from the transmission of economic impacts through global markets, depends on a number of factors. We refer to this as the global exposure to SARS. The speed of spread is likely to depend on (i) tourist flows, (ii) geographical distance to China, (iii) health expenditures and sanitary conditions, (iv) government response, (v) climate, (vi) per capita income, (vii) population density, and so on. Table 2-1 presents indicators on health expenditures, tourist arrivals, and sanitary conditions for selected countries. There are more than 33 million annual visitors to mainland China. Hong Kong (SAR) has annual tourist arrivals that are more than 200 percent of the local population. Overall health expenditure as a ratio to GDP is not small in Asian countries, but health expenditure per capita is only $45 in China.

With more data we could do some econometric estimation to capture these influences. Lacking that data, for the purposes of this paper we construct a rough

**TABLE 2-1** Health Expenditures, Tourist Arrivals, and Sanitation Indicators for Selected Countries

| | Health Expenditure, Total (% of GDP) | Health Expenditure per Capita (current US$) | Tourist Arrivals (million) | Tourist Arrivals Arrivals/ Population (%) | Improved Sanitation Facilities (% of population |
|---|---|---|---|---|---|
| China | 5.3 | 45 | 33.2 | 3 | 29 |
| Hong Kong | 4.4 | 950 | 13.7 | 203 | 100 |
| India | 4.9 | 23 | 2.5 | 0 | 16 |
| Indonesia | 2.7 | 19 | 5.2 | 2 | 47 |
| North Korea | 2.1 | 18 | n.a. | n.a. | 99 |
| South Korea | 6.0 | 584 | 5.1 | 14 | 63 |
| Malaysia | 2.5 | 101 | 12.8 | 53 | n.a. |
| Philippines | 3.4 | 33 | 1.8 | 4 | 74 |
| Singapore | 3.5 | 814 | 6.7 | 163 | 100 |
| Thailand | 3.7 | 71 | 10.1 | 16 | 79 |
| Vietnam | 5.2 | 21 | 1.4 | 2 | 29 |
| United States | 13.0 | 4,499 | n.a. | n.a. | 100 |
| Japan | n.a. | n.a. | 4.8 | 4 | n.a. |
| High-income OECD | 10.2 | 2,771 | 377.6 | n.a. | n.a. |
| World | 9.3 | 482 | 696.5 | n.a. | 55 |

SOURCE: CEIC, World Development Indicators. Recited from Hanna and Huang (2003).

measure of the intensity of exposures to SARS, based on the above information and the cumulative number of cases of SARS for each country. This index of "global exposure to SARS" is contained in Figure 2-1. This will be used to scale down the country risk shocks calculated for all other countries. For example, if a country has an index of 0.5, the country risk premium shock will be the Chinese shock of 2 percent adjusted by the "global exposure to SARS" index, which gives a shock of 1 percent.

For the shocks to the service industries, before applying the global exposure index to each country, we need to adjust the sector-specific shocks. Because we only have an aggregate service sector in the model, we need to take account for structural differences within the service sectors of each country. We do this by creating an "index of sectoral exposure to SARS." This index is assumed to be proportional to the share of industries affected by SARS within the service sector. Industries such as tourism, retail trade, and airline travel have been impacted severely. We use the GTAP5 database to calculate the share of exposed sectors to total services for each country.[7] We define the exposed sectors based on GTAP definitions as wholesale and retail trade (TRD, including hotels and restaurants), land transport (OTP), and air transport (ATP). The "index of sectoral exposure to SARS" is shown in Figure 2-2. This index is applied to the sector-specific shocks we developed for the Chinese economy. We then apply the "global exposure to SARS" to the resulting shocks.

The direct impact on any economy will be a function of a number of factors. An important aspect of the impact will be the size of the service sector in the economy as well as the relative indexes of exposure. Figure 2-3 shows the size of the service sector relative to total output in each economy in the model.

## Simulation Results

We apply the shocks outlined in the previous section to the global economy. We begin the simulation in 2003, assuming in 2003 that the SARS outbreak was completely unanticipated. Both the temporary and persistent shocks are assumed to be understood by the forward-looking agents in the model. Clearly this is problematic when it comes to a new disease like SARS, when there is likely to be a period of learning about the nature of the shock. In this case, rational expectations might not be a good way to model expectations. Yet an alternative approach is not clear. In our defense, it is worth pointing out that only 30 percent of agents have rational expectations and 70 percent of agents are using a rule of thumb in adjusting to contemporaneous information about the economy. Table 2-2 contains results for the percentage change in GDP in 2003 as a result of the temporary and permanent

---

[7]For more information on this database, see the website of the Global Trade Analysis Project at http://www.gtap.agecon.purdue.edu/.

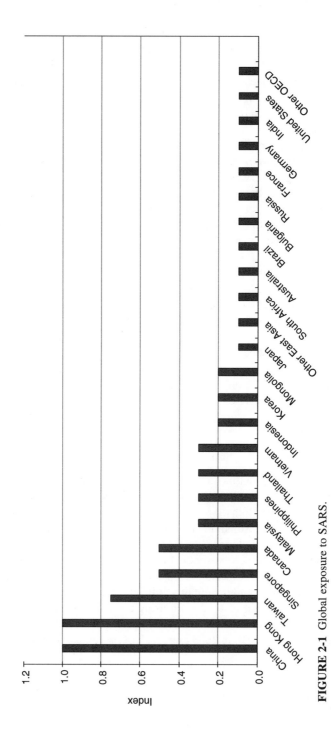

**FIGURE 2-1** Global exposure to SARS.

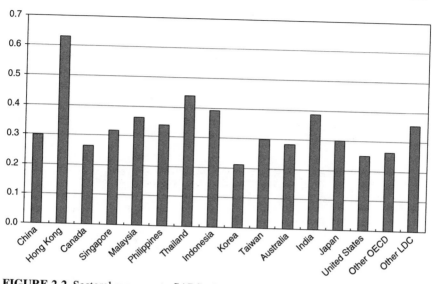

**FIGURE 2-2** Sectoral exposure to SARS: share of retail sale and travel industry in service sector.

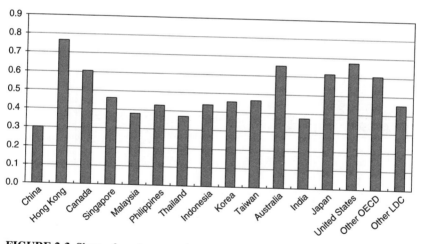

**FIGURE 2-3** Share of service sector in total output.

SARS shocks as well as the contribution of each component (i.e., demand decline for services, cost increase for services, and country risk premium).

The full dynamics of adjustment will be outlined shortly. Focusing on the GDP results, it is clear that there are interesting differences among the various components of the overall shock as well as between the temporary and permanent shocks. The temporary shock has its largest impact on China and Hong Kong

**TABLE 2–2** Percentage Change in GDP in 2003 Due to SARS

| | Temporary Shock | | | | Persistent Shock over 10 years | | | |
|---|---|---|---|---|---|---|---|---|
| | Total Effects | Demand Shift | Cost Rise | Country Risk | Total Effects | Demand Shift | Cost Rise | Country Risk |
| United States | -0.07 | -0.01 | -0.06 | 0.00 | -0.07 | -0.01 | -0.06 | 0.00 |
| Japan | -0.07 | -0.01 | -0.06 | 0.00 | -0.06 | -0.01 | -0.06 | 0.01 |
| Australia | -0.07 | 0.00 | -0.06 | 0.00 | -0.06 | 0.00 | -0.06 | 0.01 |
| New Zealand | -0.08 | 0.01 | -0.08 | 0.00 | -0.08 | 0.00 | -0.08 | 0.00 |
| Indonesia | -0.08 | 0.01 | -0.09 | 0.00 | -0.07 | 0.01 | -0.08 | 0.00 |
| Malaysia | -0.15 | 0.01 | -0.16 | 0.00 | -0.17 | 0.01 | -0.15 | -0.02 |
| Philippines | -0.10 | 0.04 | -0.14 | 0.00 | -0.11 | 0.03 | -0.13 | -0.02 |
| Singapore | -0.47 | -0.02 | -0.45 | 0.00 | -0.51 | -0.01 | -0.44 | -0.05 |
| Thailand | -0.15 | 0.00 | -0.15 | 0.00 | -0.15 | 0.00 | -0.15 | 0.00 |
| China | -1.05 | -0.37 | -0.34 | -0.33 | -2.34 | -0.53 | -0.33 | -1.48 |
| India | -0.04 | 0.00 | -0.04 | 0.00 | -0.04 | 0.00 | -0.04 | 0.00 |
| Taiwan | -0.49 | -0.07 | -0.41 | -0.01 | -0.53 | -0.07 | -0.39 | -0.07 |
| Korea | -0.10 | -0.02 | -0.08 | 0.00 | -0.08 | -0.01 | -0.08 | 0.00 |
| Hong Kong | -2.63 | -0.06 | -2.37 | -0.20 | -3.21 | -0.12 | -2.37 | -0.71 |
| ROECD | -0.05 | 0.00 | -0.05 | 0.00 | -0.05 | 0.00 | -0.05 | 0.00 |
| Non-oil developing countries | -0.05 | -0.01 | -0.04 | 0.00 | -0.05 | 0.00 | -0.04 | 0.00 |
| Eastern Europe and Russia | -0.06 | -0.01 | -0.05 | 0.00 | -0.05 | -0.01 | -0.05 | 0.00 |
| OPEC | -0.07 | -0.01 | -0.05 | 0.00 | -0.09 | -0.01 | -0.06 | -0.02 |

SOURCE: G–Cubed (Asia Pacific) Model version 50n.

(SAR), as expected. The loss to Hong Kong of 2.63 percent of GDP, however, is much larger than that of 1.05 percent for the remainder of mainland China. This primarily reflects the larger role of the service sector in Hong Kong, the larger share of impacted industries within the service sector in Hong Kong, and the greater reliance on trade within the Hong Kong region. Taiwan is the next most affected area, losing 0.49 percent of GDP in 2003, followed closely by Singapore, with a loss of 0.47 percent of GDP.

For Hong Kong, the increase in costs in the service sector is by far the largest contributing factor to the loss of GDP. In the rest of mainland China it is evenly spread across the three factors. The temporary increase in the country risk premium of 200 basis points is estimated to lower GDP by 0.33 percent for China and by 0.20 percent for Hong Kong. Interestingly, the risk premium shock has very negligible impacts, of less than 0.01 percent of GDP, on Taiwan and Singapore, which adopt floating exchange rate regimes, although they are also subject to a substantial rise in the country risk premium by 150 and 100 basis points, respectively. The difference comes from the fact that exchange rate depreciation helps Taiwan and Singapore to avoid a rise in real interest rate and subsequent output decline.

The calculations when expressed as a percent of each country's GDP may appear to be small. However, when translated into an absolute dollar amount, these figures imply that the global economic loss from SARS was close to $US 40 billion in 2003. This is a figure much greater than any calculation of the medical costs of treating SARS patients.

The persistent SARS shock is also much more serious for China and Hong Kong. The primary impact is from the persistence in the rise of the country risk premium. Although the same in 2003 as for the temporary shock, the persistence of the country risk premium causes much larger capital outflow from China and Hong Kong. This impacts on short-run aggregate demand through a sharp contraction in investment, as well as a persistent loss in production capacity through a resulting decline in the growth of the capital stock, which reduces the desirability of investment. The extent of capital outflow will be discussed below.

Interestingly, the difference in GDP loss in 2003 when SARS is expected to be more persistent distinguishes between two regions. China, Hong Kong (SAR), Malaysia, the Philippines, Singapore, and Taiwan experience a larger loss in 2003, whereas the OECD economies and others experience a lower GDP loss. This reflects the greater capital outflow from the most affected countries into the least affected countries, which tends to lower the GDP of those countries losing capital and raise the GDP of those countries receiving capital. The countries in the first group that are less affected by SARS are nonetheless worse off with a more persistent disease because of their trade links with China, Hong Kong, and Singapore. The expectation of a more persistent problem with SARS leads to a total GDP loss of roughly $US 54 billion in 2003 alone (this ignores any future years' losses).

The results for GDP illustrate how the costs of SARS can be very different in 2003, depending on expectations of how the disease will unfold. It is also interesting to examine the change in economic impacts over time.

We present two sets of figures containing six charts within each figure. These results are all expressed as deviation from the underlying baseline of the model projections (which is described in more detail in the annex at the end of this paper). They show how key variables change relative to what would have been the case without SARS. Figures 2-4 and 2-5 describe simulation outcomes for the temporary SARS shock in the three panels on the left and simulation outcomes for the more persistent SARS shock in the three panels on the right. This enables a comparison between the two for the impacts on the real economy and trade flows.

Figure 2-4 contains results for real GDP, investment, and exports for both the temporary and persistent SARS shock. The loss in GDP from the temporary shock is largely confined to 2003. The persistent shock not only has a larger impact on GDP in 2003—because of expectations about future developments—but has a persistent impact on real GDP for a number of years afterward. Investment falls more sharply in 2003, which is the source of the larger GDP loss.

The results for exports are also interesting. In the case of the temporary shock, exports from Hong Kong fall sharply. Yet, in the more persistent case, exports from Hong Kong rise in 2003. The reason for this difference is that the more persistent the shock, the larger the capital outflow from affected economies. A capital outflow will be reflected in a current account surplus and a trade balance surplus. For this to occur, either exports must rise or imports must fall or both. This can be seen clearly in Figure 2-5.

In the case of the temporary SARS shock, the net capital outflow from China and Hong Kong (relative to base) is around 0.3 percent of GDP. However, when the shock is more persistent, this capital outflow rises sharply (top right panel of Figure 2-5), to 1.4 percent of GDP for Hong Kong and 0.8 percent of GDP for China. This capital outflow is reflected in the trade balance surplus in both. This shift in the trade balance is achieved by the capital outflow depreciating the real exchange rate of both China and Hong Kong substantially.

All of these linkages have many dimensions, but a global model is able to help untangle some of the more important factors. Under this model, the SARS outbreak is predicted to have widespread economic impacts beyond the regions immediately infected with the disease and beyond the decline in the most affected service industries.

## Conclusion

The impact of SARS is estimated to be large on the affected economies of China and Hong Kong (SAR). This impact is due not to the consequence of the disease itself for the affected people, but to the impact of the disease on the be-

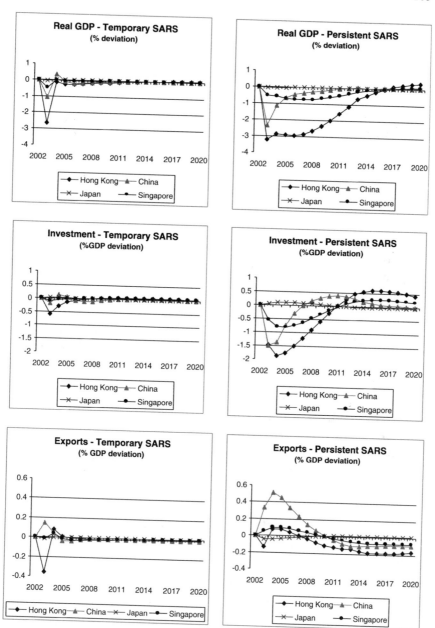

**FIGURE 2-4** Real impacts of temporary versus persistent SARS shock.

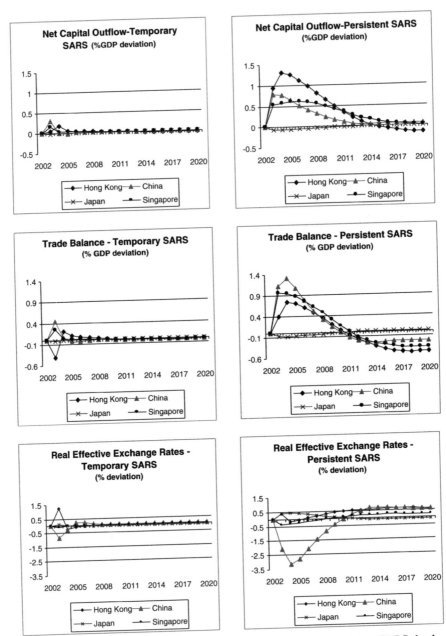

**FIGURE 2-5** Trade and captial flow impacts of temporary versus persistent SARS shock.

havior of many people within these economies. It also depends on the disease-associated adjustment of expectations reflected in integrated real and financial markets. The more persistent SARS is expected to be, the larger the negative economic impacts in 2003 in affected economies, but the smaller the impact in countries outside the core countries. The calculations above suggest that the cost in 2003 of SARS for the world economy as a whole are close to $US 40 billion in the case where SARS is expected to be a single event, versus costs of close to $US 54 billion in 2003 if SARS is expected to recur (this does not include the actual costs of later years if in fact SARS did recur). The higher costs from a persistent shock relate to the loss of investment and the impact on confidence and therefore spending in 2003.

These results illustrate that the true cost of disease is far greater than the cost to a health budget of treatment of the cases involved. The more persistent shock in this paper can be thought of as SARS lasting longer than anyone hopes, but it can also be interpreted as a recurring series of annual epidemics emerging from China and infecting the world through increased globalization. This is not a new phenomenon, since influenza viruses have been emanating from China since at least the 1918–1919 Spanish flu. Fortunately, most have been less devastating than the well-known major outbreaks. A key point of this paper is an attempt to evaluate the true underlying global cost of these diseases. If the threat of recurring SARS or SARS-like diseases from China is real, then the estimated risk to economic activity in this region and the world, as calculated in this paper, might be very large. The estimates in this paper suggest that there is a strong economic case for direct intervention in improving public health in China and other developing countries where there are inadequate expenditures on public health and insufficient investments in research into disease prevention.

As we observed from the Asian financial flu in 1997 and SARS in 2003, there is an important role for global monitoring and coordination mechanisms in containing both economic and microbial epidemics.

## Annex 2-1—Characteristics of the G-Cubed (Asia Pacific) Model

Some of the principal features of the G-Cubed (Asia Pacific) model are as follows:

- The model is based on explicit *intertemporal* optimization by the agents (consumers and firms) in each economy.[8] In contrast to static computable general equilibrium (CGE) models, time and dynamics are of fundamental importance in the G-Cubed model.
- In order to track the macro time series, however, the behavior of agents is modified to allow for short-run deviations from optimal behavior either due to

---

[8]See Blanchard and Fischer (1989) and Obstfeld and Rogoff (1996).

myopia or to restrictions on the ability of households and firms to borrow at the risk-free bond rate on government debt. For both households and firms, deviations from intertemporal optimizing behavior take the form of rules of thumb, which are consistent with an optimizing agent that does not update predictions based on new information about future events. These rules of thumb are chosen to generate the same steady-state behavior as optimizing agents, so that in the long run there is only a single intertemporal optimizing equilibrium of the model. In the short run, actual behavior is assumed to be a weighted average of the optimizing and the rule-of-thumb assumptions. Thus aggregate consumption is a weighted average of consumption based on wealth (current asset valuation and expected future after-tax labor income) and consumption based on current disposable income. Similarly, aggregate investment is a weighted average of investment based on Tobin's q (a market valuation of the expected future change in the marginal product of capital relative to the cost) and investment based on a backward-looking version of Q.

- There is an explicit treatment of the holding of financial assets, including money. Money is introduced into the model through a restriction that households require money to purchase goods.
- The model also allows for short-run nominal wage rigidity (by different degrees in different countries) and therefore allows for significant periods of unemployment depending on the labor market institutions in each country. This assumption, when taken together with the explicit role for money, is what gives the model its "macroeconomic" characteristics. (Here again, the model's assumptions differ from the standard market-clearing assumption in most CGE models.)
- The model distinguishes between the stickiness of physical capital within sectors and within countries and the flexibility of financial capital, which immediately flows to where expected returns are highest. This important distinction leads to a critical difference between the *quantity of physical capital* that is available at any time to produce goods and services, and the *valuation of that capital* as a result of decisions about the allocation of financial capital.

As a result of this structure, the G-Cubed model contains rich dynamic behavior, driven on the one hand by asset accumulation, and on the other by wage adjustment to a neoclassical steady state. It embodies a wide range of assumptions about individual behavior and empirical regularities in a general equilibrium framework. The interdependencies are solved out using a computer algorithm that solves for the rational expectations equilibrium of the global economy. It is important to stress that the term "general equilibrium" is used to signify that as many interactions as possible are captured, not that all economies are in a full market-clearing equilibrium at each point in time. Although it is assumed that market forces eventually drive the world economy to a neoclassical steady state growth equilibrium, unemployment does emerge for long periods due to wage stickiness, to an extent that differs between countries on account of differences in labor market institutions.

## Baseline Business-as-Usual Projections for G-Cubed Model Simulations

To solve the model, we first normalize all quantity variables by each economy's endowment of effective labor units. This means that in the steady state, all real variables are constant in these units, although the actual levels of the variables will be growing at the underlying rate of growth of population plus productivity. Next, we must make base-case assumptions about the future path of the model's exogenous variables in each region. In all regions we assume that the long-run real interest rate is 5 percent, tax rates are held at their 1999 levels, and fiscal spending is allocated according to 1999 shares. Population growth rates vary across regions as per the 2000 World Bank population projections.

A crucial group of exogenous variables are productivity growth rates by sector and country. The baseline assumption in G-Cubed (Asia Pacific) is that the pattern of technical change at the sector level is similar to the historical record for the United States (where data are available). In regions other than the United States, however, the sector-level rates of technical change are scaled up or down in order to match the region's observed average rate of aggregate productivity growth over the past 5 years. This approach attempts to capture the fact that the rate of technical change varies considerably across industries while reconciling it with regional differences in overall growth. This is clearly a rough approximation; if appropriate data were available, it would be better to estimate productivity growth for each sector in each region.

Given these assumptions, we solve for the model's perfect-foresight equilibrium growth path over the period 2002–2081. This a formidable task: the endogenous variables in *each* of the 80 periods number over 7,000 and include, among other things: the equilibrium prices and quantities of each good in each region, intermediate demands for each commodity by each industry in each region, asset prices by region and sector, regional interest rates, bilateral exchange rates, incomes, investment rates and capital stocks by industry and region, international flows of goods and assets, labor demanded in each industry in each region, wage rates, current and capital account balances, final demands by consumers in all regions, and government deficits.[9] At the solution, the budget constraints for all agents are satisfied, including both intra-temporal and intertemporal constraints.

---

[9]Because the model is solved for a perfect-foresight equilibrium over an 80-year period, the numerical complexity of the problem is on the order of 80 times what the single-period set of variables would suggest. We use software summarized in McKibbin and Sachs (1991), Appendix C, for solving large models with rational expectations on a personal computer.

# SARS: POLITICAL PATHOLOGY OF THE FIRST POST-WESTPHALIAN PATHOGEN[10]

*David P. Fidler*

Professor of Law and *Ira C. Batman* Faculty Fellow

Indiana University School of Law—Bloomington

The World Health Organization (WHO) has asserted that severe acute respiratory syndrome (SARS) was "the first severe infectious disease to emerge in the twenty-first century" and posed "a serious threat to global health security, the livelihood of populations, the functioning of health systems, and the stability and growth of economies" (WHO, 2003a). This paper argues that SARS was also the first post-Westphalian pathogen, and it constructs a political pathology of the outbreak to advance this claim.

In some respects, the SARS outbreak was nothing new. The great cliché of international infectious disease control—germs do not recognize borders—applies to SARS as it applied to earlier outbreaks. SARS joins a long list of infectious diseases that have not recognized borders. For my purposes, what makes SARS interesting is not its germ (SCoV); rather, SARS is important because of the political context in which the germ did not recognize borders. Put another way, I am interested in the borders SARS did not recognize. SARS is the first post-Westphalian pathogen because its nonrecognition of borders transpired in a public health governance environment radically different from what previous border-hopping bugs encountered.

## Westphalian and Post-Westphalian Public Health

### Of Germs and Borders

Principles for public health governance between countries traditionally derived from the structure for international relations known as the "Westphalian system": a system composed of principles guided by national sovereignty and nonintervention (Harding and Lim, 1999). "Westphalian public health" refers to public health governance structured by Westphalian principles. "Post-Westphalian public health" describes public health governance that departs from the Westphalian template and responds to increasing forces of globalization that include the interests of both multinational corporations and multilateral organizations. SARS is the first post-Westphalian pathogen because it highlights public health's transition from a Westphalian to a post-Westphalian governance context.

---

[10]This document summarizes Fidler DP. 2003. SARS: Political pathology of the first post-Westphalian pathogen, *Journal of Law, Medicine & Ethics*. This article served as the basis for Fidler DP. 2004. *SARS, Governance, and the Globalization of Disease*, London: Palgrave Macmillan.

The concepts that characterize post-Westphalian public health began to appear before SARS, but SARS still represents the first post-Westphalian pathogen for two reasons. First, the SARS outbreak was the first epidemic since HIV/AIDS to pose a truly global threat. Other new and not previously recognized microbes that emerged in the past 20 years had more limited capacity to threaten international public health because of inefficient human-to-human transmission or dependence on food or insects as vectors or on specific geographical conditions (WHO, 2003b). SARS posed a greater threat because of its more efficient person-to-person transmission and its fatality rate—comparable to some of history's greatest infectious disease foes, smallpox and influenza.

Second, because of the nature of the SARS threat, the epidemic seriously challenged the emerging post-Westphalian governance system. SARS was a global public health emergency (WHO, 2003c), and the sternest measure of governance systems is their performance in times of crisis. The SARS outbreak provided the first opportunity to evaluate how the new governance approach for infectious diseases would fare under serious microbial attack on a global basis.

## Westphalian Public Health

The Westphalian system is a system dominated by states (Scholte, 2001). The key principle of the Westphalian structure is sovereignty (Brownlie, 1998; Scholte, 2001). The sovereignty principle spins off corollary principles: (i) the principle of nonintervention (Jackson, 2001); and (ii) rules governing interactions among states arose from the states themselves and were not binding unless states consented to be bound (i.e., international law) (Brownlie, 1998; The SS Lotus, 1927). The combination of sovereignty, nonintervention, and consent-based international law meant that Westphalian governance was horizontal in nature, so that governance (i) involved only states; (ii) primarily addressed the mechanics of state interaction; and (iii) did not penetrate sovereignty to address how a government treated its people or ruled over its territory. The Westphalian system exhibited another characteristic—the great powers dominated Westphalian politics (Bull, 1977).

Infectious disease control became a diplomatic issue in the mid-19th century (Fidler, 1999). The regime that developed for international infectious disease control bore the imprint of all the characteristics of the Westphalian system. The International Health Regulations (IHR) (WHO, 1983), promulgated by WHO, illustrate the essence of Westphalian public health. The regulations are the only set of international legal rules binding on WHO members concerning infectious diseases (WHO, 2002), and they are are classically Westphalian in structure and content.

The IHR's objective is to ensure maximum security against the international spread of disease with minimal interference with world traffic (WHO, 1983). The regulations seek to achieve maximum security against the international spread of disease by requiring governments to (i) notify WHO of outbreaks of diseases subject to the Regulations; and (ii) maintain certain public health capabilities at ports and airports (WHO, 1983). The regulations seek to achieve minimum interference with world traffic by regulating the trade and travel restrictions WHO members can impose against countries suffering outbreaks of diseases subject to the Regulations (WHO, 1983).

In keeping with Westphalian principles, the regulations are consent-based rules of international law binding on states. The IHR's disease notification rules mandate that only information from governments can be used in surveillance (WHO, 1983). The regulations respect the principle of nonintervention by addressing only aspects of infectious diseases that relate to the intercourse among states. They do not address aspects of public health that touch on how a government prevents and controls infectious diseases within its sovereign territory. The IHR's limited governance scope is also clear from the small number of diseases subject to IHR rules—currently only cholera, plague, and yellow fever (WHO, 1983).

As a regime on international infectious disease control, the IHR proved to be a failure. WHO members routinely violated the IHR (e.g., not reporting disease outbreaks and applying excessive trade- and travel-restricting measures to other countries suffering disease outbreaks) (Fidler, 1999), and the IHR was irrelevant as a matter of international law to the emergence of the worst infectious disease epidemic in the 20th century, HIV/AIDS, because HIV/AIDS was not a disease subject to the IHR (Fidler, 1999).

The IHR's failure combined with other developments in international health policy to suggest that Westphalian public health governance was fundamentally bankrupt. After its creation, WHO began to concentrate less on horizontal public health strategies (such as those in the IHR) in order to focus more on vertical public health strategies that addressed infectious diseases at their sources inside states (e.g., disease eradication campaigns) (Arhin-Tenkorang and Conceico, 2003). Another way to sense this change in policy is to compare the IHR's horizontal approach and WHO's Health for All strategy announced at the end of the 1970s, which stressed universal access to primary health care (WHO, 1978). Or, compare the IHR's state-centric focus and lack of rules regulating domestic public health systems with the emphasis on the right to health proclaimed in the WHO Constitution (WHO, 1994) and implemented through the Health for All strategy.

### Post-Westphalian Public Health

The considerable challenges presented by emerging and re-emerging infectious diseases in the 1990s and early 2000s stimulated thinking on strategies different from the IHR's Westphalian approach. Two key post-Westphalian concepts were "global health governance" (a new kind of political process) (Dodgson et al., 2002) and "global public goods for health" (a new kind of substantive policy goal) (Smith et al., 2003). Global health governance (GHG) includes nonstate actors in the governance process. One of the best examples can be found in the Global Fund to Fight AIDS, Tuberculosis, and Malaria (Global Fund, 2003). Its board of directors includes nongovernmental organization representatives as voting members.

Global public goods for health (GPGH) are goods or services, the consumption of which is nonexcludable and nonrival across national boundaries and involving countries and peoples that are in different regional groupings (e.g., North America and sub-Saharan Africa) (Smith et al., 2003). Under the GPGH concept, public health governance should not serve the interests of the great powers, but should produce globally accessible health goods and services. The explosion of so-called public–private partnerships in global public health provide the best illustration of attempts to produce GPGH (e.g., ventures to develop new antimicrobial drugs for malaria and tuberculosis) (Reich, 2002).

The post-Westphalian strategies of GHG and GPGH can be seen in WHO's attempts to revise the IHR in the latter half of the 1990s and early 2000s. WHO proposed changes to the IHR that would create GHG and produce GPGH and that were, from the perspective of the Westphalian approach, radical. Two critical proposed changes sought to improve global infectious disease surveillance: (i) moving away from disease-specific reporting to notifications of "public health emergencies of international concern"; and (ii) allowing WHO to incorporate nongovernmental sources of information into its surveillance activities (WHO, 2002). Revising the IHR in these ways would: (i) produce GHG by including nonstate actors in the process of global infectious disease surveillance; and (ii) produce the GPGH of better infectious disease surveillance information for use by states and nonstate actors.

The development of GHG and GPGH strategies indicate that post-Westphalian public health governance had started to form in the late 1990s and early 2000s, before SARS emerged. But, prior to SARS, the post-Westphalian strategies, particularly in the context of the Global Fund and HIV/AIDS, were showing signs of severe stress, generating skepticism about the new governance approaches. The IHR revision process was not progressing well and was obscure and ignored in much of the ferment happening in global public health circles in the latter half of the 1990s and early 2000s (Fidler, 2003). If post-Westphalian public health could not handle the strain that existing diseases created, what would happen when the next infectious disease crisis broke in the world?

## China, SARS, and Post-Westphalian Public Health

SARS proved to be the next crisis. Instead of failure, the global campaign against SARS achieved a victory that will go down in the annals of public health and international relations history. In SARS, the world confronted a virus never before found in humans that was transmitted from person to person, that had a relatively high fatality rate, and against which public health practitioners had neither adequate diagnostic technologies nor effective treatments or vaccines. The last time the world confronted a virus with this disturbing profile was when HIV emerged in the early 1980s, and HIV triggered one of the worst disease epidemics in human history that is still raging globally. SARS was a crisis of the first order for global public health. Yet, unlike with HIV/AIDS, victory was achieved. How?

## China Confronts Public Health's "New World Order"

We answer this question by focusing on what happened with China's response to the SARS outbreak. China was the epicenter of the SARS outbreak; thus, it was the governance epicenter. What happened to China during its response to SARS illustrated the power of the GHG and GPGH strategies of post-Westphalian public health. China's initial responses to SARS followed the Westphalian template because China was under no international legal obligation to report SARS cases to any state or international organization, nor did it have an express duty to cooperate with WHO on the outbreak. China made the mistake, however, of acting Westphalian in a post-Westphalian world. In its confrontation with public health's "new world order," China miscalculated and lost.

GHG mechanisms—especially WHO's access to nongovernmental sources of information for surveillance purposes—trumped Chinese attempts to exercise its sovereignty through control of epidemiological information about SARS. China's initial handling of SARS demonstrated that it had not grasped the new context for public health governance—epidemiological information about disease does not recognize borders. At the outset of the SARS epidemic, China played the sovereignty card, only to retreat when its sovereignty was seen as a deliberate attempt to hide an outbreak—one that was already indicating serious consequences for the rest of the world.

The need for producing GPGH for the SARS battle—especially accurate surveillance data on the outbreak in China—swept aside China's narrow construction of its national interest vis-à-vis the outbreak. China behaved as if its national interest in preserving flows of trade and investment into China and the image of the Communist Party could simply ignore the legitimate concerns of other states and nonstate actors, such as multinational corporations. China's conception of its national interest broke apart in the post-Westphalian public health atmosphere of SARS.

In the SARS outbreak, the world did not witness China enjoying the Westphalian privileges normally accorded powerful countries, but rather saw post-Westphalian public health governance humble a rising great power in the international system for disease control.

## Beyond China: SARS and Post-Westphalian Public Health

The SARS outbreak contains other interesting features that support the emergence of post-Westphalian public health governance. The most amazing involved WHO's issuance of geographically specific travel advisories that recommended that people not travel to locations experiencing local chains of SARS transmission (e.g., Guangdong Province, Beijing, Toronto). These travel advisories were revolutionary developments in international policy on infectious diseases because, in issuing the alerts, WHO exercised independent power over its member states without express authority in international law to do so. The approval by WHO member states at the May 2003 World Health Assembly meeting of these radical acts (WHO, 2003a,d) confirms the existence of an entirely new governance context for infectious disease control.

Other aspects of the outbreak's handling also illustrated the power and promise of GPGH, including the unprecedented nature of the global collaborative efforts to create, analyze, and disseminate information on (1) the SARS virus; (2) clinical management of SARS cases; and (3) public health strategies for breaking the chain of transmission. The SARS outbreak was also post-Westphalian in how it elevated public health as a matter of national political priority in many countries (National Intelligence Council, 2003) and reinforced the linkage between infectious disease control and international human rights through the widespread use of quarantine and isolation (McNeil, 2003).

### SARS and the Vulnerabilities of Post-Westphalian Public Health

The political pathology of SARS also reveals vulnerabilities that post-Westphalian public health governance faces in light of the SARS outbreak. SARS was a victory for post-Westphalian public health, but serious problems continue to exist, including the presence of public health infrastructures in China and many other countries that remain inadequately prepared for severe infectious disease threats. Repeated warnings that SARS may return in the winter months of 2003–2004 stress the necessity of sustaining the kind of national and international commitment witnessed during the SARS outbreak, but whether sufficient political, financial, and public health commitment will be forthcoming remains unclear.

### Conclusion

The political pathology of SARS constructed in the paper suggests that governance innovations used to move public health into a post-Westphalian context contributed to the successful global response to a severe infectious disease threat. The global containment of SARS represents a historic triumph that will enter the annals of history as one of the most significant achievements in global infectious disease control since the eradication of smallpox.

Commenting on SARS, WHO's executive director for communicable diseases, Dr. David Heymann, argued that "[i]n the 21st century there is a new way of working"(Heymann, 2003). Against the global health emergency of SARS, the "new way of working" proved effective, which constitutes a victory for the emerging framework of post-Westphalian public health.

Although victory should be savored, everyone should remember that germs do not recognize victories or defeats. The challenge for post-Westphalian public health is to create the conditions necessary for the governance innovations successfully deployed in the SARS outbreak to be refined, improved, expanded, and sustained to meet the ongoing threat that pathogenic microbes present. The germs will keep coming. The great task for the global community that answered the initial challenge from SARS is to ensure that the "new way of working" continues to work far into the 21st century.

## THE SARS EPIDEMIC AND ITS AFTERMATH IN CHINA: A POLITICAL PERSPECTIVE

*Yanzhong Huang\**
John C. Whitehead School of Diplomacy and International Relations,
Seton Hall University

In November 2002, a form of atypical pneumonia called severe acute respiratory syndrome (SARS) began spreading rapidly around the world, prompting the World Health Organization (WHO) to declare the ailment "a worldwide health threat." At the epicenter of the outbreak was China, where the outbreak of SARS infected more than 5,300 people and killed 349 nationwide (Ministry of Health, 2003). History is full of ironies: the epidemic caught China, at first, unprepared to defeat the disease 45 years after Mao Zedong bade "Farewell to the God of Plagues."

The SARS epidemic was not simply a public health problem. Indeed, it caused the most severe socio-political crisis for the Chinese leadership since the 1989 Tiananmen crackdown. Outbreak of the disease fueled fears among economists that China's economy was headed for a serious downturn. A fatal period of hesitation regarding information-sharing and action spawned anxiety, panic, and rumor-mongering across the country and undermined the government's efforts to create a milder image of itself in the international arena. As Premier Wen Jiabao pointed out in a cabinet meeting on the epidemic, "the health and security of the people, overall state of reform, development, and stability, and China's national

---

*This paper is adapted from The Politics of China's SARS Crisis. *Harvard Asia Quarterly* (Autumn 2003). An earlier version of the article appeared in "Dangerous Secrets: SARS and China's Healthcare System," Roundtable before the Congressional-Executive Commission on China, May 12, 2003, www.cecc.gov.

interest and international image are at stake (Zhongguo xinwen wang, 2003a)." In the weeks that followed, the Chinese government launched a crusade against SARS, effectively bringing the disease under control in late June and eliminating all known cases by mid-August.

While clearly a test for the public health infrastructure of China, the course of the epidemic also raised crucial questions about the capacity and dynamics of the Chinese political structure and its ability to address future outbreaks. What accounted for the initial government decisions to withhold information from the public and take little action against the disease, and then the subsequent dramatic shift in government policy toward SARS? Why was the government able to contain the spread of SARS in a relatively short period? What lessons has the government drawn from the crisis? A political analysis of the crisis not only demonstrates crucial linkages between China's political system and its pattern of crisis management but also sheds light on the government's ability to handle the next disease outbreak. While problems in the formal institutional structure and bureaucratic capacity accounted for the initial official denial and inaction, the institutional forces unleashed from the terrain of state-society relations led to dramatic changes in the form and content of government policy toward SARS. Through mass mobilization, the government successfully brought the disease under control. While these developments are encouraging, China's capacity to effectively prevent and contain future infectious disease outbreaks remains uncertain. Prevention and control programs are still troubled by problems in agenda-setting, policy making, and implementation which, in turn, can be attributed to its political system. A healthier China therefore demands some fundamental changes in the political system.

## The Making of a Crisis

With hindsight, China's health system seemed initially to respond relatively well to the emergence of the illness. The earliest case of SARS is thought to have occurred in Foshan, a city southwest of Guangzhou in Guangdong province, in mid-November 2002. It was later also found in Heyuan and Zhongshan in Guangdong. This "strange disease" alerted Chinese health personnel as early as mid-December. On January 2, a team of health experts was sent to Heyuan and diagnosed the disease as an infection caused by a certain virus (Hai and Hua, 2003). A Chinese physician, who was in charge of treating a patient from Heyuan in a hospital in Guangzhou, quickly reported the disease to a local anti-epidemic station (Renmin ribao, 2003a). We have reason to believe that the local anti-epidemic station alerted the provincial health bureau about the disease, with the bureau in turn reporting to the provincial government and the Ministry of Health shortly afterwards, since the first team of experts sent by the Ministry arrived at Guangzhou on January 20, and the new provincial government (who took over on January 20) ordered an investigation of the disease almost at the same time

(Renmin wang, 2003a). A combined team of health experts from the Ministry and the province was dispatched to Zhongshan and completed an investigation report on the unknown disease. On January 27, the report was sent to the provincial health bureau and, presumably, to the Ministry of Health in Beijing. The report was marked "top secret," which meant that only top provincial health officials could open it.

Further government reaction to the emerging disease, however, was delayed by the problems of information flow within the Chinese hierarchy. For 3 days, there were no authorized provincial health officials available to open the document. After the document was finally read, the provincial bureau distributed a bulletin to hospitals across the province. However, few health workers were alerted by the bulletin because most were on vacation for the Chinese New Year (Pomfret, 2003a). In the meantime, the public was kept uninformed about the disease. According to the Implementing Regulations on the State Secrets Law regarding the handling of public health–related information, any occurrence of infectious diseases should be classified as a state secret before they are "announced by the Ministry of Health or organs authorized by the Ministry." In other words, until such time as the Ministry chose to make information about the disease public, any physician or journalist who reported on the disease would risk being persecuted for leaking state secrets (Li et al., 1999). A virtual news blackout about SARS thus continued well into February.

The initial failure to inform the public heightened anxieties, fear, and widespread speculation. On February 8, reports about a "deadly flu" began to be sent via short messages on mobile phones in Guangzhou. In the evening, words like bird flu and anthrax started to appear on some local Internet sites (South China Morning Post, 2003). On February 10, a circular appeared in the local media that acknowledged the presence of the disease and listed some preventive measures, including improving ventilation, using vinegar fumes to disinfect the air, and washing hands frequently. Responding to the advice, residents in Guangzhou and other cities cleared pharmacy shelves of antibiotics and flu medication. In some cities, even the vinegar was sold out. The panic spread quickly in Guangdong, and was felt even in other provinces.

On February 11, Guangdong health officials finally broke the silence by holding press conferences about the disease. The provincial health officials reported a total of 305 atypical pneumonia cases in the province. The officials also admitted that there were no effective drugs to treat the disease and that the outbreak was only tentatively contained (Nanfang zhoumu, 2003). From then on, information about the disease was reported to the public through the news media. Yet in the meantime, the government played down the risk of the illness. Guangzhou city government on February 11 went so far as to announce the illness was "comprehensively" under effective control (Renmin wang, 2003b). As a result, while the panic was temporarily allayed, the public also lost vigilance about the disease. When some reports began to question the government's handling of the outbreak, the provincial propaganda bureau again halted reporting on the disease on February 23. This news blackout continued during the run-up to the National People's Congress in March, and government authorities shared little information with the World Health Organization until early April.

The continuing news blackout not only restricted the flow of information to the public but contributed to the government's failure to take further actions to address the looming catastrophe. Here it is worth noting that the Law on Prevention and Treatment of Infectious Diseases (enacted in September 1989) contains a number of significant loopholes. First, provincial governments are obliged to publicize epidemics in a timely and accurate manner only after being authorized by the Ministry of Health (Article 23). Second, atypical pneumonia was not listed in the law as an infectious disease under surveillance, and thus local government officials legally were not accountable for reporting the disease. While the law allows for the addition of new items to the list, it does not specify the procedures through which new diseases can be added. Both of these factors provided disincentives for the government to effectively respond to the crisis. In fact, the Chinese Center for Disease Control and Prevention did not issue a nationwide bulletin to hospitals on how to prevent the ailment from spreading until April 3, and it was not until mid-April that the government formally listed SARS as a disease to be closely monitored and reported on a daily basis under the Law of Prevention and Treatment of Infectious Diseases.

Evidence also indicates that the provincial government, in deciding whether to publicize the event, considered not only the public health implications of the outbreak, but also the effect such information might have on local economic development (Garrett, 2003; Pomfret, 2003a). In part, this correlates with a significant shift in China's national agenda, which makes economic growth the key to solving the nation's problems and makes social stability the prerequisite to development (Development, 2000). In the words of the late paramount leader Deng Xiaoping, "the overwhelmingly important issue for China is stability, without which nothing can be achieved (Renmin Rabao, 2001)." Such concerns were only complicated by the fact that during some of the most crucial period of the disease outbreak, party elites were busy preparing for the National People's Congress (NPC) in March, which would mark the beginning of a new government (following the selection of new leaders to the Politburo Standing Committee in November). To publicly acknowledge the outbreak at this critical juncture might have risked not only causing socioeconomic instability but sullying the party's image among the people.

In fairness here, it should be noted that officials in any nation or region of the world would likely face a similar dilemma in attempting to consider its obligations to protect the public's health while at the same time considering how to maintain equally important aspects of social stability and economic development. In addition, the media blackout and the government's slow response were not the sole factors leading to the crisis. With little knowledge about the true cause of the disease and its rate and modes of transmission, the top-secret document submitted to the provincial health bureau did not even mention that the disease showed signs of being considerably contagious. Neither did it call for rigorous preventive measures, which may explain why by the end of February, nearly half of Guangzhou's 900 cases were health care workers (Pomfret, 2003a). Indeed, even countries like Canada were having difficulty controlling SARS. In this sense, SARS is a natural disaster, not a humanmade one.

Nevertheless, there is no doubt that government inaction paralleled by the absence of an effective response to the initial outbreak resulted in a crisis. To begin with, the security designation for the top-secret document meant that Guangdong health authorities could not discuss the situation with other provincial health departments in China. Consequently, hospitals and medical personnel in most localities were completely unprepared for the outbreak. When the first SARS case in northern China was admitted to the PLA 301 Hospital in Beijing on March 2, doctors in charge of the treatment had little information about the disease (Zhongguo qingnian bao, 2003). Even as the traffic through emergency rooms began to escalate, major hospitals in Beijing took few measures to reduce the chances of cross-infection. Likewise, Inner Mongolia's first SARS patient, who sought treatment in the Hohhot Hospital around March 20, was not correctly diagnosed until early April (Kahn and Rosenthal, 2003). The security designation of the Guangdong report also prevented health authorities in neighboring Hong Kong from receiving information about the disease, and consequently they were denied the knowledge they needed to prepare (Pomfret, 2003a). Soon after, the illness developed into an epidemic in Hong Kong, which proved to be a major international transit route for SARS.

*Beyond Guangdong: The Ministry of Health and Beijing*

The Ministry of Health learned about SARS in January and informed WHO and provincial health bureaus about the outbreak in Guangdong around February 7, and yet no further action was taken. It is safe to assume that Zhang Wenkang, the health minister, brought the disease to the attention of Wang Zhongyu (secretary general of the State Council) and Li Lanqing (the vice premier in charge of public health and education). We do not know what happened during this period of time, but it is likely that the leaders were so preoccupied preparing for the National People's Congress that no explicit directive was issued from the top until April 2. By March 1, the epidemic was raging in Beijing. For fear of disturbance during the NPC meeting, however, city authorities kept information about its scope not only from the public but also from the Party Center. According to Dr. Jiang Yanyong, medical staff in Beijing's military hospitals were briefed about the dangers of SARS in early March, but were told not to publicize what they had learned lest it interfere with the NPC meeting (Jakes, 2003). Similar communication obstacles hampered cooperation between China and the World

Health Organization. WHO experts were invited to China by the Ministry of Health but were not allowed to have access to Guangdong until April 2, 8 days after their arrival. It was not until April 9 that they were allowed to inspect military hospitals in Beijing.

Such obstructions to information flow and the lack of interdepartmental cooperation during the crisis provide a reference point for the "fragmented authoritarianism" model of the Chinese political system, which posits that authority below the very peak of the Chinese system is fragmented and disjointed, leading to a bogged-down policy process which is characterized by extensive bargaining (Lampton, 1987; Lieberthal and Lampton, 1992). While this model offers only a static description of how the core state apparatus works (Oksenberg, 2001), it correctly points out the coordination problems in China's policy process. Medical personnel in the city of Guangzhou blamed poor communication between the province's health bureau and the city's health authorities for the failure to control the spread of the disease (Pomfret, 2003a). In addition to the tensions among different levels of health authorities, coordination problems existed between functional departments and territorial governments, as well as between civilian and military institutions. As one senior health official admitted, before anything could be done, the Ministry of Health had to negotiate with other ministries and government departments (Pomfret, 2003b). In the public health domain, territorial governments like Beijing and Guangdong maintain primary leadership over the provincial health bureau, with the former determining the size, personnel, and funding of the latter. This constitutes a major problem for the Ministry of Health, which is bureaucratically weak, not to mention that its minister is just an ordinary member of the Chinese Communist Party (CCP) Central Committee and not represented in the powerful Politburo. A major policy initiative from the Ministry of Health, even issued in the form of a central document, is mainly a guidance document (*zhidao xin wenjian*) that has less binding power than one that is issued by territorial governments. Whether it will be honored hinges on the "acquiescence" (*liangjie*) of the territorial governments. This helps explain the continuous lack of effective response by Beijing city authorities until April 17 (when an anti-SARS joint team was established).

At one level, Beijing's municipal government apparently believed that it could handle the situation by itself and thus refused assistance from the Ministry of Health. At another, the Ministry did not have control over all available health facilities. Of Beijing's 175 hospitals, 16 are under the control of the army, which maintains a relatively independent health system. Having admitted a large number of SARS patients, military hospitals in Beijing withheld SARS statistics from the Ministry until mid-April. Organizational barriers also delayed the process of correctly identifying the cause of the disease. According to government regulations, only the Chinese CDC is the legal holder of virus samples. As a result, researchers affiliated with other government organizations had been to Guangdong many times in search of virus samples and returned empty handed

(Chinese Scientists, 2003). In addition, even the Chinese CDC in Beijing had to negotiate with local disease-control centers to obtain the samples (Garrett, 2003). After an examination of just two available samples, its chief virologist rushed to announce chlamydia as the etiological agent of SARS on February 18 (Huailing, 2003).

The presence of such a fragmented and disjointed bureaucracy within an authoritarian political structure means that policy immobility can only be overcome with the intervention of an upper-level government that has the authority to aggregate conflicting interests. However, this tends to encourage lower-level governments to shift their policy overload to the upper levels in order to avoid assuming responsibilities. As a consequence, a large number of agenda items compete for the upper level government's attention. In addition, the drive toward economic growth in the post-Mao era has marginalized public health issues (Ruan, 1992). Compared to economic issues, a public health problem often needs an attention-focusing event (e.g., a large-scale outbreak of a contagious disease) to be finally recognized, defined, and formally addressed (Kingdon, 1995). Not surprisingly, SARS did not raise the eyebrows of top decision makers until it had developed into a nationwide epidemic.

By early April, it was evident that SARS was being taken very seriously at the top level. Yet the government's ability to formulate a sound policy against SARS was hampered as lower-level government officials intercepted and distorted the upward information flow. For fear that any mishap reported in their jurisdiction might be used as an excuse to pass them over for promotion, government officials at all levels tended to distort the information they pass up to their political masters in order to place themselves in a good light. While this is not unique to China, the problem is alleviated in democracies through "decentralized oversight," which enables citizen interest groups to check up on administrative actions. Because the general public in China is not enfranchised to oversee the activities of government agencies, however, lower-level officials can fool higher authorities more easily than their counterparts in liberal democracies (Shirk, 1993). This exacerbates the information asymmetry problems inherent in a hierarchical structure. Beijing municipal authorities, for example, kept hiding the actual SARS situation in the city from the Party Center until April. Initial deception by lower-level officials in turn led the central leaders to misjudge the situation. On April 2, Premier Wen Jiabao chaired an executive meeting of the State Council to discuss SARS prevention and control. Based on the briefing given by the Ministry of Health, the meeting declared that SARS had "already been brought under effective control."

The growing dispersal of political power at the highest level in the post-Mao era further reduced the autonomy of the top leaders in responding to the crisis in a timely manner. Instead of having a personalized leadership unconstrained by laws and procedures, the post-Mao regime features collective leadership, with the Party general secretary acting as the first among equals. Political power at the national level has been further diluted since the 16th Party Congress, which expanded the membership of the Politburo Standing Committee and allowed former president Jiang Zemin (who is not a member of the CCP Central Committee) to retain the position of Chairman of the Central Military Commission. Because China's decision making emphasizes consensus, the involvement of more actors with equal status in decision making only increases the time and effort needed for policy coordination and compromise.

## The Government Crusade Against SARS

As the virus continued to spread, China's political leadership came under growing domestic and international pressures (Pomfret, 2003d). Despite the prohibition against public discussion of the epidemic, 40.9 percent of the urban residents had already heard about the disease through unofficial means (Haiyan, 2003). As mentioned above, news of the disease reached residents in Guangzhou through mobile-phone text messages in early February, forcing the provincial government to hold a news conference admitting to the outbreak. Starting on February 11, the Western news media began to aggressively report on SARS in China and the government's cover-up of the outbreak. On March 15, the WHO issued its first global warning about SARS. While China's government-controlled media was prohibited from reporting on the warning, the news circulated via mobile phones, e-mail, and the Internet. On March 25, 3 days after the arrival of a team of WHO experts, the government for the first time acknowledged the spread of SARS outside of Guangdong. The State Council held its first meeting to discuss the SARS problem 2 days after the *Wall Street Journal* published an editorial calling for other countries to suspend all travel links with China until it implemented a transparent public health campaign. The same day, the WHO issued the first travel advisory in its 55-year history advising people not to visit Hong Kong and Guangdong, prompting Beijing to hold a news conference in which the health minister promised that China was safe and SARS was under control. Enraged by the minister's false account, Dr. Jiang Yanyong, a retired surgeon at Beijing's 301 military hospital, sent an e-mail to two TV stations, accusing the minister of lying. While neither station followed up on the e-mail, *Time* magazine picked up the story and posted it on its website on April 9, which triggered a political earthquake in Beijing.

The aforementioned events are revealing examples of how evolving state-society relations can significantly influence the trajectory of public policy development in post-Mao China. Economic reform and globalization provide more Chinese with the information, connections, resources and incentives to act on their own for their personal security and personal fulfillment. In the words of Thomas Friedman, these empowered, even superpowered individuals become more demanding of the government and will get angry when their leaders fail to meet their aspirations (Friedman, 2000). The torrent of messages sent through cell phones or the Internet and Dr. Jiang Yanyong's exposure of the cover-up thus challenged the state's monopoly on information. Furthermore, while party leaders are not formally accountable to their people, they may have to take into account mass reactions of the population when they make policies, or otherwise risk a lack of cooperation with their programs from below. As a result of the strategic interaction between the state with increasing legitimacy concerns and social forces with more political and economic resources, the state may have more incentives to take seriously the people's interests and demands (Huang, forthcoming).

The growing epidemic, combined with pressures from inside and outside the country, ultimately engendered a strong and effective action by the government to contain the disease and end the crisis. On April 2, the State Council held a meeting to discuss the SARS problem, the first of three meetings held within the space of a month. This was followed by an urgent meeting of the Standing Committee of the CCP Politburo on April 17. Meanwhile, the government also showed a new level of candor. Premier Wen Jiabao on April 13 said that although progress had been made, "the overall situation remains grave" (Business Week, 2003). In hindsight, one of the strengths of party-state dualism in China is the Party's ability to push the government by signaling its priorities loudly and clearly. This helps explain why the April 2 meeting held by the State Council did not generate any serious response from the lower level, whereas the system was fully mobilized after April 17, when the Politburo's Standing Committee explicitly warned against covering up SARS cases and demanded accurate and timely reporting of the disease. After the April 17 meeting, government media began to publicize the number of SARS cases in each province, updating on a daily basis. An order from the Ministry of Health formally listed SARS as a disease to be monitored under the Law of Prevention and Treatment of Infectious Diseases and made it clear that every provincial unit should report the number of SARS cases on a given day by 12 noon on the following date. The party and government leaders around the country were now to be held accountable for the overall SARS situation in their jurisdictions.

On April 20, Health Minister Zhang Wenkang and Beijing mayor Meng Xuenong were ousted for their mismanagement of the crisis. While they were not the first ministerial-level officials since 1949 to be dismissed mid-crisis on a policy matter, the case was a signal of political innovation from China's new leadership. As an article in *The Economist* remarked, the unfolding of the event—minister presides over policy bungle; bungle is exposed and there is public outcry; minister resigns to take the rap— "almost looks like the way that politics works in a democratic, accountable country" (China's Chernobyl, 2003). The crisis also led the government to take measures to strengthen fundamental authority links within the system. As part of a nationwide mobilization campaign, the State Council sent out inspection teams to 26 provinces to scour government records for unreported cases and to fire officials for lax prevention efforts. According to the official media, by May 8 China had fired or penalized more than 120 officials for their "slack" response to the SARS epidemic (Tak-ho, 2003). It was estimated that by the end of

May, nearly 1,000 government officials had been disciplined for the same reason (Lianhe zaobao, 2003). These actions shook the complacency of local government officials, who then abandoned their initial hesitation and jumped onto the anti-SARS bandwagon. Driven by political zeal, they sealed off villages, apartment complexes, and university campuses, quarantined tens of thousands of people, and set up checkpoints to take temperatures. By May 7, 18,000 people had been quarantined in Beijing. The Maoist "Patriotic Hygiene Campaign" was revitalized. In Guangdong, 80 million people were mobilized to clean houses and streets (Renmin ribao, 2003b). In the countryside, virtually every village was on SARS alert, with roadside booths installed to examine all those who entered or left.

The crisis also improved interdepartmental and interagency coordination and speeded up the process of institutionalizing China's emergency response system to be able to handle public health contingencies. On April 17, an anti-SARS joint team was created for the city of Beijing, which included leading members from the Ministry of Health and the military (Xinhua News, 2003a). On April 23, a task force known as the SARS Control and Prevention Headquarters of the State Council was established to coordinate national efforts to combat the disease. Vice Premier Wu Yi was appointed as commander-in-chief of the task force, and similar arrangements were made at the provincial, city, and county levels. On May 12, China issued a set of Regulations on Public Health Emergencies. According to these regulations, the State Council shall set up an emergency headquarters to deal with any public health emergencies, which are referred to as serious epidemics, widespread unidentified diseases, mass food and industrial poisoning, and other serious public health threats (Xinhua News, 2003b).

Direct involvement of the political leadership also increased program resources and mobilized resources from other systems. On April 23, a national fund of 2 billion *yuan* ($US 250 million) was created for SARS prevention and control. The fund was to be used to upgrade county-level hospitals, to finance the treatment of farmers and poor urban residents infected with SARS, and to purchase SARS-related medical facilities in central and western China. This central government funding was complemented by an additional 7 billion *yuan* ($US 875 million) from local governments (Renmin wang, 2003c). Free treatment was offered to SARS sufferers anywhere in the country.

These momentous measures appeared to have worked. The epidemic started to lose its momentum in late May, and on June 24, the World Health Organization lifted its advisory against travel to Beijing. On August 16, with the last two SARS patients discharged from the Beijing Ditan Hospital, China for the time being was free from SARS.

## Improvements Resulting from the SARS Crisis

The weaknesses and strengths demonstrated by the government during the crisis raised questions regarding its capacity to respond to other disease outbreaks.

With the SARS outbreak wreaking havoc and shaving an estimated seven-tenths of a percentage point off China's gross domestic product for 2003, the government appears to have drawn some important lessons from the crisis, including the need for coordinated development. When interviewed by the executive editor of the *Washington Post*, Premier Wen Jiabao said that "one important inspirational lesson" the new Chinese leadership learned from the SARS crisis was that "uneven development between the urban and rural areas, and imbalance between economic development and social progress" were "bound to stumble and fall (Renmin ribao, 2003d)." On various occasions since the crisis, central leaders have emphasized the importance of public health, especially rural health care (Renmin ribao, 2003e,f,g; Ministry of Health, 2003). The government has also provided more funding to public health. It earmarked billions of dollars to SARS prevention and control, and recently it invested 6.8 billion *yuan* ($US 850 million) for the construction of a three-tiered network of disease control and prevention (Guangming ribao, 2003). While a nationwide SARS training program is underway, the government has initiated an Internet-based disease reporting system which allows local hospitals to directly report suspected SARS cases to the Chinese CDC and the Ministry of Health (Zhongguo xinwen wang, 2003b).

Moreover, as China emerges from the shadow of SARS, Chinese leaders appear to be showing a new, more proactive attitude toward AIDS. Since summer 2003, the government has started offering free treatment for poor people with HIV/AIDS, and it plans to expand the program next year until free treatment is available for all poor HIV carriers and AIDS patients (Chang, 2003; Yardley, 2003). The government has also allocated 11.4 billion *yuan* ($US 1.42 billion) for strengthening the AIDS medical assistance system and training more health personnel for AIDS prevention and treatment (Jiankang bao, 2003). On December 1, Premier Wen Jiabao appeared on state television shaking hands with AIDS patients and called on the nation to treat them with "care and love." This event was significant because until then, no senior Chinese leader had even discussed the disease in public.

These measures reflected the increased efforts of the Party to cultivate a new image for its leadership. It wants citizens to see the leaders as being in touch with the people and committed to their best interests. More attention has thus been paid to the basic needs of China's farmers and workers. On August 17, the government promulgated Regulations on the Management of Village Doctors, promising more professional training for rural health personnel (Xinhua news, 2003c). In September, Premier Wen indicated that a majority of the increased health funding will be used to support rural public health. He also reaffirmed his commitment to a new medical insurance scheme in the countryside (Renmin ribao, 2003h). Given that rural areas were viewed as the weakest link in containing the spread of SARS, such measures are expected to strengthen the ability of the public health system to respond to a future disease outbreak.

Equally important, the government seems to have learned that in an era of the Internet and cell phones, a complete information blackout is not only impossible but also counterproductive. There are signs suggesting that the crisis is forcing the government to take steps to establish an image of a more open and transparent government. For example, an April 28 Politburo meeting obviously made the decision to publicize a submarine accident that same month that cost 70 lives. News of the tragedy was reported by the official Xinhua news agency on May 2. This marks a significant departure from the traditionally secretive approach taken to the nation's military disasters. If this new openness continues in the post-SARS era, it will not only create conditions for a government that is more accountable to its people but might also provide considerable incentives for sharing knowledge of an outbreak with the international community as early as possible.

As evidenced by the government campaign against SARS, an infectious disease can potentially trigger the party-state to organize a political campaign to reach deep into the hinterlands and snap people into action. This government capacity to mobilize against a disease outbreak is enhanced by a more institutionalized crisis management system. The Regulations on Public Health Emergencies issued by the State Council in mid-May, for example, require setting up an emergency headquarters right after a public health emergency is identified. It has also been reported that the government plans to set up an Emergency Response Bureau, which would draw on the example of the U.S. Federal Emergency Management Administration to tackle future health crises and natural disasters (Wiest, 2003).

*Problems and Concerns*

These changes are worth applauding, but will they suffice to effectively contain future epidemics? Here, one of the major problems is a public health system in China that has been compromised by a lack of sufficient state funding. The portion of total health spending financed by the government has fallen from 34 percent in 1978 to less than 20 percent now (Huang, 2003), and a lack of adequate facilities and medical staff shortages compromised early government efforts to contain SARS. For example, hospitals in Guangdong reportedly faced shortages in hospital beds and ambulances, and even among the 66,000 health care workers in Beijing, less than 3,000 (or 4.3 percent) were familiar with respiratory diseases (Renmin ribao, 2003c). Apart from imposing severe constraints on the government's ability to respond to a public health crisis, the shortage of affordable health care also impacted the ability and willingness of patients to seek out treatment. The *Washington Post* reported a SARS patient who fled quarantine in Beijing because he did not believe that the government would treat his disease free of charge, and some hospitals are reported to have refused to accept patients who had affordability problems (Washington Post, 2003). More broadly, according to a recent report by the Chinese Consumer's Association, about 50 percent of people who are sick do not see a doctor because of the extremely high out-of-pocket payments (Zhongguo jingji shibao, 2003). All of these factors sow the seeds for a larger and more catastrophic disease attack.

We should also keep in mind that SARS is not the sole microbial threat confronting China. The country faces challenges from other major infectious diseases such as the plague, cholera, HIV/AIDS, other sexually transmitted diseases, tuberculosis, viral hepatitis, and endemic schistosomiasis (Renmin ribao, 2003i). These multiple public health challenges require China to build on the anti-SARS momentum and integrate a comprehensive epidemic control plan into the national socioeconomic development agenda. While the health sector is now receiving increased attention at high levels, the government so far has placed top priority only on preventing the return of SARS. The top leaders have been generally silent on other major infectious diseases. Despite official recognition of the seriousness of HIV/AIDS, China does not have a comprehensive national program for disease prevention and control to help stop the epidemic. In rural areas hard-hit by AIDS, local governments continue to harass public health activists, devote few resources to educating people about the disease, and sometimes even meet the demands of the villagers with violence (Pan, 2003). Furthermore, there has been no fundamental change in the government's development agenda. The central government still equates development with economic growth and uses that as a yardstick in measuring local government performance.

In addition, it is worth noting that the apparent policy transparency has not been accompanied by significant state relaxation of media control. On May 12, the very same day that Premier Wen Jiabao released the new regulations to promote openness, the *Beijing Morning News* carried an article on how people who spread "rumors" about SARS could be jailed for up to 5 years. While the newly promulgated Regulations on Public Health Emergencies stipulate that government officials make timely and truthful reports about any such emergencies, they do not enshrine the public's right to be informed in the same manner. Indeed, a recent speech by Vice Premier Wu Yi reiterated state control over the media in order to "strictly prohibit the spread of rumors and other harmful information (Wu Yi, 2003)."

While feedback from the public may matter more for the government than it used to, government officials ultimately remain responsible not to the public but to the higher authorities. Hence, the government will always be more sensitive to pressure that comes top down, rather than bottom up. Ironically, the likelihood of deception has increased as a result of the spread of some government measures in fighting SARS, such as the practice of holding bureaucratic officials personally accountable for local SARS cases through a "responsibility pledge" (*junling zhuang*) without giving due consideration of actual local conditions (e.g., the public health infrastructure). If indeed an outbreak is imminent, a local government official concerned about his post may well choose to lie. Manipulation of SARS-related data remained a serious problem even after April 17—among other things, a pattern could be easily identified in the government war against SARS in which when upper-level leaders demanded a reduction of SARS cases, their orders would be reflected in statistics afterwards (Wong, 2003).

To the extent that upward accountability and performance-based legitimacy will cause problems in agenda setting and policy making, the lack of effective civil society participation reduces government effectiveness in policy enforcement. In initiating many anti-SARS projects during the crisis, the government did nothing to consult or inform the local people. Chinese non-governmental organizations (NGOs), if anything, were absent in the war against SARS (21st Century Economic Herald, 2003). Instead, the government relied on the extensive array of mobilization vehicles installed in the Mao era—village party branches, street sub-district offices, former barefoot doctors—to take temperatures, quarantine people, trace infections and round up laggards. To be sure, party leaders undertaking the anti-SARS measures differed from their predecessors by emphasizing "science" and "rule by law." Yet the absence of genuinely engaged civil society groups as a source of oversight and information, coupled with the increasing pressure from higher authorities, easily created a results-oriented implementation structure that made nonscientific, heavy-handed measures more appealing to local government officials. They found it safer to be overzealous than to be seen as "soft." Until June 2, for example, Shanghai was quarantining people from the regions hard hit by SARS (such as Beijing) for 10 days even if they had no symptoms (Pomfret, 2003c).

The government's heavy reliance on quarantine during the epidemic also raises a question about the impact of future disease control measures and the worsening of the human rights situation in China. This question, of course, is not unique to China—even countries like the United States are debating whether it is necessary to apply mandatory approaches to confront health risks more effectively. The Model Emergency Health Powers pushed by the Bush administration would permit state governors in a health crisis to impose quarantines, limit people's movements and ration medicine, and seize anything from dead bodies to private hospitals (Kristof, 2003). While China's Law on Prevention and Treatment of Infectious Disease did not until recently explicate that quarantines apply to the SARS epidemic, Articles 24 and 25 authorize local governments to take emergency measures that may compromise personal freedom. The problem is that unlike democracies, China in applying these measures excludes the input of civil associations. Official reports suggested that innocent people were dubbed rumor spreaders and arrested simply because they relayed some SARS-related information to their friends or colleagues (Xinhua News, 2003d). According to the Ministry of Public Security, public security departments have investigated 107 cases in which people used Internet and cell phones to spread SARS-related "rumors (Renmin wang, 2003d)." Some Chinese legal scholars have already expressed concerns that the government, in order to block information about epidemics, may turn to more human rights violations (ChineseNewsNet, 2003).

The lack of engagement by civil society in the policy process could deplete the social capital that would be so important for future government outbreak control efforts. In the case of SARS, the government's failure to publicize the outbreak in a timely and accurate manner and the ensuing rapid policy turnaround eroded the public's trust and contributed to the spread of rumors even after the government adopted a more open stance toward information on the epidemic. In late April, thousands of residents of a rural town of Tianjin ransacked a building, believing it would be used to house ill patients with confirmed or suspected SARS, even though officials insisted that it would be used only as a medical observation facility to accommodate people who had close contacts with SARS patients and for travelers returning from SARS hot spots. Opposition to official efforts to contain SARS was also found in a coastal Zhejiang province, where several thousand people took part in a violent protest against six people being quarantined after returning from Beijing (Kuhn, 2003). Here again, the lack of active civilian participation exacerbated existing problems of trust. In initiating the project in Tianjin, the government had done nothing to consult or inform the local people (Eckholm, 2003).

Finally, the mobilization model for confronting public health crises also suffers from a problem of sustainability in the post-Mao era. By placing great political pressure on local cadres in policy implementation, mobilization is a convenient bureaucratic tool for overriding fiscal constraints and bureaucratic inertia while promoting grassroots cadres to behave in ways that reflect the priorities of their superiors. Direct involvement of the local political leadership increases program resources, helps ensure they are used for program purposes, and mobilizes resources from other systems, including free manpower transferred to program tasks. Yet in doing so, a bias against routine administration is built into its implementation structure. While personal rewards of private life (e.g., medals, higher pay, extra credits for medical workers' children attending the college entrance exam) were provided for activism in the anti-SARS campaign, decades of reforms have eroded state control and increased the opportunity cost of participation. While the government demonstrated in this case a continued ability to spur people to action in even the most remote villages, in a post-totalitarian context it is generally difficult to sustain a state of high alert across the country for an extended period.

## Conclusions

The pattern of the Chinese government's response to SARS was shaped by the institutional dynamics of the country's political system. A deeply ingrained authoritarian impulse to maintain secrecy, in conjunction with a performance-based legitimacy and an obsession with development and stability during political succession, contributed to China's initial failure to publicize the outbreak. Meanwhile, an upwardly directed system of accountability, a fragmented bureaucracy, and an oligarchic political structure hampered any effective government response to the outbreak. In spite of these problems, interactions between the state and society unleashed dynamics that prompted the central party-state to intervene on society's behalf. The direct involvement of the Party strengthened authority links, increased program resources, and maximized the potential for interdepartmental and intergovernmental cooperation. In this manner, the party-state remains capable of implementing its will throughout the system without serious institutional constraints. The government's capacity for crisis management has been further enhanced by a series of measures taken in the post-SARS era. However, this does not mean that the government is ready for the next disease outbreak. In the absence of fundamental changes in the political system and a comprehensive epidemic control plan, not only is the same pattern of cover-up and inaction likely to be repeated, but the government will find it increasingly difficult to control the multiple public health challenges it is now facing.

The above analysis clearly points to a need for the Chinese government to significantly enhance its capacity to combat future outbreaks of SARS and other infectious diseases. Given that a public health crisis reduces state capacity just when ever-increasing capacity is needed to tackle the challenges, purely endogenous solutions to build capacity are unlikely to be successful, and capacity will have to be imported from exogenous sources such as massive foreign aid (Price-Smith, 2002). In this sense, building state capability also means building more effective partnerships and institutions internationally. International actors can play an important role in creating a more responsible and responsive government in China (Huang, 2003). First, aid from international organizations opens an alternative source of financing for health care, increasing the government's financial capacity in the health sector. Second, international aid can strengthen bureaucratic capacity through technical assistance, policy counseling, and personnel training. Third, while international organizations and foreign governments provide additional health resources in policy implementation, the government increasingly has to subject its agenda-setting regime to the donors' organizational goals, which can make the government more responsive to its people. The agenda shift for SARS to a large extent was caused by strong international pressures exerted by the international media, international organizations, and foreign governments. There are also indications that the Internet is increasingly used by the new leadership to solicit policy feedback, collect public opinions, and mobilize political support. Starting February 11, Western news media were aggressively reporting about SARS and about government cover-ups of the number of cases in China. It is very likely that Hu Jintao and Wen Jiabao, both Internet users, made use of international information in making decisions concerning the epidemic. In other words, external pressures can be very influential because Chinese governmental leaders are aware of weaknesses in the existing system for effectively responding to a crisis and therefore have incentives to seek political resources exogenous to the system.

From the perspective of international actors, helping China to fight future epidemics also helps themselves. Against the background of a global economy, diseases originating in China can be spread and transported globally through trade, travel, and population movements. Moreover, an unsustainable economy or state collapse spawned by poor health will deal a serious blow to the global economy. As foreign companies shift manufacturing to China, the country is becoming a workshop to the world. A world economy that is so dependent on China as an industrial lifeline can become increasingly vulnerable to a major supply disruption caused by disease epidemics. Perhaps equally important, if future epidemics in China result in truly global health crises, the unwanted social and political changes will be felt by even the most powerful nations. As every immigrant or visitor from China or Asia is viewed as a potential Typhoid Mary, minorities and immigration could become a sensitive domestic political issue in countries such as the United States and Canada. An incident in New Jersey during the SARS outbreak, in which artists of Chinese background were denied access to a middle school, suggests that when SARS becomes part of a national lexicon, fear, rumor, suspicion, and misinformation can jeopardize racial harmony in any country (Newman and Zhao, 2003).

Given the international implications of China's public health, it is in the interest of the United States and other industrialized nations to expand cooperation with China in the areas of information exchange, research, personnel training, and improvement of public health facilities. Meanwhile, these countries could send clear signals to the Chinese leadership that reform-minded leaders in the forefront of fighting epidemic diseases and supporting public health will be supported. The world's interests will be well served by continuing to support a Chinese government that is increasingly more open and interested in international engagement. It should also not miss this unique opportunity to help create a healthier China.

## REFERENCES

Arhin-Tenkorang D, Conceiçao P. 2003. Beyond communicable disease control: health in the age of globalization. In: Kaul I, Conceiçao P, Le Goulven K, and Mendoza RU, eds., *Providing Global Public Goods: Managing Globalization*. New York, NY: Oxford University Press. Pp. 484-515.

Australian Treasury. 2003 (Winter). *Economic Roundup*. Canberra, Australia: Commonwealth Government.

Bagnoli P, McKibbin W, Wilcoxen P. 1996. Future projections and structural change. In: Nakicenovic N, Nordhaus W, Richels R, Toth F, eds., *Climate Change: Integrating Economics and Policy*. CP 96–1. Laxenburg, Austria: International Institute for Applied Systems Analysis. Pp. 181-206.

Barro R, Sala-I-Martin X. 1995. *Economic Growth*. New York, NY: McGraw-Hill.

Beech H. 2003. Unhappy returns. *Time* 162(22). [Online] Available: http://www.time.com/time/asia/magazine/article/0,13673,501031208-552154,00.html.

Blanchard O, Fischer S. 1989. *Lectures on Macroeconomics*. Cambridge, MA: MIT Press.

Bloom DE, Canning D, Sevilla J. 2001. *The Effect of Health on Economic Growth: Theory and Evidence*. NBER Working Paper #8587. Cambridge, MA: National Bureau of Economic Research.

Bloom DE, Mahal AS. 1997. AIDS, flu, and the Black Death: impacts on economic growth and well-being. In: Bloom DE, Godwin P, eds., *The Economics of HIV and AIDS: The Case of South and South East Asia*. Oxford, UK: Oxford University Press. Pp. 22-52.

Brainerd E, Siegler MV. 2002. The Economic Effects of the 1918 Influenza Epidemic. CEPR Discussion Paper #3791. London, UK: Center for Economic Policy Research.

Brownlie I. 1998. *Principles of Public International Law*, 5th ed. Oxford: Clarendon Press.

Bull H. 1977. *The Anarchical Society: A Study of Order in World Politics.* London, UK: Macmillan.

*BusinessWeek.* April 28, 2003.

Chang L. 2003. China may apply lessons from SARS to fight AIDS. *The Wall Street Journal.* August 4, 2003.

ChineseNewsNet. 2003. [Online] Available: http://www.duoweinews.com [accessed on May 10, 2003].

China's Chernobyl? 2003. *Economist.* 00130613, April 26, 2003. 367(8321).

Chinese Scientists Defeated by SARS. 2003. *People's Daily.* [Online] Available: http://english. peopledaily.com.cn/200306/09/eng20030609_117919.shtml

Chou J, Kuo N, Peng S. 2003 (May). *The Potential Impacts on the Taiwanese Economy of the Outbreak of SARS.* Paper presented at Asian Economic Panel, Keio University, Tokyo.

Commission on Macroeconomics and Health. 2002. *Macroeconomics and Health: Investing in Health for Economic Development.* Report of the Commission on Macroeconomics and Health to WHO. Geneva: WHO.

Development: key to China's solutions of all issues. 2003. *People's Daily.* [Online] Available: http://fpeng.peopledaily.com.cn/200003/06/eng20000306A104.html.

Dodgson R, Lee K, Drager N. 2002. *Global Health Governance: A Conceptual Review.* Key Issues in Global Health Governance Discussion Paper No. 1. London, UK: World Health Organization and Centre for Global Change and Health.

Eckholm E. April 28, 2003. Thousands riot in rural Chinese town over SARS. *New York Times.* P. A14.

Fewsmith J. 2003. China and the politics of SARS. *Current History.* P. 252.

Fidler DP. 1999. *International Law and Infectious Diseases.* Oxford, UK: Clarendon Press.

Fidler DP. 2003. Emerging trends in international law concerning global infectious disease control. *Emerging Infectious Diseases* 9:285-90.

Friedman TL. 2000. A Russian dinosaur. *New York Times.* [Online] Available: http://www.nytimes. com/library/opinion/friedman/090500frie.html [accessed February 19, 2004].

Garrett L. 2003. A Chinese lab's race to ID and halt SARS: politics and rivalry mix with research. *Newsday.* [Online] Available: http://www.aegis.com/news/newsday/2003/ND030501.html [accessed February 19, 2004].

Global Fund to Fight AIDS, Tuberculosis, and Malaria. 2003. [Online] Available: http:// www.globalfundatm.org.

Guangming ribao (Bright daily). September 25, 2003. [Online] Available: http://news.sina.com.cn/o/ 2003-09-25/1036816387s.shtml.

Guangzhou is fighting an unknown virus. February 13, 2003. *Southern Weekly.*

Haacker M. 2002. *The Economic Consequences of HIV/AIDS in South Africa.* IMF Working Paper, WP/02/38.

Hai C, Hua J. 2003. Guangzhou kangji buming bingdu (Guangzhou is fighting an unknown virus). *Nanfang zhoumu* (Southern Weekly).

Haiyan Z. 2003. Bu pingjing de chuntian (Unquiet spring). *Nanfang Zhoumu* (Southern Weekly).

Hanna D, Huang Y. 2003 (May). *SARS Impact on Asian Economies.* Paper presented at Asian Economic Panel, Keio University, Tokyo.

Harding C, Lim CL. 1999. The significance of Westphalia: an archaeology of the international legal order. In: Harding C, Lim CL, eds., *Renegotiating Westphalia.* The Hague: M. Nijhoff Publishers. Pp. 1-23.

Hertel T, ed. 1997. *Global Trade Analysis: modeling and Applications.* Cambridge, UK: Cambridge University Press.

Heymann D. April 7, 2003. Testimony on Severe Acute Respiratory Syndrome Threat (SARS), Hearing Before the Senate Committee on Health, Education, Labor and Pensions, 108th Congress.

Huailing L. 2003. Chengshi de shengli (The triumph of honesty), *Nanfeng chuang* (Southern wind window). [Online] Available: http://www.szonline.net/content/2003/200305/20030516/175335.html.

Huang Y. (Forthcoming). Bringing the local state back in: the political economy of public health in rural China. *Journal of Contemporary China.*

Huang Y. 2003 (May). *Mortal Peril: Public Health in China and Its Security Implications.* CBACI Health and Security Series, Special Report 6. Washington, DC: CBACI.

Jackson RH. 2001. The Evolution of International Society. In: Baylis J, Smith S, eds., *The Globalization of World Politics*, 2nd ed. Oxford, UK: Oxford University Press. Pp. 35-50.

Jakes S. April 8, 2003. Beijing's SARS attack. *Time.* [Online] Available: http://www.time.com/time/asia/news/daily/0,9754,441615,00.html.

*Jiankang bao* (Health news). November 7, 2003.

Kahn J, Rosenthal E. 2003. New health worry for China as SARS hits the hinterland. *New York Times.* Section A, P. 1, Column 6.

Kingdon JW. 1995. *Agendas, Alernatives, and Public Policies.* 2nd ed. New York, NY: Harper Collins College Publishers.

Kristof ND. May 2, 2003. Lock 'em up. *New York Times.* P. 33.

Kuhn A. 2003. China's fight against SARS spawns backlash. *Los Angeles Times.* P. A5.

Lampton DM. 1987. *Policy Implementation in Post-Mao China.* Berkeley and Los Angeles, CA: University of California Press.

Lee JW, McKibbin W. 2004. Globalization and Disease: The Case of SARS. *Asian Economic Papers.* Cambridge, MA: MIT Press.

Li Z et al. 1999. *Zhonghua renmin gonghe guo baomifa quanshu* (Encyclopedia on the PRC State Secrets Law). Changchun: Jilin renmin chubanshe. Pp. 372-4.

Lieberthal KG, David M. Lampton. 1992. *Bureaucracy, Politics, and Decision Making in Post-Mao China.* California: University of California Press.

Lianhe zaobao online. 2003. [Online] Available: http://www.zaobao.com/special/pneumonia/pages2/pneumonia250603.html.

McKibbin W. 1998. Risk re-evaluation, capital flows and the crisis in Asia. In: Garnaut R, McLeod R, eds., *East Asia in Crisis: From Being a Miracle to Needing One?* New York, NY: Routledge. Pp. 227-44.

McKibbin WJ, Sachs J. 1991. *Global Linkages: Macroeconomic Interdependence and Co-operation in the World Economy.* Washington, DC: Brookings Institution.

McKibbin WJ, Stoeckel A. 2003. *The SARS Outbreak: How Bad Could it Get?* Issue #5. [Online] Available: http://www.economicscenarios.com.

McKibbin WJ, Vines D. 2000. Modelling reality: The need for both intertemporal optimization and stickiness in models for policymaking. *Oxford Review of Economic Policy* 16(4):106-37.

McKibbin W, Wilcoxen P. 1998. The theoretical and empirical structure of the G-Cubed Model. *Economic Modelling* 16(1):123-48.

McNeil, DG. 2003. Health officials wield a big stick, carefully, against SARS. *New York Times.* P. A12.

Ruan. 1992. *Chronicle of an Empire.* Translated and edited by Liu N, Rand P, Sullivan LR. Boulder, CO: Westview Press. P. 189.

Ministry of Health. 1999. *National Health Service Research.* Beijing, China: Ministry of Health.

Ministry of Health. 2003. [Online] Available: http://www.moh.gov.cn/zhg1/yqfb/1200308160002.htm.

*Nanfang zhoumu* (Southern Weekly). February 13, 2003.

National Intelligence Council. 2003. *SARS: Down But Still a Threat* (Intelligence Community Assessment 2003-09). Washington, DC: National Intelligence Council.

Newman M, Zhao Y. 2003. Fear, not SARS, rattles south Jersey school. *New York Times.* P. B1.

Obstfeld M, Rogoff K. 1996. *Foundations of International Macroeconomics*. Cambridge, MA: MIT Press.

Oi J. 1989. *State and Peasant in Contemporary China*. Berkeley: University of California Press. P. 228.

Oksenberg M. 2001. China's political system: challenges of the twenty-first century. *The China Journal* 4:28.

Pan PP. 2003. China meets AIDS crisis with force. *The Washington Post*. P. A01.

Pei M. April 7, 2003. A country that does not take care of its people. *Financial Times*.

Pomfret J. 2003a. China's slow reaction to fast-moving illness. *The Washington Post*. P. A18.

Pomfret J. April 27, 2003b. China's crisis has a political edge. *The Washington Post*. P. A33.

Pomfret J. 2003c. China feels side effects from SARS. *The Washington Post*. P. A01.

Pomfret J. 2003d. Outbreak gave China's Hu an opening. *The Washington Post*. P. A1.

Price-Smith AT. 2002 (September). *Pretoria's Shadow: The HIV/AIDS Pandemic and National Security in South Africa*. Special Report No. 4, CBACI Health and Security Series. Washington, DC: CBACI. P. 27.

Reich M. 2002. *Public-Private Partnerships for Public Health*. Cambridge, MA: Harvard University Press.

*Renmin ribao* (People's daily). June 26, 2001. [Online] Available: http://past.people.com.cn/GB/shizheng/252/5303/5304/20010626/497648.html.

*Renmin ribao* (People's Daily), overseas edition. April 22, 2003a.

*Renmin ribao*, overseas edition. April 9, 2003b.

*Renmin ribao*, overseas edition. May 1, 2003c.

*Renmin ribao*, overseas edition. November 24, 2003d.

*Renmin ribao*, overseas edition. August 26, 2003e.

*Renmin ribao*, overseas edition. September 3, 2003f.

*Renmin ribao*, overseas edition. November 3, 2003g.

*Renmin ribao*, overseas edition. September 12, 2003h.

*Renmin ribao*, overseas edition. August 26, 2003i.

Renmin wang (People). 2003a. [Online] Available: http://www.people.com.cn/GB/shehui/47/20030211/921420.html.

Renmin wang (People). February 11, 2003b. [Online] Available: http://www.people.com.cn/GB/shehui/47/20030211/921422.html.

Renmin wang (People). May 21, 2003c. [Online] Available: http://past.people.com.cn/GB/shizheng/252/17/1853/20030521/997636.html.

Renmin wang (People). May 8, 2003d. [Online] Available: http://www.people.com.cn/GB/shehui/44/20030508/987610.html [accessed May 8, 2003].

Sachs J, Malaney P. 2002. The economic and social burden of malaria. Nature 415(6872): 680-685.

Scholte JA. 2001. The Globalization of World Politics. In: Baylis J, Smith S, eds., *The Globalization of World Politics*, 2nd ed. Oxford, UK: Oxford University Press. Pp. 12-32.

Shirk SL. 2003. *The Political Logic of Economic Reform in China*. Berkeley, CA: University of California Press. P. 57.

Siu A, Wong R. 2003 (May). *Ravaged by SARS: The Case of Hong Kong SARS*. Paper presented at Asian Economic Panel, Keio University, Tokyo.

Smith R, Beaglehole R, Woodward D, Drager N, eds. 2003. *Global Public Goods for Health: Health Economic and Public Health Perspectives*. Oxford, UK: Oxford University Press.

*South China Morning Post*. February 11, 2003.

Tak-ho F. 2003. Leaders get tough with local officials. *South China Morning Post*.

*The SS Lotus (France v. Turkey)*. 1927. Permanent Court of International Justice, Series A, No. 10.

Treadway A. 1969. On rational entrepreneurial behavior and the demand for investment. *Review of Economic Studies* 36(106):227-39.

*Washington Post*. April 14, 2003.

Wen H. 2003 (May). *China in the Eye of the Storm.* Paper presented at Asian Economic Panel, Keio University, Tokyo.

Wiest NC. 2003. Powerful disaster agency is unveiled. *South China Morning Post.*

Wong KW. 2003. SARS: What happened to April 20? *AsiaTimes* online.

WHO (World Health Organization). July 22, 1946. In: World Health Organization. 1994. *Basic Documents,* 40th ed. Geneva: WHO. Pp. 1-18.

WHO. 1978. Declaration of Alma-Ata, adopted at the International Conference on Primary Health Care. Alma Ata, USSR.

WHO. 1983. *International Health Regulations,* 3rd ann. ed. Geneva: WHO.

WHO. 2002. *Global Crises—Global Solutions: Managing Public Health Emergencies of International Concern Through the Revised International Health Regulations.* Geneva: WHO.

WHO. 2003a. World Health Assembly, Severe Acute Respiratory Syndrome (SARS), WHA56.29.

WHO. 2003b. *Severe Acute Respiratory Syndrome (SARS): Status of the Outbreak and Lessons for the Immediate Future.* Geneva: WHO.

WHO. 2003c. Severe Acute Respiratory Syndrome (SARS)—Multi-Country Outbreak. [Online] Available: http://www.who.ing.csr/don/2003_03_15/en/html.

WHO. 2003d. Revision of the International Health Regulations, WHA56.28.

Wu Yi. October 9, 2003. [Online] Available: http://www.people.com.cn/GB/shizheng/1026/2126148.html.

Xinhua News. April 24, 2003a.

Xinhua News. 2003b. [Online] Available: http://news.xinhuanet.com/newscenter/2003-05/12/content_866362.htm.

Xinhua News. August 17, 2003c.

Xinhua News. April 26, 2003d. [Online] Available: http://www.cecc.gov/pages/roundtables/051203/huang.php and [Online] Available: http://www.people.com.cn/GB/shehui/47/20030426/980282.html.

Yardley J. 2003. China begins giving free H.I.V./AIDS drugs to the poor. *New York Times.* P. A3.

Zhongguo jingji shibao (China economic times). November 5, 2003.

Zhongguo qingnian bao (China Youth Daily), in Renmin wang (People). June 6, 2003. [Online] Available: http://www.people.com.cn/GB/shehui/47/20030606/1009738.html.

Zhongguo xinwen wang (China News Service). April 13, 2003a. [Online] Available: www.chinanews.com.cn/n/2003-04-13/26/293925.html.

Zhongguo xinwen wang (China News Service). September 23, 2003b. [Online] Available: http://news.sina.com.cn/o/2003-09-23/0934803130s.shtml.

# 3

# Microbiology, Ecology, and Natural History of Coronaviruses

## OVERVIEW

Coronaviruses cause a substantial fraction of human colds and a host of common respiratory infections in many other animals, including economically important diseases of livestock, poultry, and laboratory rodents. Moreover, although these viruses were not known for producing more than mild infections in humans prior to the SARS epidemic, veterinary coronavirologists have long been aware of their potential for producing lethal infections in animals, as Linda Saif describes in this chapter's first paper. For this reason, there is already an extensive amount of research on animal coronaviruses that can be drawn from for understanding the life cycle and pathogenicity of the SARS virus, and veterinary scientists are now being called on to join the research response to the epidemic and share their knowledge of coronaviruses with a broader audience. Mark Denison's paper describes the current state of research on animal coronaviruses and discusses how results from these animal models suggest promising directions for future research on SARS and other emerging zoonoses.

Animal coronaviruses tend to follow one of two basic pathogenic models, producing either enteric or respiratory infections. Both models show parallels to the clinical features of SARS patients, the majority of whom presented with respiratory infections but in some cases also suffered from enteric complications. In adult animals, coronavirus infections of a respiratory nature have shown increased severity in the presence of several factors, including high exposure doses, respiratory coinfections, stress related to shipping or commingling with animals from different farms, and treatment with corticosteroids. In young, seronegative animals, enteric coronaviruses can cause fatal infections. Although coronaviruses generally cause disease in a single animal species, some have been demonstrated to cross species barriers.

Considerable effort has already been applied toward uncovering an animal source of the SARS virus. This has been sought primarily through the genetic characterization of viral isolates from suspected animal sources and comparison with human SARS coronavirus samples. In the past, however, epidemiological detective work has identified the source of many outbreaks of infectious disease, and one workshop participant suggested that a case control study of the first 50 to 100 SARS patients from China's Guangdong Province, where the earliest cases of the disease were detected, might prove similarly fruitful. While a natural reservoir for the SARS virus has not yet been identified, the combination of such genomic and epidemiological techniques is already yielding suggestive results. For example, the last paper in this chapter by Yi Guan et al. describes the presence of coronaviruses closely related to SARS among live animals sold in Guangdong markets. Similar epidemiological principles may yet provide valuable direction for further laboratory surveys of animal viruses aimed at finding the original source and reservoir of the SARS coronavirus.

Coronaviruses have been classified into three major categories based on their genetic characteristics. While the SARS virus has been linked with Group II coronaviruses, whose members include human and bovine respiratory viruses and the mouse hepatitis virus, there is still some debate over whether its genetic features might be sufficiently distinct to warrant classification within a separate, fourth class of coronaviruses. Studies of coronavirus replication at the molecular level reveal several mechanisms that account for the repeated, persistent infections typical of coronaviral disease. High rates of mutation and RNA-RNA recombination produce viruses that are able to adapt to acquire and regain virulence. Although researchers have identified several potential targets for antiviral therapies, the ability of the virus to mutate and recombine represents a major challenge to vaccine development. A vaccine that can provide highly effective, long-term protection against respiratory coronavirus infections has not yet been developed, nor have appropriate animal models been developed to test potential vaccines against SARS. It was noted by several workshop participants that a coordinated, multidisciplinary research effort, drawing on expertise in both the veterinary and biomedical sciences, will likely be needed to meet these goals.

## ANIMAL CORONAVIRUSES: LESSONS FOR SARS

*Linda J. Saif*
Department of Food Animal Health Research Program, Ohio Agricultural Research and Development Center

The emergence of severe acute respiratory syndrome (SARS) illustrates that coronaviruses (CoVs) may quiescently emerge from possible animal reservoirs and can cause potentially fatal disease in humans, as previously recognized for animals. Consequently the focus of this review will be on the emergence of new CoV strains and the comparative pathogenesis of SARS CoV with those CoVs that cause enteric and respiratory infections of various animal hosts. A review of animal CoV vaccines recently has been compiled (Saif, in press), so this topic will not be addressed.

## Emergence of New Coronaviruses

The medical community was amazed by the emergence of a new coronavirus associated with SARS in healthy adults in 2003 (Drosten et al., 2003; Ksiazek et al., 2003; Peiris et al., 2003b; Poutanen et al., 2003). Historically human CoV infections (229E and OC43 CoV strains) were mild and associated with only common cold symptoms although reinfections, even with the same strain, occur (Callow et al, 1990; Holmes, 2001). However, veterinary coronavirologists had previously recognized the potential for coronaviruses to cause fatal enteric or respiratory infections in animals and for new CoV strains to emerge from unknown reservoirs, often evoking fatal disease in naïve populations. For example, the porcine epidemic diarrhea CoV (PEDV) first appeared from an unknown source in Europe and Asia in the 1970s and 1980s, causing severe diarrhea and widespread deaths in baby pigs before becoming endemic in swine (Pensaert, 1999). The PEDV is absent in U.S. swine. Interestingly, PEDV is genetically more closely related to human CoV 229E than to the other animal group I CoV (Duarte et al., 1994), and unlike the other group I CoV, it grows in Vero cells like SARS CoV (Hoffman and Wyler, 1988). These observations raise intriguing, but unanswered, questions about its origin.

Alternatively new CoV strains differing in tissue tropism and virulence may arise from existing strains. The less virulent porcine respiratory coronavirus (PRCV) evolved as a spike (S) gene deletion mutant of the highly virulent enteric CoV, transmissible gastroenteritis virus (TGEV) ( reviewed in Laude et al., 1993; Saif and Wesley, 1999). Curiously, differences in the sizes of the $5'$ end S gene deletion region (621–681 nucleotides) between European and U.S. PRCV strains provided evidence for their independent origin on two continents within a similar time frame (1980s). Deletion of this region (or in combination with deletions in ORF 3a) presumably accounted for altered tissue tropism from enteric to respiratory and reduced virulence of the PRCV strains (Ballesteros et al., 1997; Sanchez et al., 1999). The ability of certain CoVs to persist in their host also provides a longer opportunity for new mutants to be selected with altered tissue tropisms and virulence from among the viral RNA quasispecies (or swarm of viruses). An example is the virulent systemic variant, the feline infectious peritonitis virus (FIPV), which likely arises from persistent infection of cats with the less virulent feline enteric CoV (Herrewegh et al., 1997; Vennema et al., 1995).

Furthermore, animal CoVs may acquire new genes via recombination, as exemplified by the acquisition of an influenza C-like hemagglutinin by bovine

CoV or its ancestor CoV (Brian et al., 1995). Recombination events among CoVs may also generate new strains with altered tissue or host tropisms. For example, targeted recombination between feline and mouse S proteins enables feline CoV to infect mice (Haijema et al., 2003). Recent phylogenetic analysis suggests that SARS CoV may have evolved from a past recombination event between mammalian-like and avian-like parent strains with the S gene representing a mammalian (group 1)–avian origin mosaic (Stavrinides and Guttman, 2004). This recognition that CoVs can further evolve in a host population to acquire new tissue tropisms or virulence via mutations or recombination suggests that similar events may occur if SARS CoV persists in humans.

## Interspecies Transmission of Coronaviruses

The genus *coronavirus* is composed of at least three genetically and autigenically distinct groups of CoV that cause mild to severe enteric, respiratory, or systemic disease in domestic and wild animals, poultry, rodents, and carnivores and mild colds in humans (Table 3-1) The SARS CoV is genetically distantly related to known CoVs and comprises a provisional new group (IV) (Drosten et al., 2003; Marra et al., 2003; Rota et al., 2003) or alternatively, using rooted tree phylogenetic analysis, belongs to a subgroup of group II (Snijder et al., 2003). Coronaviruses from two wild animal species (civet cats and raccoon dogs) recently have been characterized genetically as members of the SARS CoV group (Guan et al., 2003). Coronaviruses within each group share various levels of genetic and antigenic relatedness and several show cross-species transmission. Thus the likelihood that SARS CoV is a zoonotic infection potentially transmitted from wild animals to humans is not unprecedented based on previous research on interspecies transmission of animal CoV and wildlife reservoirs for CoV. As examples, the porcine CoV, TGEV, and canine and feline CoVs can cross-infect pigs, dogs, and cats with variable disease expression and levels of cross-protection in the heterologous host (Saif and Wesley, 1999; Saif and Heckert, 1990). These three related CoVs appear to be host range mutants of an ancestral CoV. Wildlife reservoirs for CoVs were recognized prior to SARS. Captive wild ruminants harbor CoVs antigenically closely related to bovine CoV and CoV isolates from the wild ruminants experimentally infected domestic calves (Tsunemitsu et al., 1995; Majhdi et al., 1997). The promiscuousness of bovine CoV is evident by infection of dogs and also humans by genetically similar (>97 percent identity) CoV strains (Erles et al., 2003; Zhang et al., 1994). Even more dramatic than infection of mammalian hosts by bovine CoV is the finding that bovine CoV can experimentally infect and cause disease (diarrhea) in phylogenetically diverse species such as avian hosts, including baby turkeys, but not baby chicks (Ismail et al., 2001b). It is notable that in the latter study, the bovine CoV-infected baby turkeys also transmitted the viruses to unexposed contact control birds. The reasons for the broad host range of bovine CoV are unknown, but may relate to the

**TABLE 3-1** Coronavirus Groups, Target Tissues, and Diseases

| Genetic Group | Virus | Host | Disease/Infection Site | | |
|---|---|---|---|---|---|
| | | | Respiratory | Enteric[a] | Other[b] |
| I | HCoV-229E | Human | X upper | X S1 | |
| | TGEV | Pig | X upper | X S1 | Vitremia |
| | PRCV | Pig | X upper/lung | | |
| | PEDV | Pig | | X SL, colon | |
| | FIPV | Cat | X upper | X | Systemic |
| | FCoV | Cat | | X S1 | |
| | CCoV | Dog | | X S1 | |
| | RaCoV | Rabbit | | | Systemic |
| 11 | HCoV-OC43 | Human | X upper | ?? (BCoV?) | |
| | NUN | Mouse | | X | Hepatitis, CNS, systemic |
| | RcoV (sialodocry-adenitis) | Rat | X | | Eye, salivary glands |
| | BEV | Pig | X | | CNS |
| | BCoV | Cattle | X upper/lung | X S1, colon | |
| III | IBV | Chicken | X upper | X | Kidney, oviduct |
| IV?? | TCoV (TECoV) | Turkey | | X S1 | |
| IIA? | SARS | Human | X lung | X (?) | Viremia, kidney? |
| | Civet cat CoV | Himalayan palm civet | X | X | Subclinical? |
| | Raccoon dog CoV | Raccoon dog | ? | X | Subclinical? |

[a]SI = small intestine; ?? = BCoV-like CoV from a child, Zhang et al. (1994); ? = unknown.
[b]CNS = central nervous system.

presence of a hemagglutinin on bovine CoV and its possible role in binding to diverse cell types.

Recent data suggest that SARS CoV may also have a broad host range besides humans. Genetically similar CoVs were isolated from civet cats and raccoon dogs (Guan et al., 2003). In experimental studies, the SARS CoV infected and caused disease in macaques and ferrets and infected cats subclinically (Fouchier et al., 2003; Martina et al., 2003). In the latter two species, the SARS CoV was further transmitted to exposed contacts, documenting transmission within the new host species. Consequently, although previous data document the emergence of new animal CoV strains and the broad host range of several CoVs, the determinants for host range specificity among CoVs are undefined. In addition, we understand little about CoVs circulating in wildlife and relatively few animal CoV strains have been fully sequenced for comparative phylogenetic analysis to trace their evolutionary origins.

## Pathogenesis of Animal Enteric and Respiratory Coronaviruses

*Pathogenesis of Group I TGEV and PRCV CoV: Models of Enteric and Respiratory Infections*

Because both pneumonia and diarrhea occur in SARS patients, an understanding of the tissue tropisms and pathogenesis of respiratory and enteric animal CoVs should contribute to our understanding of similar parameters for SARS. The TGEV targets the small intestinal epithelial cells leading to severe villous atrophy, malabsorptive diarrhea, and a potentially fatal gastroenteritis (Table 3-1). The virus also infects the upper respiratory tract with transient nasal shedding (Van Cott et al., 1993), but infection or lesions in the lung are less common. In adults, TGEV is mild with transient diarrhea or inappetence, but pregnant or lactating animals develop more severe clinical signs and agalactia (Saif and Wesley, 1999).

The PRCV, an S gene deletion mutant of TGEV, has an altered tissue tropism (respiratory) and reduced virulence (Laude et al., 1993; Saif and Wesley, 1999). Like SARS, PRCV spreads by droplets and has a pronounced tropism for the lung, replicating to titers of $10^7$-$10^8$ $TCID_{50}$ and producing interstitial pneumonia affecting 5 to 60 percent of the lung (Cox et al., 1990; Halbur et al., 1993; Laude et al., 1993; Saif and Wesley, 1999). Although many uncomplicated PRCV infections are mild or subclinical, lung lesions are invariably present. Like SARS, clinical signs of PRCV include fever with variable degrees of dyspnea, polypnea, anorexia, and lethargy, and less coughing and rhinitis (Cox et al., 1990; Halbur et al., 1993; Hayes, 2000; Laude et al., 1993; Saif and Wesley, 1999). Further resembling SARS, PRCV replicates in lung epithelial cells, although viral antigen is also detected in type I and II pneumocytes and alveolar macrophages. In lungs, bronchiolar infiltration of mononuclear cells, lymphohistiocytic exudates, and epithelial cell necrosis leads to interstitial pneumonia. PRCV induces transient viremia with virus also detected from nasal swabs and in tonsils and trachea, similar to SARS (Drosten et al., 2003; Ksiazek et al., 2003; Peiris et al., 2003b). The PRCV further replicates in undefined cells in the gut lamina propria, but without inducing villous atrophy or diarrhea and with limited fecal shedding (Cox et al., 1990; Saif and Wesley, 1999). Recently, however, fecal isolates of PRCV were detected with consistent, minor point mutations in the S gene compared to the nasal isolates from the same pig (Costantini et al., in press). Such observations suggest the presence of CoV quasispecies in the host with some strains more adapted to the intestine, a potential corollary for the fecal shedding of SARS CoV (Drosten et al., 2003; Ksiazek et al., 2003; Peiris et al., 2003a). Of further relevance to SARS was the displacement of the virulent TGEV infections by the widespread dissemination of PRCV in Europe and the disappearance of PRCV from swine herds in summer with its reemergence in older pigs in winter (Laude et al., 1993; Saif and Wesley, 1999).

## Group II Bovine CoV (BCoV): Models of Pneumoenteric Infections

The shedding of SARS in feces of many patients and the occurrence of diarrhea in 10 to 27 percent of patients (Peiris et al., 2003a), but with a higher percentage (73 percent) in the Amoy Gardens, Hong Kong, outbreak (Chim et al., 2003) suggests that SARS may be pneumoenteric like BCoV. BCoV causes three distinct clinical syndromes in cattle: calf diarrhea; winter dysentery with hemorrhagic diarrhea in adults; and respiratory infections in cattle of various ages, including cattle with shipping fever (Table 3-1) (Clark, 1993; Lathrop et al., 2000a; Lathrop et al., 2000b; Saif and Heckert, 1990; Storz et al., 1996, 2000a, Tsunemitsu et al., 1995). Based on BCoV antibody seroprevalence, the virus is ubiquitous in cattle worldwide. All BCoV isolates from both enteric and respiratory infections are antigenically similar in virus neutralization (VN) tests, comprising a single serotype, but with two to three subtypes identified by VN or using monoclonal antibodies (MAbs) (Clark, 1993; Hasoksuz et al., 1999a; Hasoksuz et al., 1999b; Saif and Heckert, 1990; Tsunemitsu and Saif, 1995). In addition, genetic differences (point mutations but not deletions) have been detected in the S gene between enteric and respiratory isolates, including ones from the same animal (Chouljenko et al., 2001; Hasoksuz et al., 2002b). Nevertheless, inoculation of gnotobiotic or colostrum-deprived calves with calf diarrhea, winter dysentery, or respiratory BCoV strains led to both nasal and fecal CoV shedding and cross-protection against diarrhea after challenge with a calf diarrhea strain (Cho et al., 2001b; El-Kanawati et al., 1996). However, subclinical nasal and fecal virus shedding detected in calves challenged with the heterologous BCoV strains (Cho et al., 2001b; El-Kanawati et al., 1996) confirmed field studies showing that subclinically infected animals may be a reservoir for BCoV (Heckert et al., 1990, 1991). Cross-protection against BcoV-induced respiratory disease has not been evaluated.

## Calf Diarrhea and Calf Respiratory BCoV Infections

Calf diarrhea BCoV strains infect the epithelial cells of the distal small and large intestine and superficial and crypt enterocytes of the colon, leading to villous atrophy and crypt hyperplasia (Saif and Heckert, 1990; Van Kruiningen et al., 1987). One- to 4-week-old calves develop a severe, malabsorptive diarrhea, resulting in dehydration and often death. Concurrent fecal and nasal shedding often occur. BCoV are also implicated as a cause of mild respiratory disease (coughing, rhinitis) or pneumonia in 2- to 24-month-old calves and are detected in nasal secretions, lungs, and often the intestines (Clark, 1993; Heckert et al., 1990; Heckert et al., 1991; Saif and Heckert, 1990). In studies of calves from birth to 20 weeks of age, Heckert and colleagues (1990, 1991) documented both fecal and nasal shedding of BCoV, with repeated respiratory shedding episodes in the same animal with or without respiratory disease, and subsequent increases in their serum antibody titers consistent with these reinfections. These findings suggest a lack of long-term mucosal immunity in the upper respiratory tract after natural CoV infection, confirming similar observations for human respiratory CoV (Callow et al., 1990; Holmes, 2001).

### Winter Dysentery BCoV Infections

Winter dysentery (WD) occurs in adult cattle during the winter months and is characterized by hemorrhagic diarrhea, frequent respiratory signs, and a marked reduction in milk production in dairy cattle (Saif, 1990; Saif and Heckert, 1990; Van Kruiningen et al., 1987). Intestinal lesions and BCoV-infected cells in the colonic crypts resemble those described for calf diarrhea. The BCoV isolates from WD outbreaks at least partially reproduced the disease in BCoV seropositive nonlactating cows (Tsunemitsu et al., 1999) and in BCoV seronegative lactating cows (Traven et al., 2001). Interestingly, in the later study, the older cattle were more severely affected than similarly exposed calves, mimicking the milder SARS cases seen in children versus adults (Kamps and Hoffmann, 2003a).

### Shipping Fever BCoV Infections

More recent studies done in 1995 have implicated BCoV in association with respiratory disease (shipping fever) in feedlot cattle (Lathrop et al., 2000a, Storz et al., 1996). BCoV was isolated from nasal secretions and lungs of cattle with pneumonia and from feces (Hasoksuz et al., 1999a, 2002a; Storz et al., 2000a, b). In a subsequent study, a high percentage of feedlot cattle (45 percent) shed BCoV both nasally and in feces by ELISA (Cho et al., 2001a). Application of nested RT-PCR detected higher BCoV nasal and fecal shedding rates of 84 percent and 96 percent, respectively (Hasoksuz et al., 2002a).

## Cofactors That Exacerbate CoV Infections, Disease, or Shedding

Underlying disease or respiratory coinfections, dose and route of infection, and immunosuppression (corticosteroids) are all potential cofactors related to the severity of SARS. These cofactors can also exacerbate the severity of BCoV, TGEV, or PRCV infections. In addition, these cofactors may play a role in the superspreader cases seen in the SARS epidemic (Kamps and Hoffmann, 2003b) by enhancing virus transmission.

## Impact of Respiratory Co-Infections on CoV Infections, Disease, and Shedding

Shipping fever is recognized as a multifactorial, polymicrobial respiratory disease complex in young adult feedlot cattle with several factors exacerbating respiratory disease, including BCoV infections (Lathrop et al., 2000a,b; Storz et al., 1996; Storz et al., 2000a; Storz et al., 2000b). Shipping fever can be precipitated by several viruses, alone or in combination, including viruses similar to common human respiratory viruses (BCoV, bovine resiratory syncytial virus, parainfluenza-3 virus), bovine herpesvirus, and viruses capable of mediating immunosuppression (bovine viral diarrhea virus, etc.). The shipping of cattle long distances to feedlots and the commingling of cattle from multiple farms creates physical stresses that overwhelm the animal's defense mechanisms and provides close contact for exposure to new pathogens or strains not previously encountered. Such factors are analogous to the physical stress of long airplane trips with close contact among individuals from diverse regions of the world, both of which may play a role in enhancing an individual's susceptibility to SARS. For shipping fever, various predisposing factors (viruses, stress) allow commensal bacteria of the nasal cavity (*Mannheimia haemolytica*, *Pasteurella* spp., *Mycoplasma* spp., etc.) to infect the lungs, leading to fatal fibrinous pneumonia (Lathrop et al., 2000a,b; Storz et al., 1996, 2000a,b). Like PRCV or SARS infections, it is possible that antibiotic treatment of such individuals with massive release of bacterial lipopolysaccharides (LPS) could precipitate induction of proinflammatory cytokines, which may further enhance lung damage. For example, Van Reeth et al. (2000) showed that pigs infected with PRCV followed by a subclinical dose of *E. coli* LPS within 24 hours developed enhanced fever and more severe respiratory disease compared to each agent alone. They concluded that the effects were likely mediated by the significantly enhanced levels of proinflammatory cytokines induced by the bacterial LPS. Thus there is a need to examine both LPS and lung cytokine levels in SARS patients as possible mediators of the severity of SARS. Bacteria (*Chlamydia* spp.) have been isolated from SARS patients, but their role in enhancing the severity of SARS is undefined (Poutanen et al., 2003).

Interactions between PRCV and other respiratory viruses may also parallel the potential for concurrent or preexisting respiratory viral infections to interact with SARS CoV (such as metapneumoviruses, influenza, reoviruses, respiratory syncytial virus [RSV], OC43 or 229E CoV). Hayes (2000) showed that sequential dual infections of pigs with the arterivirus (order Nidovirales, like CoV) PRRSV followed in 10 days by PRCV significantly enhanced lung lesions and reduced weight gains compared to each virus alone. The dual infections also led to more pigs shedding PRCV nasally for a prolonged period and surprisingly, to fecal shedding of PRCV. The lung lesions observed resembled those in SARS victims (Nicholls et al., 2003).

In another study, Van Reeth and Pensaert (1994) inoculated pigs with PRCV followed in 2 to 3 days by swine influenza A virus (SIV). They found that SIV lung titers were reduced in the dually compared to the singly infected pigs, but paradoxically the lung lesions were more severe in the dually infected pigs. They postulated that the high levels of IFN-alpha induced by PRCV may mediate interference with SIV replication but may also contribute to the enhanced lung lesions. Such studies are highly relevant to potential dual infections with SARS CoV and influenza virus and potential treatments of SARS patients with IFN alpha.

## Impact of Route (Aerosols) and Dose on CoV Infections

Experimental inoculation of pigs with PRCV strains showed that administration of PRCV by aerosol compared to the oronasal route, or in higher doses, resulted in higher virus titers shed and longer shedding (Van Cott et al., 1993). In other studies, high PRCV doses induced more severe respiratory disease. Pigs given $10^{8.5}$ TCID$_{50}$ of PRCV had more severe pneumonia and deaths than pigs exposed by contact (Jabrane et al., 1994), and higher intranasal doses of another PRCV strain (AR310) induced moderate respiratory disease whereas lower doses produced subclinical infections (Halbur et al., 1993). By analogy, hospital procedures that could potentially generate aerosols or exposure to higher initial doses of SARS CoV may enhance SARS transmission or lead to enhanced respiratory disease (Kamps and Hoffman, 2003a,b).

## Impact of Treatment with Corticosteroids on CoV Infections of Animals

Corticosteroids are known to induce immunosuppression and reduce the numbers of CD4 and CD8 T cells and certain cytokine levels (Giomarelli et al., 2003). Many hospitalized SARS patients were treated with steroids to reduce lung inflammation, but there are no data to assess the outcome of this treatment on virus shedding or respiratory disease. A recrudescence of BCoV fecal shedding was observed in one of four winter dysentery BCoV infected cows treated with dexamethasone (Tsunemitsu et al., 1999). Similarly, treatment of older pigs with dexamethasone prior to TGEV challenge led to profuse diarrhea and reduced lymphoproliferative responses in the treated pigs (Shimizu and Shimizu, 1979). These data raise issues for corticosteroid treatment of SARS patients related to possible transient immunosuppression leading to enhanced respiratory disease or increased and prolonged CoV shedding (superspreaders). Alternatively, corticosteroid treatment may be beneficial in reducing proinflammatory cytokines if found to play a major role in lung immunopathology (Giomarelli et al., 2003).

## Group I Feline CoV (FCoV): Model for Systemic and Persistent CoV Infection

The spectrum of disease evident for FCoV (feline infectious peritonitis virus) exemplifies the impact of viral persistence and macrophage tropism on CoV disease progression and severity. Historically, two types of FCoVs have been recognized: feline enteric CoV (FECoV) and FIPV. Current information suggests that the FECoV that causes acute enteric infections in cats establishes persistent infections in some cats, evolving into the systemic virulent FIPV in 5 to 10 percent of cats (deGroot and Horzinek, 1995; Herrewegh et al., 1997; Vennema et al., 1995). The relevance of this model to SARS is whether similar persistent CoV infections might occur in some patients, leading to the emergence of macrophage-tropic mutants of enhanced virulence and precipitating systemic or immune-mediated disease. The initial site of FCoV replication is in the pharyngeal, respiratory, or intestinal epithelial cells (deGroot and Horzinek, 1995; Olsen, 1993), and clinical signs include anorexia, lethargy, and mild diarrhea. The prolonged incubation period for FIPV and its reactivation upon exposure to immunosuppressive viruses or corticosteroids suggested that FCoVs could cause chronic enteric infections in cats (deGroot and Horzinek, 1995; Olsen, 1993). Recent reports of chronic fecal shedding and persistence of FCoV mRNA or antigen in infected cats confirm this scenario (Herrewegh et al., 1997).

A key pathogenetic event for development of FIPV is productive infection of macrophages followed by cell-associated viremia and systemic dissemination of virus (deGroot and Horzinek, 1995; Olsen, 1993). Stress (immunosuppressive infections, transport to new environments, cat density) leading to immune suppression may trigger FIP in chronically infected cats, similar to its role in shipping fever CoV infections of cattle. Two major forms of FIP occur: (1) effusive, with a fulminant course and death within weeks to months, and (2) noneffusive, progressing more slowly (deGroot and Horzinek, 1995; Olsen, 1993). The effusive form is characterized by fibrin-rich fluid accumulation in peritoneal, pleural, pericardial, or renal spaces, with fever, anorexia, and weight loss. Noneffusive FIP involves pyogranulomatous lesions with thrombosis, central nervous system, or ocular involvement. Fulminant FIP with accelerated early deaths appears to be immune mediated in FCoV seropositive cats. At least two mechanisms implicating IgG antibodies to FCoV S protein in FIP immunopathogenesis have been described. In the first, circulating immune complexes (IC) with C' depletion in sera and IC in lesions are evident in cats with terminal FIP (deGroot and Horzinek, 1995). In the second, antibody dependent enhancement (ADE) of FCoV infection of macrophages in vitro is mediated by neutralizing IgG MAbs to the S protein of

FIPV, or of interest, to the antigenically-related CoV, TGEV (Olsen et al., 1993). Similar accelerated disease was seen in vivo in cats inoculated with recombinant vaccinia virus expressing the S protein (but not the M or N proteins) of FIPV (deGroot and Horzinek, 1995; Olsen et al., 1993). Thus the FIPV model provides a frightening glimpse of the severity and potential complications associated with a persistent, systemic CoV infection.

*Group III CoVs: Infectious Bronchitis Virus (IBV): Model for Respiratory CoV Infection with Other Target Tissues*

The IBV is a highly contagious respiratory disease of chickens, like SARS, spread by aerosol or possibly fecal-oral transmission, and distributed worldwide (Cavanagh and Naqi, 2003; Cook and Mockett, 1995). Genetically and antigenically closely related CoV have been isolated from pheasants and turkeys (Guy et al., 1997; Ismail et al., 2001a), but in young turkeys, they cause mainly enteritis. Respiratory infections of chickens are characterized by tracheal rales, coughing, and sneezing, with the disease most severe in chicks (Cavanagh and Naqi, 2003; Cook and Mockett, 1995). The IBV also replicates in the oviduct, causing decreased egg production. Nephropathogenic strains can cause mortality in young birds. In broilers, severe disease or death ensues from systemic *E. coli* co-infections after IBV damage to the respiratory tract or *Mycoplasma* sp. co-infections with IBV. The IBV is recovered intermittently from the respiratory tract for about 28 days after infection and from the feces after clinical recovery, with the cecal tonsil being a possible reservoir for IBV persistence, similar to the persistence of FCoV in the intestine of cats (Herrewegh et al., 1997). The IBV was recovered from both tracheal and cloacal swabs in chickens at onset of egg production, suggesting re-excretion of IBV from chronically infected birds, as also demonstrated for fecal shedding of FCoV or BCoV after induction of immunosuppression (Olsen, 1993; Tsunemitsu et al., 1999).

The IBV replicates in epithelial cells of the trachea and bronchi, intestinal tract, oviduct, and kidney, causing necrosis and edema with small areas of pneumonia near large bronchi in the respiratory tract and interstitial nephritis in the kidney (Cavanagh and Naqi, 2003; Cook and Mockett, 1995). Of interest for SARS is the persistence of IBV in the kidney and its prolonged fecal shedding because SARS CoV is detected in urine and shed longer term in feces. However, it is unclear if SARS CoV shedding in urine is a consequence of viremia or a kidney infection like IBV. Both diagnosis and control of IBV are complicated by the existence of multiple serotypes and the occurrence of IBV recombinants (Cavanagh and Naqi, 2003; Cook and Mockett, 1995). This is unlike the scenario for most group 1 or 2 respiratory CoVs in which only one or two (FCoV) serotypes are known. Also relevant to SARS CoV is the finding that IBV strains also replicate in Vero cells, but only after passage in chicken embryo kidney cells (Cavanagh and Nagi, 2003).

In summary, studies of animal CoV infections in the natural host provide enteric and respiratory disease models that enhance our understanding of both the similarities and divergence of CoV disease pathogenesis and targets for control. Unanswered questions for SARS pathogenesis, but highly relevant to the design of strategies for prevention and control, include the following: What is the initial site of viral replication? Is SARS CoV pneumoenteric like BCoV, with variable degrees of infection of the intestinal and respiratory tracts and disease precipitated by the co-factors discussed or unknown variables? Alternatively, is SARS primarily targeted to the lung like PRCV, with fecal shedding of swallowed virus and with undefined sequelae contributing to the diarrhea cases? Does SARS CoV infect the lung directly or via viremia after initial replication in another site (oral cavity, tonsils, upper respiratory tract) and does it productively infect secondary target organs (intestine, kidney) via viremia after replication in the lung?

Finally, the persistent, macrophage tropic, systemic FIPV CoV infection of cats presents yet another CoV disease model and a dilemma for attempted control strategies. In this disease scenario, induction of neutralizing IgG antibodies to the FIPV S protein not only fails to prevent FIPV infections, but actually potentiates the immunopathogenesis of FIPV (Olsen, 1993).

The suspected zoonotic origin of SARS CoV (Guan et al., 2003) and the recognized propensity of several CoV to cross species barriers illustrate the need for additional animal studies of the mechanisms of interspecies transmission of CoVs and adaptation to new hosts. The possible animal reservoir for SARS remains undefined. At present we understand very little about CoVs or other viruses circulating in wildlife or their potential to emerge or recombine with existing CoVs (Stavrinides and Guttman, 2004) as public or animal health threats. Hopefully the SARS epidemic will generate new interest and funding for these fundamental research questions applicable not only to SARS CoV, but also to the estimated 75 percent of newly emerging human diseases arising as zoonoses (Taylor, 2001).

## CORONAVIRUS RESEARCH: KEYS TO DIAGNOSIS, TREATMENT, AND PREVENTION OF SARS

*Mark R. Denison, M.D.*
Department of Pediatrics, Department of Microbiology & Immunology, Elizabeth B. Lamb Center for Pediatric Research, Vanderbilt University Medical Center, Nashville, TN

For coronavirus investigators, the recognition of a new coronavirus as the cause of severe acute respiratory syndrome (SARS) was certainly remarkable, yet perhaps not surprising (Baric et al., 1995). The cadre of investigators who have worked with this intriguing family of viruses over the past 30 years are familiar with many of the features of coronavirus biology, pathogenesis, and disease that manifested so dramatically in the worldwide SARS epidemic. Advances in the biology of coronaviruses have resulted in greater understanding of their capacity for adaptation to new environments, transspecies infection, and emergence of new diseases. New tools of cell and molecular biology have led to increased understanding of intracellular replication and viral cell biology, and the advent in the past five years of reverse genetic approaches to study coronaviruses has made it possible to begin to define the determinants of viral replication, transspecies adaptation, and human disease. This summary will discuss the basic life cycle and replication of the well-studied coronavirus, mouse hepatitis virus (MHV), identifying the unique characteristics of coronavirus biology and highlighting critical points where research has made significant advances, and which might represent targets for antivirals or vaccines. Areas where rapid progress has been made in SCoV research will be described. Finally, areas of need for research in coronavirus replication, genetics, and pathogenesis will be summarized.

## Coronavirus Life Cycle

The best studied model for coronavirus replication and pathogenesis has been the group 2 murine coronavirus, mouse hepatitis virus, and much of what is known of the stages of the coronavirus life cycle has been determined in animals and in culture using this virus. Thus this discussion will focus on MHV with comparisons to SCoV and other coronaviruses. This is appropriate because bioinformatics analyses suggest that SCoV, while a distinct virus, has significant similarities in organization, putative protein functions, and replication to the group II coronaviruses, particularly within the replicase gene (Snijder et al., 2003). Excellent, detailed reviews of MHV and coronavirus replication are available elsewhere (Holmes and Lai, 1996; Lai and Cavanagh, 1997).

The coronavirus virion is an enveloped particle containing the spike (S), membrane (M), and envelope (E) proteins. In addition, some strains of coronaviruses, but not SCoV, express a hemagglutinin protein (HE) that is also incorporated in the virion. The genome of coronaviruses is a linear, single-stranded RNA molecule of positive (mRNA) polarity, and from 28 to 32 kb in length (Bonilla et al., 1994; Drosten et al., 2003; Lee et al., 1991). Within the virion, the genome is encapsidated by multiple copies of the nucleocapsid protein (N), and has the conformation of a helical RNA/nucleocapsid structure. The S protein has been a focus of pathogenesis studies in mice because it appears to be the critical determinant of cell tropism, species specificity, host selection, cell tropism, and disease (Navas and Weiss, 2003; Navas et al., 2001; Rao and Gallagher, 1998).

Virus replication is initiated by binding of the S protein to specific receptors on the host cell surface. For MHV, the primary receptor has been shown to be the carcino-embryonic antigen–cell adhesion molecule (CEACAM) (Dveksler et al., 1991; 1996; Holmes and Lai, 1996; Yokomuri and Lai, 1992), and for the human coronavirus, HCoV-229E, and other group 1 coronaviruses, the receptor is aminopeptidase N (Yeager et al., 1992). The precise mechanisms of entry and uncoating have yet to be defined, but likely occur by either fusion from without or viroplexis through endocytic vesicles. For wildtype MHV, entry and uncoating constitute a pH independent process that is probably direct fusion mediated by a fusion peptide in the S protein (Gallagher et al., 1991). The understanding of the region of the S1 component of coronavirus that binds to receptors was the basis for studies leading to the very recent and very rapid identification of angiotensin converting enzyme 2 (ACE 2) as a receptor for SCoV (Li et al., 2003).

The next discrete stage in the life cycle is translation and proteolytic processing of viral replicase proteins from the input genome RNA, followed by formation of cytoplasmic replication complexes in association with cellular membranes (Denison et al., 1999; Gosert et al., 2002; Shi et al., 1999; van der Meer et al., 1999). Replication complexes are thought to be sites of all stages of viral RNA transcription and replication, and possibly assembly of nascent viral nucleocapsids. Viral assembly occurs both temporally and physically distinct from viral replication complexes in the endoplasmic-reticulum-Golgi-intermediate compartment (ERGIC), a transitional zone between late ER and Golgi (deVries et al., 1997; Klumperman et al., 1994; Krijnse-Locker et al., 1994; Rottier and Rose, 1987). Although the mechanisms by which replication products are delivered to sites of assembly remain to be determined, it has been shown that subpopulations of replicase proteins and the structural nucleocapsid (N) translocate from replication complexes to sites of assembly and may mediate the process in association with cellular membrane/protein trafficking pathways (Bost et al., 2000). Virus assembly in the ERGIC involves interactions of genome RNA, N, the membrane protein (M), and the small membrane protein (E), resulting in budding of virions into the lumen of ER/Golgi virosomes (Opstetten et al., 1995). Further maturation of virus particles occurs during movement through the Golgi, resulting in virosomes filled with mature particles (Salamuera et al., 1999). Trafficking of the virosomes to the cell surface has not been well characterized, but is presumed to occur via normal vesicle maturation and exocytic processes. The outcome is the nonlytic release of the vast majority of mature virions into the extracellular space. For MHV and several other coronaviruses that can directly fuse with cells, there is a characteristic and rapidly detectable cytopathic effect of cell-cell fusion into multinucleated syncytia. Production of infectious virus continues even after the majority of cells are fused. Syncytia were recently reported as a readout of SCoV receptor expression and cell infection (Li et al., 2003).

## Viral Replication Complex Formation and Function

Following entry and uncoating, the 5′ most replicase gene of the input positive strand RNA genome is translated into two co-amino terminal replicase polyproteins that are co- and post-translationally processed by viral proteinases to yield 15 to 16 mature replicase proteins, as well as intermediate precursors. The nascent replicase polyproteins and intermediate precursors likely mediate the formation of viral replication complexes in the host cell cytoplasm. Interestingly, coronavirus replication requires continuous replicase gene translation and processing throughout the life cycle to maintain productive infection (Kim et al., 1995; Perlman et al., 1987; Sawicki and Sawicki, 1986). Replication complexes of MHV are associated with double-membrane vesicles (Gosert et al., 2002), and all tested MHV replicase proteins have been shown to colocalize to replication complexes at the earliest time of detection, likely both by membrane integration and by protein-protein and protein-RNA interactions (Bost et al., 2000; Denison et al., 1999; Prentice and Denison, in press; Shi et al., 1999; Sims et al., 2000; van der Meer et al., 1999). Further, replicase proteins likely mediate the process of double-membrane vesicle formation, likely by induction of cellular autophagy pathways (E. Prentice, unpublished results).

Coronavirus replication complexes are sites for replicase gene translation and replicase polyprotein processing, and also for viral RNA synthesis. Replicase gene proteins likely mediate positive-strand, negative-strand, subgenomic, and genomic RNA synthesis, as well as processes of capping, polyadenylation, RNA unwinding, template switching during viral RNA synthesis, and discontinuous transcription and transcription attenuation. The coronavirus replicase polyproteins and mature replicase proteins represent the largest and most diverse repertoire of known and predicted distinct enzymatic functions of any positive-strand RNA virus family. Until recently, of the 15 or more mature replicase proteins, only the proteinase, RNA helicase, and RNA-dependent RNA polymerase activities had been predicted or experimentally confirmed (Brockway et al., 2003; Heusipp et al., 1997; Lee et al., 1991; Ziebuhr et al., 2000). With the advent of SARS, more extensive bioinformatics analyses have resulted in predictions of several additional functions involved in RNA processing, including methyltransferase and exonuclease activities (Snijder et al., 2003; Thiel et al., 2003). Even with inclusion of distant predicted relationships, up to eight of the replicase proteins remain without predicted or confirmed functions. In summary, it is likely that coronaviruses have exploited their genetic capacity to encode proteins in the replicase gene with distinct functions in RNA synthesis and processing, as well as proteins with specific roles in induction or modification in host cellular membrane biogenesis and trafficking, delivery of replication products to sites of assembly, and possibly virus assembly. Thus replicase translation, replicase polyprotein processing, and mature replicase proteins constitute important targets for interference with coronavirus replication, virus-cell interactions, or viral pathology.

## Coronavirus Replicase Protein Expression and Processing

The proteinase activities for all coronaviruses include both papain-like proteinase (PLP) and picornavirus 3C-like proteinase activities that are encoded within the replicase polyproteins and mediate both cis and trans cleavage events (Ziebuhr et al., 2000). Because of the parallel evolution of the proteinases, their cleavage sites, and the hierarchical cleavage processes, the proteolytic processing of the coronavirus replicase proteins may serve as distinct regulatory and genetic elements (Ziebuhr et al., 2001). Specifically, there are both conserved and divergent regions of the replicase polyproteins by amino acid identity and similarity, with the sequences and predicted mature proteins beginning with the 3C-like proteinases through the carboxy terminus of the replicase polyprotein retaining higher identity and similarity across the predicted proteins. In contrast, the amino-terminal third of the replicase demonstrates the most variation in proteins, cleavage site locations, and the number of proteinases that mediate maturation processing. SCoV appears to have the general organization of, and similar protein sizes to, the group 2 coronaviruses such as MHV in this part of the genome (Snijder et al., 2003). However, SCoV likely uses only one PLP to mediate the cleavages, similar to the group 3 coronavirus infectious bronchitis virus (IBV). Thus this region of the replicase may experience the most variability, suggesting either the encoding of accessory functions that are flexible and tolerant of changes, or conversely group or host-specific roles that are subject to pressure for more rapid change.

## Expression of Structural and Accessory Genes

Only the 5' most replicase gene is translated from the input positive-strand genome RNA. The genome contains multiple other genes for the known structural proteins S, E, M, and N, as well as other genes for expression of proteins that have been labeled as "nonstructural" or "accessory" because they have been presumed to not be required for replication, and are not thought to be incorporated into virions. MHV encodes six of these genes, while SCoV encodes possibly up to 11 structural and accessory genes, which are expressed from subgenomic mRNAs (Snijder et al., 2003). Subgenomic RNA transcription occurs during minus-strand RNA synthesis by acquisition of the antileader RNA sequences from the 5' end of the genome via homology to a transcriptional regulatory sequence (TRS, also known as an intergenic sequence), and requiring a discontinuous activity of the nascent minus-strand template and polymerase complex to acquire the leader (Sawicki and Sawicki, 1998). The outcome of transcription is the generation of a "nested set" of subgenomic negative-strand RNAs that all contain the antileader sequences that serve as templates for similar size subgenomic mRNAs. This transcriptional strategy exposes different genes as the 5' ORF in different mRNAs, all of which also contain the 3' sequence downstream of the gene, including the 3' nontranslated region of the genome.

For MHV, genes 3, 5b, 6, and 7 encode S, E, M, and N, respectively. Genes 2, 4, and 5a are not required for replication in culture, and have been mutated to block expression, deleted, or substituted with noncoronavirus genes such as GFP (de Haan et al., 2002; Ortego et al., 2003; Sarma et al., 2002). Because all coronaviruses retain these genes in various combinations in the face of presumed pressure for genetic economy and apparent lack of functions in RNA synthesis, it is presumed that these genes serve roles in modification of host cells, pathogenesis, or interactions with the immune system. SCoV encodes a larger and more complex array of these genes than MHV or other coronaviruses, which may reflect its evolution in its original animal host (Ksiazek et al., 2003; Marra et al., 2003; Snijder et al., 2003; Thiel et al., 2003). In addition, the report of a deletion within one of the accessory genes in human isolates of SCoV suggests that this may be a gene involved in host range or adaptation for replication and transmission in humans (Guan et al., 2003).

## Coronavirus Genetics

Until recently, the genetics of coronavirus replication and pathogenesis have largely been studied using natural variants, host range mutants, passaged virus, and mutagenized viruses selected for temperature sensitivity and specific phenotypes. Classical complementation of functions made it possible to define at least eight genetic groups for MHV, with most of the complementation groups localized to the replicase gene (Stalcup et al., 1998). Taking advantage of naturally high rates of homologous RNA-RNA recombination and of host range determinants in the S protein, the development of targeted recombination has allowed more defined and detailed studies of the accessory and structural genes of MHV, transmissible gastroenteritis virus (TGEV), and feline infectious peritonitis virus (FIPV) (Haijema et al., 2003; Kuo et al., 2000; Masters et al., 1994). Studies with natural variants and targeted recombination genetic studies have demonstrated that the S protein is the major determinant of host range, tropism, and pathogenesis; other genetic elements, possibly in the replicase, may influence these characteristics of different coronaviruses (Navas and Weiss, 2003). The capacity of coronaviruses to change host range, transmission, pathogenesis, and disease has been established in the laboratory using cell adaptation and virus passage (Baric et al., 1997, 1999; Chen and Baric, 1995, 1996), and has been demonstrated in nature by natural variants of MHV, TGEV, and bovine coronavirus (BCoV), as well as by studies using heterologous viruses such as canine coronavirus (CcoV) to immunize cats against FIPV (Enjuanes et al., 1995; Tresnan et al., 1996). Further, targeted recombination studies have confirmed the genetic flexibility of the coronavirus genome and the ability of coronaviruses to recover wild-type replication following deletions, mutations, substitutions, and gene order rearrangements in the structural and accessory genes (de Haan et al., 2002).

Challenges for genetic studies using natural variants and mutants, particularly in defining the precise changes responsible for altered phenotypes, has limited progress in genetic studies. Targeted recombination, while a robust system with powerful selection, has been limited to studies of the 3′ 10 kb of the MHV genome, and is limited to selection of viable recombinants. Recently, the establishment of "infectious clone" reverse genetic strategies for the coronaviruses TGEV (Transmissible Gastroenteritis Coronavirus), HCoV-229E, IBV, and MHV has made it theoretically possible to study the genetics of the entire genome and all of the structural, accessory, and replicase genes. Approaches to "infectious cloning" have included full-length cDNA clones of TGEV genome in bacterial artificial chromosomes (Gonzalez et al., 2001), recombinant vaccinia viruses containing full-length cDNA clones of HCoV-229E and IBV genomes (Casais et al., 2001; Thiel et al., 2001), and in vitro assembly strategies for TGEV, MHV, and most recently, SCoV (Yount, 2000; Yount et al., 2002, 2003).

The in vitro assembly approach was developed to overcome the challenge of full-length cDNA cloning of the TGEV and MHV genomes, which contained "toxic" regions in the replicase gene, resulting in unstable or toxic clones in *E. coli* (Yount, 2000; Yount et al., 2002). Subcloning of the regions required splitting the toxic domains into separate clones. The result of this strategy was the cloning of the MHV genome into seven fragments (A through G). To recover viable virus, the following strategy is pursued: (1) cloned cDNA fragments are excised from plasmid using class 2 restriction enzymes that remove the recognition site and leave overhanging genomic sequence; (2) excised fragments are ligated (assembled) in vitro; (3) transcription of full-length genomic RNA is driven in vitro using a T7 promoter on the 5′ fragment A; (4) full-length genome RNA is electroporated into competent cells that are then plated on a monolayer of naturally permissive cells; and (5) cells are monitored for cytopathic effect or plaques, and virus is recovered from plaques or media supernatant.

In vitro assembly has many advantages for genetic studies of such a large and complex genome RNA. First, genetic changes can be introduced and confirmed in stable small fragments without the need for a ~30kb genomic clone. Second, the cloned fragments make it possible to develop libraries of mutations that can rapidly be tested in different combinations. Furthermore, identification of putative second-site reversion mutations for deleterious introduced changes can be introduced with the original mutation to confirm their reversion potential. In combination with biochemical and cell imaging approaches, it also is possible to study highly defective or lethal mutations in electroporated cells, in order to define critical determinants of replication. The in vitro assembly approach has been used to introduce marker mutations that are silent for replication in culture (Yount et al., 2003). In addition, we have engineered mutations in the MHV replicase gene to define the requirements for polyprotein processing and to determine the role of specific replicase proteins in replication in culture and in pathogenesis in animals. Using this approach we have recovered viruses with mutations at polyprotein cleavage sites and proteinase catalytic residues, all of which have distinct phenotypes in protein processing, viral growth, and viral RNA synthesis (unpublished results). Thus, direct reverse genetic studies of the critical replicase gene functions can be performed using in vitro assembly of infectious clones.

## Advances in SCoV Research

The rapid progress in the identification and characterization of SCoV as the etiologic agent of SARS was made possible by the fact that the virus grows well in culture, and by the foundational research in coronaviruses that has been supported by the National Institutes of Health, the Multiple Sclerosis Foundation, the U.S. Department of Agriculture, and other organizations over the past two decades. The application of knowledge concerning virus structure, genetics, receptor binding, virus entry, and viral pathogenesis has made it possible to target the spike protein for studies of SCoV replication, pathogenesis, and immune response (Xiao et al., 2003). The remarkably rapid identification of ACE 2 as a receptor for SARS has demonstrated the foundational importance of studies of other coronaviruses (Li et al., 2003). Similarly, understanding of replicase gene expression, processing, and predicted functions has identified possible targets for structure/function studies and possible therapeutic intervention. The studies of coronavirus proteinase activities, cleavage site, and structures were the basis for studies leading to the rapid determination of SCoV replicase polyprotein cleavage sites and 3CLpro crystal structure (Anand et al., 2003; Campanacci et al., 2003; Snijder et al., 2003; Thiel et al., 2003).

## Application of Reverse Genetics to Studies of SCoV

Because of the potential for reemergence of SARS, it is important to move forward with research in diagnostics, vaccines, and therapeutics for SCoV. Experience with the development and use of reverse genetics to study other coronaviruses resulted in establishment of reverse genetics for SCoV within months of the onset of the worldwide epidemic (Yount et al., 2003). How should the understanding of other coronaviruses, the rapid advances in research with SCoV, and the development of reverse genetics for SCoV be harnesssed to achieve these goals and attack these critical questions in SCoV replication, pathogenesis, and disease? Certainly, the use of SCoV reverse genetics, along with robust tissue culture systems and emerging animal models, creates the potential to rapidly answer questions concerning: (1) determinants of virus growth in culture; (2) potential mechanisms of transpecies adaptation; (3) sensitivity to and escape from biochemical and immune interference with replication; (4) determinants of virulence and pathogenesis; (5) mechanisms of genome recombination and mutation; (6) functions of and requirements for replicase, structural, and accessory proteins; and (7) development of stably attenuated viruses for use as seed stocks for inactivated vaccine or testing as live-attenuated vaccines.

How then should these critical issues be investigated while recognizing the potential of SCoV to cause severe disease, as well as the potential for rapid spread? First, there is significant experience with other coronaviruses in attenuation of virus replication and pathogenesis, both using virus passage and by direct engineering of changes. Although coronavirus genome organization, proteins, and replication appear more tolerant of changes then previously thought, all changes of gene order, gene deletion, insertion, or mutagenesis so far reported have led to viruses impaired in replication, pathogenesis, or both. Many of the attenuating changes in MHV and other coronaviruses are conserved in SCoV and thus could be tested for likely attenuation in SCoV culture and animal models. Second, where there is clear conservation of sequences, motifs, proteins, or putative functions between SCoV and model viruses such as MHV, new or untested changes might be most rapidly analyzed under BSL2 conditions in those model viruses, and then directly applied to SARS once their phenotypes are determined. Third, all work with SCoV will be performed only under BSL3 conditions. This would also apply to chimeric viruses, whether engineered by introduction into the SCoV background, or by introducing SCoV proteins or sequences with known or predicted pathogenic consequences into other coronavirus backgrounds. Finally, it is important to develop strains of SCoV that are attenuated and stabilized against reversion and recombination, to be used as the basis for studies of other replication and pathogenesis determinants and construction of virus chimeras. Such attenuated variants would provide additional safeguards while allowing application of powerful genetic tools to the study of SCoV emergence, biology, disease, treatment, and prevention. Overall, newly invigorated programs in other human and animal coronaviruses, combined with the new research in SCoV, will shed important new light on this important virus family and perhaps lead to better understanding of the potential for resurgence of SCoV or the emergence of other coronaviruses into human populations.

## ISOLATION AND CHARACTERIZATION OF VIRUSES RELATED TO THE SARS CORONAVIRUS FROM ANIMALS IN SOUTHERN CHINA

*Y. Guan,*[1] *B. J. Zheng,*[1] *Y. Q. He,*[2] *X. L. Liu,*[2] *Z. X. Zhuang,*[2] *C. L. Cheung,*[1] *S. W. Luo,*[1] *P. H. Li,*[1] *L. J. Zhang,*[1] *Y. J. Guan,*[1] *K. M. Butt,*[1] *K. L. Wong,*[1] *K. W. Chan,*[3] *W. Lim,*[4] *K. F. Shortridge,*[1] *K. Y. Yuen,*[1] *J. S. M. Peiris,*[1] *and L. L. M. Poon*[1,5]
Reprinted with permission from Guan et al., 2003. Copyright 2003 AAAS.

A novel coronavirus (SCoV) is the etiological agent of severe acute respiratory syndrome (SARS). SCoV-like viruses were isolated from Himalayan palm civets

[1]Department of Microbiology, The University of Hong Kong, University Pathology Building, Queen Mary Hospital, Hong Kong Special Administrative Region (S.A.R.), of the People's Republic of China (China).

[2]Center for Disease Control and Prevention, Shenzhen, Guangdong Province, China.

[3]Department of Pathology, The University of Hong Kong, University Pathology Building, Queen Mary Hospital, Hong Kong S.A.R., China.

[4]Government Virus Unit, Department of Health, Hong Kong S.A.R., China.

[5]We thank the Department of Health and Department of Agriculture of Shenzhen Government for facilitating the study. We gratefully acknowledge the encouragement and support of L.C. Tsui, Vice-Chancellor, The University of Hong Kong. We thank X.Y. Zhao from the Department of Microbiol-

found in a live-animal market in Guangdong, China. Evidence of virus infection was also detected in other animals (including a raccoon dog, *Nyctereutes procyonoides*) and in humans working at the same market. All the animal isolates retain a 29-nucleotide sequence that is not found in most human isolates. The detection of SCoV-like viruses in small, live wild mammals in a retail market indicates a route of interspecies transmission, although the natural reservoir is not known.

Severe acute respiratory syndrome (SARS) recently emerged as a human disease associated with pneumonia (WHO, 2003c). This disease was first recognized in Guangdong Province, China, in November 2002. Subsequent to its introduction to Hong Kong in mid-February 2003, the virus spread to more than 30 countries and caused disease in more than 7900 patients across five continents (WHO, 2003d). A novel coronavirus (SCoV) was identified as the etiological agent of SARS (Ksiazek et al., 2003; Peiris et al., 2003a), and the virus causes a similar disease in cynomolgous macaques (Fouchier et al., 2003). Human SCoV appears to be an animal virus that crossed to humans relatively recently. Thus, identifying animals carrying the virus is of major scientific interest and public health importance. This prompted us to examine a range of domestic and wild mammals in Guangdong Province.

Because the early cases of SARS in Guangdong reportedly occurred in restaurant workers handling wild mammals as exotic food (Zhong et al., 2003), our attention focused on wild animals recently captured and marketed for culinary purposes. We investigated a live-animal retail market in Shenzhen. Animals were held, one per cage, in small wire cages. The animals sampled included seven wild, and one domestic, animal species (see Table 3-2). They originated from different regions of southern China and had been kept in separate storehouses before arrival to the market. The animals remained in the markets for a variable period of time, and each stall holder had only a few animals of a given species. Animals from different stalls within the market were sampled. Nasal and fecal samples were collected with swabs and stored in medium 199 with bovine serum albumin and antibiotics. Where possible, blood samples were collected for serology. Before sampling, all animals were examined by a veterinary surgeon and confirmed to be free of overt disease. Serum samples were also obtained, after informed consent, from traders in animals ($n = 35$) and vegetables ($n = 20$) within the market. Sera ($n = 60$) submitted for routine laboratory tests from patients

ogy, The University of Hong Kong, for the excellent technical assistance. We also thank C.C. Hon and F.C. Leung from the Department of Zoology, The University of Hong Kong, and Richard Webby from St. Jude Children's Research Hospital (Memphis, TN) for assistance in the phylogenetic analysis. We thank K.V. Holmes' laboratory from the Department of Microbiology, University of Colorado Health Sciences Center (Denver, CO) for validating the animal viral sequences. Supported by research funding from Public Health Research (Grant A195357), the U.S. National Institute of Allergy and Infectious Diseases, the Wellcome Trust (067072/D/02/Z), and SARS research funds from The University of Hong Kong.

**TABLE 3-2** Animal Species Tested for Coronavirus Detection

| Sample number | Animal | RT-PCR | | Isolation | | Titer to SZ16 |
|---|---|---|---|---|---|---|
| | | N | F | N | F | |
| SZ1 | HPC | +* | + | | | ND |
| SZ2 | HPC | + | + | | | 40 |
| SZ3 | HPC | + | + | +* | | 40 |
| SZ4 | HB | | | | | <20 |
| SZ5 | B | | | | | <20 |
| SZ6 | DC | | | | | ND |
| SZ7 | DC | | | | | <20 |
| SZ8 | CH | | | | | ND |
| SZ9 | CH | | | | | <20 |
| SZ10 | CM | | | | | <20 |
| SZ11 | CFB | | | | | 160 |
| SZ12 | CFB | | | | | <20 |
| SZ13 | RD | | + | | +* | 640 |
| SZ14 | CM | | | | | <20 |
| SZ15 | B | | | | | <20 |
| SZ16 | HPC | + | + | +* | + | <20 |
| SZ17 | HPC | | | + | | <20 |
| SZ18 | B | | | | | 640 |
| SZ19 | CH | | | | | <20 |
| SZ20 | CH | | | | | <20 |
| SZ21 | DC | | | | | <20 |
| SZ22 | DC | | | | | <20 |
| SZ23 | HB | | | | | ND |
| SZ24 | HB | | | | | ND |
| SZ25 | HPC | | | | + | ND |

NOTE: Abbreviations of animal species: B = beaver (*Castor fiber*); CFB = Chinese ferret-badger (*Melogale moschata*); CH = Chinese hare (*Lepus sinensis*); CM = Chinese muntjac (*Muntiacus reevesi*); DC = domestic cat (*Felis catus*); HB = hog-badger (*Arctonyx collaris*); HPC = Himalayan palm civet (*P. larvata*); RD = raccoon dog (*N. procyonoides*) (China species information system, 2003); N = nasal sample; F = fecal sample; titer to SZ16, neutralizing antibody titer to SZ16; + denotes positive by RT-PCR or virus isolation; *denotes the PCR product or virus isolates sequenced in the study; ND = not done.

hospitalized for nonrespiratory disease in Guangdong were made anonymous and used for comparison.

Nasal and fecal swabs from 25 animals were tested for SCoV viral nucleic acid by using reverse transcription–polymerase chain reaction (RT-PCR) for the N gene of the human SCoV. Swabs from four of six Himalayan palm civets were positive in the RT-PCR assay (see Table 3-2). All specimens were inoculated into FRhK-4 cells as previously described for virus isolation (Peiris et al., 2003a). A cytopathic effect was observed in cells inoculated with specimens from four Himalayan palm civets (*Paguma larvata*), two of which also positive for coronavirus in the original specimen by RT-PCR. A virus was also detected by virus isolation and direct RT-PCR from the fecal swab of a raccoon dog (*Nyctereutes procyonoides*). No virus was detectable in six other species sampled. Electron microscopy of one infected cell supernatant (SZ16) showed viral particles with a morphology compatible with coronavirus (see Figure S-1)[6]. Sera from five animals had neutralizing antibody to the animal coronavirus; these were from three palm civets, a raccoon dog, and a Chinese ferret badger, respectively (see Table 3-2).

To further validate the results from the neutralization test, a Western blot assay was used to detect SCoV-specific antibodies from these animal serum samples (see Figure 3-1). Indications of positive antibodies were observed from samples SZ2, SZ3, SZ11, and SZ17 (which were also positive in the neutralization assay) and from the positive control human serum. No positive signal was observed from those serum samples that were negative in the neutralization test. There was insufficient serum left over from the raccoon dog (SZ13) to be analyzed by this assay.

Sera from humans working in the market were tested for antibody to SZ16 virus by neutralization and indirect immunofluorescence assays. Although 8 out of 20 (40 percent) of the wild-animal traders and 3 of 15 (20 percent) of those who slaughter these animals had evidence of antibody, only 1 (5 percent) of 20 vegetable traders was seropositive. None of these workers reported SARS-like symptoms in the past 6 months. In comparison, none of 60 control sera from patients admitted to a Guangdong hospital for nonrespiratory diseases was seropositive (see Table 3-3).

Two of the virus isolates (SZ3 and SZ16) isolated from the nasal swabs of palm civets were completely sequenced, and the amino acid sequence was deduced. Two other viruses were partially sequenced, from the S gene to the 3' end of the virus (GenBank accession numbers AY304486 to AY304489). Viral RNA sequences from these original swab samples from animal were confirmed in an independent laboratory (Holmes K., unpublished observations). The full-length genome sequences had 99.8 percent homology to the human SCoV, which indicates that the human and animal SCoV-like viruses were closely related. Phylogenetic analysis of the S gene of both human and animal SCoV-like viruses indicated that the animal viruses are separate from the human virus cluster (see Figure 3-2 and Figure S-2)[7]. However, the viruses SZ1, SZ3, and SZ16 from palm civets were phylogenetically distinct. The viruses SZ3 and SZ16 had 18 nucleotide differences between them over the 29,709–base pair (bp) genome, whereas the human SCoV isolated from five geographically separate sites (GZ50, CUHK-W1,

---

[6]Supporting online material, www.sciencemag.org/cgi/content/full/1087139/DC1, Materials and Methods, Figures S1 and S2, and References and Notes.

[7]Supporting online material, www.sciencemag.org/cgi/content/full/1087139/DC1, Materials and Methods, Figures S1 and S2, and References and Notes.

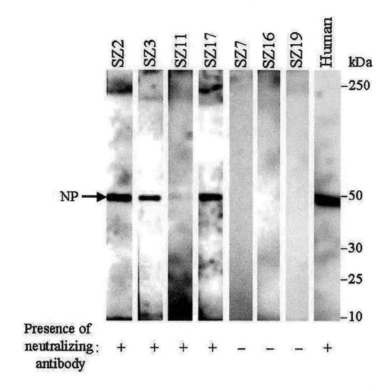

Presence of
neutralizing : + + + + – – – +
antibody

**FIGURE 3-1** Detection of antibodies against recombinant nucleocapsid protein of SCoV in animal sera by Western blot assay. Recombinant nuleocapsid protein (NP, 49.6 kD) was used as an antigen to detect anti-ScoV antibodies in animal sera. Protein A-HRP was used as a secondary antibody, and reactive bands were visualized by the enhanced chemiluminesence Western blotting system. A serum sample from a convalescent SARS patient was used as a positive control. Blots reacted with animal (SZ2, SZ3, SZ11, SZ17, SZ7, SZ16, or SZ19) or human sera are indicated. Results from the neutralization test for ScoV-specific antibodies in these serum samples are also shown.

**TABLE 3-3** Prevalence of Antibody to Animal SCoV SZ16 in Humans. Controls Are Serum Specimens from Patients Hospitalized for Nonrespiratory Diseases in Guangdong Made Anonymous

| Occupation | Sample numbers | Antibody positive (%) |
| --- | --- | --- |
| Wild-animal trader | 20 | 8 (40) |
| Slaughterer of animals | 15 | 3 (20) |
| Vegetable trader | 20 | 1 (5) |
| Control | 60 | 0 (0) |

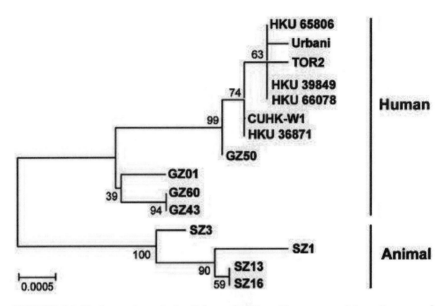

**FIGURE 3-2** Phylogenetic analysis of the nucleotide acid sequence of the spike gene of SCoV-like viruses. Nucleotide sequences of representative SCoV Sgenes (Sgene coding region 21477 to 25244, 3768 bp) were analyzed. The phylogenetic tree was constructed by the neighbor-joining method with bootstrap analysis (1000 replicates) using MEGA 2 (Kumar et al., 2001). Number at the nodes indicates bootstrap values in percentage. The scale bar shows genetic distance estimated using Kimura's two-parameter substitution model (Kimura, 1980). In addition to viruses sequenced in the present study, the other sequences used in the analysis could be found in GenBank with accession number: from AY304490 to AY304495, AY278741, AY278554 , AY278491, AY274119, and AY278489.

Tor-2, HKU-39848, and Urbani) differed by only 14 nucleotides (nt). Nevertheless, animal virus SZ13 (raccoon dog) and SZ16 (palm civet) were genetically almost identical, and transmission or contamination from one host to the other within the market cannot be excluded.

When the full genome of the animal ($n = 2$) and human ($n = 5$, see above) virus groups were compared, the most striking difference was that these human viruses have a 29-nt deletion (5'-CCTACTGGTTACCAACCTGAATG-GAATAT-3', residue 27869 to 27897) that is 246 nt upstream of the start codon of the N gene (see Figure 3-3). Of human SCoV sequences currently available in GenBank, there was only one (GZ01) with this additional 29-nt sequence. In addition to that, there were 43 to 57 nucleotide differences observed over the rest of the genome. Most of these differences were found in the S gene coding region. The existence of the additional 29-nt sequence in the animal viruses results in demolishing the open reading frames (ORFs) 10 and 11 (Marra et al., 2003) and merging these two ORFs into a new ORF encoding a putative protein of 122 amino acids (see Figure 3-3). This putative peptide has a high homology to the putative proteins encoded by ORF10 and ORF11. Because ORF11 does not have a typical transcription regulatory sequence for SCoV (Marra et al., 2003), the putative ORF11 reported by others may just be the direct result of the deletion of the 29-nt sequence. BLAST search of this peptide yields no significant match to any other known peptide. Further investigation is required to elucidate the biological significance of this finding.

When the S-gene sequences of the four animal viruses were compared with 11 human SCoV viruses, 38 nucleotide polymorphisms were noted, and 26 of them were nonsynonymous changes (see Table 3-4). The S genes among the four

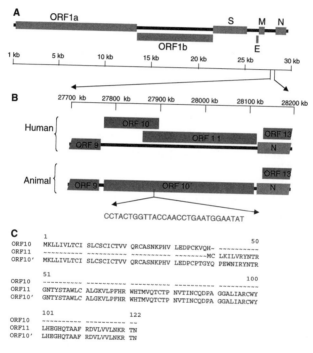

**FIGURE 3-3** A 29-nt deletion in the human SCoV genome. (A) Genetic organization of SCoV-like viruses found in humans and animals. ORFs 1a and 1b, encoding the nonstructural polyproteins, and those encoding the S, E, M, and N structural proteins are indicated (green boxes). (B) Expanded view of the SCoV genomic sequence (27700 nt to 28200 nt, based on AY278554 numbering). ORFs for putative proteins and for N in human isolates are indicated as brown and green boxes, respectively (Marra et al., 2003). An extra 29-nt sequence is present downstream of the nucleotide of 27868 of the animal SCoV (based on AY278554 numbering). The presence of this 29-nt sequence in animals isolates results in fusing the ORFs 10 and 11 (top) into a new ORF (bottom; ORF10', light blue box). (C) Protein sequence alignment of ORF10 and 11 from human isolates and ORF 10' from animal isolates.

**TABLE 3-4** Nucleotide Sequence Variation of the S Gene of Animal and Human SCoV

Nucleotide residue

| Virus | 2 1 6 2 | 2 1 6 0 | 2 1 7 0 | 2 1 7 9 | 2 1 9 0 | 2 1 9 2 | 2 2 0 5 | 2 2 4 0 | 2 2 5 7 | 2 2 9 5 | 2 2 9 7 | 2 3 0 2 | 2 3 0 7 | 2 3 1 3 | 2 3 2 7 | 2 3 3 7 | 2 3 3 6 | 2 3 5 8 | 2 3 6 8 | 2 3 7 8 | 2 3 8 6 | 2 3 8 7 | 2 3 8 8 | 2 3 9 7 | 2 3 9 7 | 2 4 1 3 | 2 4 1 5 | 2 4 3 6 | 2 4 4 7 | 2 4 5 8 | 2 4 5 7 | 2 4 6 3 | 2 4 8 2 | 2 4 9 1 | 2 4 4 3 | 2 5 0 2 |
|---|---|---|---|---|---|---|---|---|---|---|---|---|---|---|---|---|---|---|---|---|---|---|---|---|---|---|---|---|---|---|---|---|---|---|---|---|
| SZ3 | C | A | T | T | C | A | T | T | C | A | G | G | G | C | A | A | G | T | T | C | C | T | C | G | C | G | T | C | T | T | G | T | | | | |
| SZ16 | C | A | T | T | C | A | T | C | C | A | G | G | G | G | A | G | A | T | T | C | C | T | C | G | G | C | T | C | T | T | G | T | | | | |
| SZ1 | C | A | T | T | C | A | T | C | C | A | G | A | A | T | G | T | A | T | T | T | C | T | C | G | G | C | T | T | T | T | G | T | | | | |
| SZ13 | C | A | T | T | C | A | T | C | C | A | G | A | A | T | G | T | A | T | T | C | C | T | C | G | G | C | T | C | T | T | G | T | | | | |
| | | | | | | | | | | | | | | | | | | | | | | | | | | | | | | | | | | | | |
| GZ01 | C | A | T | T | C | A | C | C | C | G | T | G | T | C | A | G | T | C | C | C | A | C | A | C | G | C | C | T | A | C | G | C | T | A | | T |
| GZ43 | C | — | — | A | C | T | C | T | C | G | T | G | T | C | A | G | T | C | C | C | A | C | A | C | G | C | C | C | A | C | G | C | C | T | A | C |
| GZ60 | C | — | — | A | C | T | C | T | C | G | T | G | T | C | A | G | T | C | C | C | A | C | A | C | G | C | C | C | A | C | G | C | C | T | A | C |
| GZ50 | T | A | T | T | C | A | T | C | C | G | A | A | T | G | T | C | T | T | C | C | A | C | A | C | G | C | C | C | A | C | G | G | T | T | A | T |
| CUHK-W1 | C | A | T | T | C | A | T | C | C | G | A | A | T | G | T | C | T | T | C | C | A | C | A | C | G | C | C | C | A | C | G | T | T | A | | T |
| HKU-36871 | C | A | T | T | C | A | T | C | C | G | A | A | T | G | T | C | T | T | C | C | A | C | A | C | G | C | C | C | A | C | G | T | T | A | | T |
| HKU-39848 | C | A | T | T | C | A | T | C | C | G | A | A | T | G | T | C | T | T | C | C | A | C | A | C | G | C | C | C | A | C | G | T | T | A | | T |
| HKU-66078 | C | A | T | T | C | A | T | C | C | G | A | A | T | G | T | C | T | T | C | C | A | C | A | C | G | C | C | C | A | C | G | T | T | A | | T |
| HKU-65806 | C | A | T | T | C | A | T | C | C | G | A | A | T | G | T | C | T | T | C | C | A | C | A | C | G | C | C | C | A | C | G | T | T | A | | T |
| Urbani | C | A | T | T | C | A | T | C | C | G | A | A | T | G | T | C | T | T | C | C | A | C | A | C | G | C | C | C | A | C | G | T | C | A | | T |
| Tor2 | C | A | T | T | C | A | T | C | C | G | A | A | T | G | T | G | T | T | C | C | A | C | A | C | G | C | C | C | A | C | G | T | T | A | | T |

NOTE: The nucleotide residues are based on AY278554 numbering. Nonsilent mutations are highlighted in bold. Dash indicates a nucleotide deletion.

animal viruses had eight nucleotide differences, whereas there were 20 nucleotide differences among 11 human viruses. Thus, the animal viruses, although isolated from one market, are no less divergent than the human viruses isolated from Hong Kong, Guangdong, Canada, and Vietnam. However, whereas 14 (70 percent) of the 20 polymorphisms among the human viruses were nonsynonymous mutations, only two (25 percent) of the eight nucleotide substitutions within the animal viruses were. An amino acid deletion (nucleotide positions 21690 to 21692) was observed in two of the human viruses (GZ43 and GZ60). Of the 38 polymorphisms, there were 11 consistent nucleotide signatures that appeared to distinguish animal and human viruses. The observation that the human and animal viruses are phylogenetically distinct (see Figure 3-2) makes it highly unlikely that the SCoV-like viruses isolated in these wild animals is due to the transmission of SCoV from human to animals.

Our findings suggest that the markets provide a venue for the animal SCoV-like viruses to amplify and to be transmitted to new hosts, including humans, and this is critically important from the point of view of public health. However, it is not clear whether any one or more of these animals are the natural reservoir in the wild. It is conceivable that civets, raccoon dog, and ferret badgers were all infected from another, as yet unknown, animal source, which is in fact the true reservoir in nature. However, because of the culinary practices of southern China, these market animals may be intermediate hosts that increase the opportunity for transmission of infection to humans. Further extensive surveillance on animals will help to better understand the animal reservoir in nature and the interspecies transmission events that led to the origin of the SARS outbreak.

## REFERENCES

Anand K, Ziebuhr J, Wadhwani P, Mesters JR, Hilgenfeld R. 2003. Coronavirus main proteinase (3CLpro) structure: basis for design of anti-SARS drugs. *Science* 300(5626):1763-7.

Anonymous. 2003. Severe acute respiratory syndrome (SARS). *Weekly Epidemiological Record* 78:81-3.

Ballesteros ML, Sanchez CM, Enjuanes L. 1997. Two amino acid changes at the N-terminus of transmissible gastroenteritis coronavirus spike protein result in the loss of enteric tropism. *Virology* 227(2):378-88.

Baric RS, Fu K, Chen W, Yount B. 1995. High recombination and mutation rates in mouse hepatitis virus suggest that coronaviruses may be potentially important emerging viruses. *Advances in Experimental Medicine and Biology* 380:571-6.

Baric RS, Sullivan E, Hensley L, Yount B, Chen W. 1999. Persistent infection promotes cross-species transmissibility of mouse hepatitis virus. *Journal of Virology* 73(1):638-49.

Baric RS, Yount B, Hensley L, Peel SA, Chen W. 1997. Episodic evolution mediates interspecies transfer of a murine coronavirus. *Journal of Virology* 71(3):1946-55.

Bonilla PJ, Gorbalenya AE, Weiss SR. 1994. Mouse hepatitis virus strain A59 RNA polymerase gene ORF 1a: heterogeneity among MHV strains. *Virology* 198(2):736-40.

Bost AG, Carnahan RH, Lu XT, Denison MR. 2000. Four proteins processed from the replicase gene polyprotein of mouse hepatitis virus colocalize in the cell periphery and adjacent to sites of virion assembly. *Journal of Virology* 74(7):3379-87.

Bost AG, Prentice E, Denison MR. 2001. Mouse hepatitis virus replicase protein complexes are translocated to sites of M protein accumulation in the ERGIC at late times of infection. *Virology* 285(1):21-9.

Brian DA, Hogue BG, Kienzle TE. 1995. The Coronavirus Hemagluttinin Esterase Clycoprotein. In: Siddell SG, ed., *The Coronaviridae*. New York: Plenum Press. Pp. 165-79.

Brockway SM, Clay CT, Lu XT, Denison MR. 2003. Characterization of the expression, intracellular localization, and replication complex association of the putative mouse hepatitis virus RNA-dependent RNA polymerase. *Journal of Virology* 77(19):10515-27.

Callow KA, Parry HF, Sergeant M, Tyrrell DA. 1990. The time course of the immune response to experimental coronavirus infection of man. *Epidemiology and Infection* 105:435-46.

Campanacci V, Egloff MP, Longhi S, Ferron F, Rancurel C, Salomoni A, Durousseau C, Tocque F, Bremond N, Dobbe JC, Snijder EJ, Canard B, Cambillau C. 2003. Structural genomics of the SARS coronavirus: cloning, expression, crystallization and preliminary crystallographic study of the Nsp9 protein. *Acta Crystallographica. Section D, Biological Crystallography* 59(Pt 9):1628-31.

Casais R, Thiel V, Siddell SG, Cavanagh D, Britton P. 2001. Reverse genetics system for the avian coronavirus infectious bronchitis virus. *Journal of Virology* 75(24):12359-69.

CDC. 2003. Update: outbreak of severe acute respiratory syndrome-Worldwide, 2003. *MMWR* 52:241-8.

Chen W, Baric RS. 1995. Evolution and persistence mechanisms of mouse hepatitis virus. *Advances in Experimental Medicine & Biology* 380:63-71.

Chen W, Baric RS. 1996. Molecular anatomy of mouse hepatitis virus persistence: coevolution of increased host cell resistance and virus virulence. *Journal of Virology* 70(6):3947-60.

Chim SS, Tsui SK, Chan KC, Au TC, Hung EC, Tong YK, Chiu RW, Ng EK, Chan PK, Chu CM, Sung JJ, Tam JS, Fung KP, Waye MM, Lee CY, Yuen KY, Lo YM. 2003. Genomic characterisation of the severe acute respiratory syndrome coronavirus of Amoy Gardens outbreak in Hong Kong. *Lancet* 362(9398):1807-8.

Cho KO, Hasoksuz M, Nielsen PR, Chang KO, Lathrop S, Saif LJ. 2001. Cross-protection studies between respiratory and calf diarrhea and winter dysentery coronavirus strains in calves and Rt-Pcr and nested Pcr for their detection. *Archives of Virology* 146(12):2401-19.

Cho KO, Hoet AE, Loerch SC, Wittum TE, Saif LJ. 2001. Evaluation of concurrent shedding of bovine coronavirus via the respiratory tract and enteric route in feedlot cattle. *American Journal of Veterinary Research* 62(9):1436-41.

Chouljenko VN, Lin XQ, Storz J, Kousoulas KG, Gorbalenya AE. 2001. Comparison of genomic and predicted amino acid sequences of respiratory and enteric bovine coronaviruses isolated from the same animal with fatal shipping pneumonia. *Journal of General Virology* 82(12):2927-2933.

Clark MA. 1993. Bovine coronavirus. *British Veterinary Journal.* 149(1):51-70.

Cook J, Mockett APA. 1995. Epidemiology of infectious bronchitis virus. In: Siddell SG, ed., *The Coronaviridae*. New York: Plenum Press. Pp. 317-35.

Costantini V, Lewis P, Alsop J, Templeton C, Saif LJ. In press. Respiratory and enteric shedding of porcine respiratory coronavirus (PRCV) in sentinel weaned pigs and sequence of the partial S gene of the PRCV isolates. *Archives of Virology.*

Cox E, Hooyberghs J, Pensaert MB. 1990. Sites of replication of a porcine respiratory coronavirus related to transmissible gastroenteritis virus. *Research in Veterinary Science* 48(2):165-9.

deGroot RJ, Horzinek MC. 1995. Feline infectious peritonitis. In: Siddell SG, ed., *The Coronaviridae*. New York: Plenum Press. Pp. 293-315.

de Haan CA, Masters PS, Shen X, Weiss S, Rottier PJ. 2002. The group-specific murine coronavirus genes are not essential, but their deletion, by reverse genetics, is attenuating in the natural host. *Virology* 296(1):177-89.

de Jong JC, Claas EC, Osterhaus AD, Webster RG, Lim WL. 1997. A pandemic warning? *Nature* 389:544.

de Vries AAF, Horzinek MC, Rottier PJM, de Groot RJ. 1997. The genome organization of the nidovirales: similarities and differences between arteri-, toro-, and coronaviruses. *Seminars in Virology* 8(1):33-47.

Denison MR, Spaan WJ, van der Meer Y, Gibson CA, Sims AC, Prentice E, Lu XT. 1999. The putative helicase of the coronavirus mouse hepatitis virus is processed from the replicase gene polyprotein and localizes in complexes that are active in viral RNA synthesis. *Journal of Virology* 73(8):6862-71.

Domingo E, Holland JJ. 1997. RNA virus mutations and fitness for survival. *Annual Review of Microbiology* 51:151-78.

Drosten C, Gunther S, Preiser W, van der Werf S, Brodt HR, Becker S, Rabenau H, Panning M, Kolesnikova L, Fouchier RA, Berger A, Burguiere AM, Cinatl J, Eickmann M, Escriou N, Grywna K, Kramme S, Manuguerra JC, Muller S, Rickerts V, Sturmer M, Vieth S, Klenk HD, Osterhaus AD, Schmitz H, Doerr HW. 2003. Identification of a novel coronavirus in patients with severe acute respiratory syndrome. *New England Journal of Medicine* 348(20):1967-76.

Duarte M, Tobler K, Bridgen A, Rasschaert D, Ackermann M, Laude H. 1994. Sequence analysis of the porcine epidemic diarrhea virus genome between the nucleocapsid and spike protein genes reveals a polymorphic ORF. *Virology* 198(1):466-476.

Dveksler GS, Gagneten SE, Scanga CA, Cardellichio CB, Holmes KV. 1996. Expression of the recombinant anchorless N-terminal domain of mouse hepatitis virus (MHV) receptor makes hamster of human cells susceptible to MHV infection. *Journal of Virology* 70(6):4142-5.

Dveksler GS, Pensiero MN, Cardellichio CB, Williams RK, Jiang GS, Holmes KV, Dieffenbach CW. 1991. Cloning of the mouse hepatitis virus (MHV) receptor: expression in human and hamster cell lines confers susceptibility to MHV. *Journal of Virology* 65(12):6881-91.

El-Kanawati ZR, Tsunemitsu H, Smith DR, Saif LJ. 1996. Infection and cross-protection studies of winter dysentery and calf diarrhea bovine coronavirus strains in colostrum-deprived and gnotobiotic calves. *American Journal of Veterinary Research* 57(1):48-53.

Enjuanes L, Smerdou C, Castilla J, Anton IM, Torres JM, Sola I, Golvano J, Sanchez JM, Pintado B. 1995. Development of protection against coronavirus induced diseases: a review. *Advances in Experimental Medicine and Biology* 380:197-211.

Erles K, Toomey C, Brooks HW, Brownlie J. 2003. Detection of a group 2 coronavirus in dogs with canine infectious respiratory disease. *Virology* 310(2):216-23.

Fouchier RA, Kuiken T, Schutten M, van Amerongen G, van Doornum GJ, van den Hoogen BG, Peiris M, Lim W, Stohr K, Osterhaus AD. 2003. Aetiology: Koch's Postulates Fulfilled for Sars Virus. *Nature* 423(6937):240.

Gallagher TM, Escarmis C, Buchmeier MJ. 1991. Alteration of the pH dependence of coronavirus-induced cell fusion: effect of mutations in the spike glycoprotein. *Journal of Virology* 65(4):1916-28.

Gonzalez JM, Almazan F, Penzes Z, Calvo E, Enjuanes L. 2001. Cloning of a transmissible gastroenteritis coronavirus full-length cDNA. *Advances in Experimental Medicine and Biology* 494:533-6.

Gosert R, Kanjanahaluethai A, Egger D, Bienz K, Baker SC. 2002. RNA replication of mouse hepatitis virus takes place at double-membrane vesicles. *Journal of Virology* 76(8):3697-708.

Guan Y, Peiris JM, Lipatov AS, Ellis TM, Dyrting KC, Krauss S, Zhang LJ, Webster RG, Shortridge KF. 2002. Emergence of multiple genotypes of H5N1 avian influenza viruses in Hong Kong SAR. *Proceedings of the National Academy of Sciences* 99:8950-5.

Guan Y, Zheng BJ, He YQ, Liu XL, Zhuang ZX, Cheung CLLSW, Li PH, Zhang LJ, Guan YJ, Butt KM, Wong KLCKW, Lim W, Shortridge KF, Yuen KY, Peiris JSM, Poon LLM. 2003. Isolation and characterization of viruses related to the SARS coronavirus from animals in southern China. *Science* 302(5643):276-8.

Guangdong Public Health Office. January 21, 2003. Summary report of investigating an atypical pneumonia outbreak in Zhongshan, Document No 2.

Haijema BJ, Volders H, Rottier PJM. 2003. Switching species tropism: an effective way to manipulate the feline coronavirus genome. *Journal of Virology* 77(8):4528-38.

Hayes JR. 2000. Evaluation of dual infection of nursery pigs with U.S. strains of porcine reproductive and respiratory syndrome virus and porcine respiratory coronavirus. Master's Thesis, Food Animal Health Research Program, OARDC/The Ohio State University.

Herrewegh AA, Mahler M, Hedrich HJ, Haagmans BL, Egberink HF, Horzinek MC, Rottier PJ, de Groot RJ. 1997. Persistence and evolution of feline coronavirus in a closed cat-breeding colony. *Virology* 234(2):349-63.

Heusipp G, Harms U, Siddell SG, Ziebuhr J. 1997. Identification of an ATPase activity associated with a 71-kilodalton polypeptide encoded in gene 1 of the human coronavirus 229E. *Journal of Virology* 71(7):5631-4.

Hoffmann C, Kamps BS. 2003. Clinical presentation and diagnosis. In: Kamps BS, Hoffmann C, eds., *SARS Reference*. 3rd ed. Pp. 124-43. [Online] Available: http://www.SARSreference.com.

Hoffmann M and Wyler R. 1988. Propagation of the virus of porcine epidemic diarrhea in cell culture. *Journal of Clinical Microbiology* (26):2235-9.

Holland JJ, de la Torre JC, Clarke DK, Duarte E. 1991. Quantitation of relative fitness and great adaptability of clonal populations of RNA viruses. *Journal of Virology* 65(6):1960-2967.

Holmes KV. 2001. Coronaviruses. In: Knipe DM, Howley PM, eds. *Field Virology*, 4th ed. Philadelphia: Lippincott Williams and Wilkins. Pp. 1187-203.

Holmes KV. 2003. SARS coronavirus: a new challenge for prevention and therapy. *Journal of Clinical Investigation* 111(11):1605-9.

Holmes KV, Lai MMC. 1996. Coronaviridae: the viruses and their replication. In: Fields BN, Knipe DM, Howley PM, eds., *Virology*. Vol. 1. 3rd ed. Philadelphia: Lippincott-Raven. Pp. 1075-93.

Ismail MM, Cho KO, Hasoksuz M, Saif LJ, Saif YM. 2001. Antigenic and genomic relatedness of turkey-origin coronaviruses, bovine coronaviruses, and infectious bronchitis virus of chickens. *Avian Diseases* 45(4):978-84.

Ismail MM, Cho KO, Ward LA, Saif LJ, Saif YM. 2001. Experimental bovine coronavirus in turkey poults and young chickens. *Avian Diseases* 45(1):157-63.

Kamps BS, Hoffmann C. 2003a. Pediatric SARS. In: Kamps BS, Hoffmann C, eds., *SARS Reference*. 3rd ed. Pp. 49-60. [Online] Available: http://www.SARSreference.com.

Kamps BS, Hoffmann C. 2003b. Transmission. In: Kamps BS, Hoffmann C, eds., *SARS Reference*. 3rd ed. Pp. 49-60. [Online] Available: http://www.SARSreference.com.

Kim JC, Spence RA, Currier PF, Lu X, Denison MR. 1995. Coronavirus protein processing and RNA synthesis is inhibited by the cysteine proteinase inhibitor E64d. *Virology* 208(1):1-8.

Kimura M. 1980. A simple method for estimating evolutionary rates of base substitutions through comparative studies of nucleotide sequences. *Journal of Molecular Evolution* 16(2):111-20.

Klumperman J, Locker JK, Meijer A, Horzinek MC, Geuze HJ, Rottier PJ. 1994. Coronavirus M proteins accumulate in the Golgi complex beyond the site of virion budding. *Journal of Virology* 68(10):6523-34.

Krijnse-Locker J, Ericsson M, Rottier PJ, Griffiths G. 1994. Characterization of the budding compartment of mouse hepatitis virus: evidence that transport from the RER to the Golgi complex requires only one vesicular transport step. *Journal of Cell Biology* 124(1-2):55-70.

Ksiazek TG, Erdman D, Goldsmith CS, Zaki SR, Peret T, Emery S, Tong S, Urbani C, Comer JA, Lim W, Rollin PE, Dowell SF, Ling AE, Humphrey CD, Shieh WJ, Guarner J, Paddock CD, Rota P, Fields B, DeRisi J, Yang JY, Cox N, Hughes JM, LeDuc JW, Bellini WJ, Anderson LJ, SARS Working Group. 2003. A novel coronavirus associated with severe acute respiratory syndrome. *New England Journal of Medicine* 348(20):1953-66.

Kumar S, Tarnura K, Jakobsen IB, Nei M. 2001. MEGA2: molecular evolutionary genetics analysis software. *Bioinformatics* 17:1244-5.

Kuo L, Godeke GJ, Raamsman MJ, Masters PS, Rottier PJ. 2000. Retargeting of coronavirus by substitution of the spike glycoprotein ectodomain: crossing the host cell species barrier. *Journal of Virology* 74(3):1393-406.

Lai MM, Cavanagh D. 1997. The molecular biology of coronaviruses. *Advances in Virus Research* 48:1-100.

Laude H, Van Reeth K, Pensaert M. 1993. Porcine respiratory coronavirus: molecular features and virus-host interactions. *Veterinary Research* 24(2):125-50.

Lee N, Hui D, Wu A, Chan P, Cameron P, Joynt GM, Ahuja A, Yung MY, Leung CB, To K, Lui SF, Szeto CC, Chung S, Sung JJ. 2003. A major outbreak of severe acute respiratory syndrome in Hong Kong. *New England Journal of Medicine* 348:1986-94.

Lee HJ, Shieh CK, Gorbalenya AE, Koonin EV, La Monica N, Tuler J, Bagdzhadzhyan A, Lai MM. 1991. The complete sequence (22 kilobases) of murine coronavirus gene 1 encoding the putative proteases and RNA polymerase. *Virology* 180(2):567-82.

Li W, Moore MJ, Vasilieva N, Sui J, Wong SK, Berne MA, Somasundaran M, Sullivan JL, Luzuriaga K, Greenough TC, Choe H, Farzan M. 2003. Angiotensin-converting enzyme 2 is a functional receptor for the SARS coronavirus. *Nature* 426(6965):450-4.

Lu Y, Lu X, Denison MR. 1995. Identification and characterization of a serine-like proteinase of the murine coronavirus MHV-A59. *Journal of Virology* 69(6):3554-9.

Majhdi F, Minocha HC, Kapil S. 1997. Isolation and characterization of a coronavirus from elk calves with diarrhea. *Journal of Clinical Microbiology* 35(11):2937-42.

Marra MA, Jones SJ, Astell CR, Holt RA, Brooks-Wilson A, Butterfield YS, Khattra J, Asano JK, Barber SA, Chan SY, Cloutier A, Coughlin SM, Freeman D, Girn N, Griffith OL, Leach SR, Mayo M, McDonald H, Montgomery SB, Pandoh PK, Petrescu AS, Robertson AG, Schein JE, Siddiqui A, Smailus DE, Stott JM, Yang GS, Plummer F, Andonov A, Artsob H, Bastien N, Bernard K, Booth TF, Bowness D, Czub M, Drebot M, Fernando L, Flick R, Garbutt M, Gray M, Grolla A, Jones S, Feldmann H, Meyers A, Kabani A, Li Y, Normand S, Stroher U, Tipples GA, Tyler S, Vogrig R, Ward D, Watson B, Brunham RC, Krajden M, Petric M, Skowronski DM, Upton C, Roper RL. 2003. The genome sequence of the SARS-associated coronavirus. *Science* 300(5624):1399-404.

Masters PS, Koetzner CA, Kerr CA, Heo Y. 1994. Optimization of targeted RNA recombination and mapping of a novel nucleocapsid gene mutation in the coronavirus mouse hepatitis virus. *Journal of Virology* 68(1):328-37.

Navas S, Seo SH, Chua MM, Das Sarma J, Hingley ST, Lavi E, Weiss SR. 2001. Role of the spike protein in murine coronavirus induced hepatitis: an in vivo study using targeted RNA recombination. *Advances in Experimental Medicine and Biology* 494:139-44.

Navas S, Weiss SR. 2003. Murine coronavirus-induced hepatitis: JHM genetic background eliminates A59 spike-determined hepatotropism. *Journal of Virology* 77(8):4972-8.

Opstelten DJ, Raamsman MJ, Wolfs K, Horzinek MC, Rottier PJ. 1995. Envelope glycoprotein interactions in coronavirus assembly. *Journal of Cell Biology* 131(2):339-49.

Ortego J, Sola I, Almazan F, Ceriani JE, Riquelme C, Balasch M, Plana J, Enjuanes L. 2003. Transmissible gastroenteritis coronavirus gene 7 is not essential but influences in vivo virus replication and virulence. *Virology* 308(1):13-22.

Peiris JS, Lai ST, Poon LL, Guan Y, Yam LY, Lim W, Nicholls J, Yee WK, Yan WW, Cheung MT, Cheng VC, Chan KH, Tsang DN, Yung RW, Ng TK, Yuen KY, SARS study group. 2003a. Coronavirus as a possible cause of severe acute respiratory syndrome. *Lancet* 361(9366):1319-25.

Peiris JS, Chu CM, Cheng VC, Chan KS, Hung IF, Poon LL, Law KI, Tang BS, Hon TY, Chan CS, Chan KH, Ng JS, Zheng BJ, Ng WL, Lai RW, Guan Y, Yuen KY, HKU/UCH SARS Study Group. 2003b. Clinical progression and viral load in a community outbreak of coronavirus-associated SARS pneumonia: a prospective study. *Lancet* 361(9371):1767-72.

Peng GW, He JF, Lin JY, Zhou DH, Yu DW, Liang WJ, Li LH, Guo RN, Luo HM, Xu RH. 2003. Epidemiological study on severe acute respiratory syndrome in Guangdong province. *Chinese Journal of Epidemiology* 24:350-2.

Pensaert MB. 1999. Porcine epidemic diarrhea. In: Straw BE, D'Allaire S, Mengeling WL, Taylor D. eds., *Diseases of Swine*. 8th ed. Ames, IA: Iowa State Press. Pp. 179-85.

Perlman S, Ries D, Bolger E, Chang LJ, Stoltzfus CM. 1986. MHV nucleocapsid synthesis in the presence of cycloheximide and accumulation of negative strand MHV RNA. *Virus Research* 6(3):261-72.

Poutanen SM, Low DE, Henry B, Finkelstein S, Rose D, Green K, Tellier R, Draker R, Adachi D, Ayers M, Chan AK, Skowronski DM, Salit I, Simor AE, Slutsky AS, Doyle PW, Krajden M, Petric M, Brunham RC, McGeer AJ, National Microbiology Laboratory Canada, Canadian Severe Acute Respiratory Syndrome Study Team. 2003. Identification of severe acute respiratory syndrome in Canada. *New England Journal of Medicine* 348(20):1995-2005.

Prentice E, Denison MR. 2001. The cell biology of coronavirus infection. In: Lavi E, Weiss SR, Hingley S, eds., *The Nidoviruses.* Philadelphia, PA: Plenum.

Rao PV, Gallagher TM. 1998. Mouse hepatitis virus receptor levels influence virus-induced cytopathology. *Advances in Experimental Medicine and Biology* 440:549-55.

Rota PA, Oberste MS, Monroe SS, Nix WA, Campagnoli R, Icenogle JP, Penaranda S, Bankamp B, Maher K, Chen MH, Tong S, Tamin A, Lowe L, Frace M, DeRisi JL, Chen Q, Wang D, Erdman DD, Peret TC, Burns C, Ksiazek TG, Rollin PE, Sanchez A, Liffick S, Holloway B, Limor J, McCaustland K, Olsen-Rasmussen M, Fouchier R, Gunther S, Osterhaus AD, Drosten C, Pallansch MA, Anderson LJ, Bellini WJ. 2003. Characterization of a novel coronavirus associated with severe acute respiratory syndrome. *Science* 300(5624):1394-9.

Rottier PJ, Rose JK. 1987. Coronavirus E1 glycoprotein expressed from cloned cDNA localizes in the Golgi region. *Journal of Virology* 61(6):2042-5.

Saif LJ. In press. Comparative biology of coronaviruses: Lessons for SARS. In: Peiris M, ed., *SARS: The First New Plague of the 21st Century.* Oxford, UK: Blackwell.

Saif L, Wesley R. 1999. Transmissible gastroenteritis virus. In: Straw BE, D'Allaire S, Mengeling WL, Taylor D. eds., *Diseases of Swine.* 8th ed. Ames, IA: Iowa State University Press.

Saif LJ, Heckert RA. 1990. Enteric coronaviruses. In: Saif LJ, Thiel KW. *Viral Diarrheas of Man and Animals.* Boca Raton, FL: CRC Press. Pp. 185-252.

Salanueva IJ, Carrascosa JL, Risco C. 1999. Structural maturation of the transmissible gastroenteritis coronavirus. *Journal of Virology* 73(10):7952-64.

Sanchez CM, Izeta A, Sanchez-Morgado JM, Alonso S, Sola I, Balasch M, Plana-Duran J, Enjuanes L. 1999. Targeted recombination demonstrates that the spike gene of transmissible gastroenteritis coronavirus is a determinant of its enteric tropism and virulence. *Journal of Virology* 73 (9):7607-18.

Sarma JD, Scheen E, Seo SH, Koval M, Weiss SR. 2002. Enhanced green fluorescent protein expression may be used to monitor murine coronavirus spread in vitro and in the mouse central nervous system. *Journal of Neurovirology* 8(5):381-91.

Sawicki SG, Sawicki DL. 1986. Coronavirus minus-strand RNA synthesis and effect of cycloheximide on coronavirus RNA synthesis. *Journal of Virology* 57(1):328-34.

Sawicki SG, Sawicki DL. 1998. A new model for coronavirus transcription. *Advances in Experimental Medicine and Biology* 440:215-9.

Shi ST, Schiller JJ, Kanjanahaluethai A, Baker SC, Oh JW, Lai MM. 1999. Colocalization and membrane association of murine hepatitis virus gene 1 products and De novo-synthesized viral RNA in infected cells. *Journal of Virology* 73(7):5957-69.

Shortridge KF, Stuart-Harris CH. 1982. An influenza epicentre? *Lancet* 2:812-13.

Sims AC, Ostermann J, Denison MR. 2000. Mouse hepatitis virus replicase proteins associate with two distinct populations of intracellular membranes. *Journal of Virology* 74(12):5647-54.

Snijder EJ, Bredenbeek PJ, Dobbe JC, Thiel V, Ziebuhr J, Poon LL, Guan Y, Rozanov M, Spaan WJ, Gorbalenya AE. 2003. Unique and conserved features of genome and proteome of SARS-coronavirus, an early split-off from the coronavirus group 2 lineage. *Journal of Molecular Biology* 331(5):991-1004.

Stalcup RP, Baric RS, Leibowitz JL. 1998. Genetic complementation among three panels of mouse hepatitis virus gene 1 mutants. *Virology* 241(1):112-21.

Stavrinides J, Guttman DS. 2004. Mosaic evolution of the severe acute respiratory syndrome coronavirus. *Journal of Virology* 78(1):76-82.

Subbarao K, Klimov A, Katz J, Regnery H, Lim W, Hall H, Perdue M, Swayne D, Bender C, Huang J, Hemphill M, Rowe T, Shaw M, Xu X, Fukuda K, Cox N. 1998. Characterisation of an avian influenza A (H5N1) virus isolated from a child with a fatal respiratory illness. *Science* 279:393-6.

Thiel V, Herold J, Schelle B, Siddell SG. 2001. Infectious RNA transcribed in vitro from a cDNA copy of the human coronavirus genome cloned in vaccinia virus. *Journal of General Virology* 82(Pt 6):1273-81.

Thiel V, Ivanov KA, Putics A, Hertzig T, Schelle B, Bayer S, Weissbrich B, Snijder EJ, Rabenau H, Doerr HW, Gorbalenya AE, Ziebuhr J. 2003. Mechanisms and enzymes involved in SARS coronavirus genome expression. *Journal of General Virology* 84(Pt 9):2305-15.

Tresnan DB, Levis R, Holmes KV. 1996. Feline aminopeptidase N serves as a receptor for feline, canine, porcine, and human coronaviruses in serogroup I. *Journal of Virology* 70(12):8669-74.

Tsang KW, Ho PL, Ooi GC, et al. 2003. A cluster of cases of severe acute respiratory syndrome in Hong Kong. *New England Journal of Medicine* 348:1977-85.

Tsunemitsu H, El-Kanawati ZR, Smith DR, Reed HH, Saif LJ. 1995. Isolation of coronaviruses antigenically indistinguishable from bovine coronavirus from wild ruminants with diarrhea. *Journal of Clinical Microbiology* 33(12):3264-9.

Tsunemitsu H, Saif LJ. 1995. Antigenic and biological comparisons of bovine coronaviruses derived from neonatal calf diarrhea and winter dysentery of adult cattle. *Archives of Virology* 140(7):1303-11.

van der Meer Y, Snijder EJ, Dobbe JC, Schleich S, Denison MR, Spaan WJ, Locker JK. 1999. Localization of mouse hepatitis virus nonstructural proteins and RNA synthesis indicates a role for late endosomes in viral replication. *Journal of Virology* 73(9):7641-57.

Vennema H, Poland A, Floyd Hawkins K, Pedersen NC. 1995. A comparison of the genomes of FECVs and FIPVs and what they tell us about the relationships between feline coronaviruses and their evolution. *Feline Practice* 23:40-4.

WHO (World Health Organization). 2003a. Cumulative number of reported probable cases of severe acute respiratory syndrome (SARS). [Online] Available: http://www.who.int/csr/sarscountry/2003_07_11/en [accessed July 16, 2003].

WHO. 2003b. Case definitions for surveillance of severe acute respiratory syndrome (SARS) [Online] Available: http://www.who.int/csr/sars/casedefinition/en/ [accessed May 1, 2003].

WHO [Online] Available: www.who.int/csr/sars/en/.

WHO. Cumulative Number of reported probable cases of severe acute respiratory syndrome (SARS). [Online] Available: www.who.int/csr/sars/country/2003_05_20/en/.

Xiao X, Chakraborti S, Dimitrov AS, Gramatikoff K, Dimitrov DS. 2003. The SARS-CoV S glycoprotein: expression and functional characterization. *Biochemincal and Biophysical Research Communucations* 312(4):1159-64.

Yeager CL, Ashmun RA, Williams RK, Cardellichio CB, Shapiro LH, Look AT, Holmes KV. 1992. Human aminopeptidase N is a receptor for human coronavirus 229E. *Nature* 357(6377):420-2.

Yokomori K, Lai MM. 1992. Mouse hepatitis virus utilizes two carcinoembryonic antigens as alternative receptors. *Journal of Virology* 66(10):6194-9.

Yount B, Curtis KM, Baric RS. 2000. Strategy for systematic assembly of large RNA and DNA genomes: transmissible gastroenteritis virus model. *Journal of Virology* 74(22):10600-11.

Yount B, Curtis KM, Fritz EA, Hensley LE, Jahrling PB, Prentice E, Denison MR, Geisbert TW, Baric RS. 2003. Reverse genetics with a full-length infectious cDNA of severe acute respiratory syndrome coronavirus. *Proceedings of the National Academy of Sciences* 100(22):12995-3000.

Yount B, Denison MR, Weiss SR, Baric RS. 2002. Systematic assembly of a full-length infectious cDNA of mouse hepatitis virus strain A59. *Journal of Virology* 76(21):11065-78.

Zhang XM, Herbst W, Kousoulas KG, Storz J. 1994. Biological and genetic characterization of a hemagglutinating coronavirus isolated from a diarrhoeic child. *Journal of Medical Virology* 44 (2):152-61.

Zhong NS, Zheng BJ, Li YM, Poon, Xie ZH, Chan KH, Li PH, Tan SY, Chang Q, Xie JP, Liu XQ, Xu J, Li DX, Yuen KY, Peiris, Guan Y. 2003. Epidemiology and cause of severe acute respiratory syndrome (SARS) in Guangdong, People's Republic of China. *Lancet* 362(9393):1353-8.

Ziebuhr J, Snijder EJ, Gorbalenya AE. 2000. Virus-encoded proteinases and proteolytic processing in the Nidovirales. *Journal of General Virology* 81(Pt 4):853-79.

Ziebuhr J, Thiel V, Gorbalenya AE. 2001. The autocatalytic release of a putative RNA virus transcription factor from its polyprotein precursor involves two paralogous papain-like proteases that cleave the same peptide bond. *Journal of Biological Chemistry* 276(35):33220-32.

# 4

# Diagnostics, Therapeutics, and Other Technologies to Control SARS

## OVERVIEW

The strong possibility that SARS will return is being addressed by multiple sectors, including public health planners preparing for a broad range of challenges and contingencies (see also Chapter 1); researchers developing clinical diagnostics and technologies for infection control, as well as antiviral drugs and vaccines; and epidemiologists searching for clues from the recent SARS epidemic that could prevent a future outbreak or reduce its impact. Each of these perspectives is discussed in this chapter.

The development of a diagnostic test to rapidly detect SARS in its early stages is a top research priority. Because researchers do not know which tissues contain the highest concentrations of virus in the presymptomatic stages of infection, this task is particularly challenging. Reverse-transcription polymerase chain reaction (RT-PCR), a method to detect viral nucleic acids, is considered to be a likely platform for early SARS testing due to its high analytical sensitivity and speed. An evaluation of two RT-PCR protocols presented in this chapter found them to be highly specific for the SARS coronavirus; however, the tests were determined to be insufficiently sensitive to reliably detect the virus in respiratory specimens. Without a clinical diagnostic test, suspected cases of SARS must be confirmed in the laboratory, using RT-PCR or slower methods of detection—involving serology or viral culture, isolation, and identification by electron microscopy—thereby causing a significant increase in the time required for an accurate diagnosis.

This chapter also includes a description of an alternative diagnostic platform—the mass spectroscopic identification of microbial nucleic acid signatures—that can be adapted to detect the SARS coronavirus. Using technology originally designed for the environmental surveillance of biowarfare agents, this platform could potentially identify the SARS virus directly from a patient sample, obviating the need for time-consuming viral culture. This method is designed to distinguish between SARS and other coronaviruses, and perhaps even between genetic variants of the SARS virus; however, direct comparisons of sensitivity between this and other SARS detection systems using patient samples have yet to be conducted.

Several workshop participants expressed concern about the limited capacity in health care systems—particularly related to workforce and facilities shortages—that present a significant barrier to preparations for SARS and other threats to public health. It was suggested at the workshop by Jerome Schentag that this situation might be mitigated in some degree through the use of flexible approaches to isolating SARS patients. One such approach, discussed in this chapter, is a mobile technology that destroys viral particles and droplets in the air. These mobile units, by isolating individual patients being transported to and within hospitals, potentially could be used to protect staff during high-risk procedures such as intubation or bronchoscopy, to decontaminate larger areas such as hospital waiting rooms or airplanes, and to create air exchange systems for isolation facilities or areas within hospitals. Importantly however, it was noted during the workshop that the technologies described here must be thoroughly evaluated to determine their suitability for containing SARS in a variety of clinical settings before they are recommended for use.

Research has proceeded rapidly to develop antiviral drugs and vaccines to combat SARS. Previous antiviral discovery efforts by researchers at Pfizer on the human rhinovirus protease 3C—a functional, genetic, and structural analog to a key SARS coronavirus protease that has therefore been named "3C-like" (3CL)—are recounted in this chapter. This knowledge has aided in a search for 3CL protease inhibitors, a project undertaken by Pfizer in collaboration with scientists at the National Institute of Allergy and Infectious Diseases and the U.S. Army Medical Research Institute of Infectious Diseases (USAMRIID). Several candidate inhibitors have been selected by bioassay and are currently being evaluated for clinical development, while others are being sought through alternative strategies such as structure-based design and combinatorial chemistry. A vaccine for SARS—even if steered along a highly streamlined route to development—might still postdate a return of SARS, perhaps by several years. Nevertheless, because the medical need for developing such a vaccine and/or effective antiviral drugs is perceived to be acute, several pharmaceutical and biotechnology companies have taken up this challenge.

# EVALUATION OF REVERSE TRANSCRIPTION-PCR ASSAYS FOR RAPID DIAGNOSIS OF SEVERE ACUTE RESPIRATORY SYNDROME ASSOCIATED WITH A NOVEL CORONAVIRUS

W.C. Yam, K.H. Chan, L.L.M. Poon, Y. Guan, K.Y. Yuen,
W.H. Seto, and J.S.M. Peiris
Department of Microbiology, Queen Mary Hospital, The University of
Hong Kong, Hong Kong, People's Republic of China

The reverse transcription (RT)-PCR protocols of two World Health Organization (WHO) severe acute respiratory syndrome (SARS) network laboratories (WHO SARS network laboratories at The University of Hong Kong [WHO-HKU] and at the Bernhard-Nocht Institute in Hamburg, Germany [WHO-Hamburg]) were evaluated for rapid diagnosis of a novel coronavirus (CoV) associated with SARS in Hong Kong. A total of 303 clinical specimens were collected from 163 patients suspected to have SARS. The end point of both WHO-HKU and WHO-Hamburg RT-PCR assays was determined to be 0.1 50 percent tissue culture infective dose. Using seroconversion to CoV as the "gold standard" for SARS CoV diagnosis, WHO-HKU and WHO-Hamburg RT-PCR assays exhibited diagnostic sensitivities of 61 and 68 percent (nasopharyngeal aspirate specimens), 65 and 72 percent (throat swab specimens), 50 and 54 percent (urine specimens), and 58 and 63 percent (stool specimens), respectively, with an overall specificity of 100 percent. For patients confirmed to have SARS CoV and from whom two or more respiratory specimens were collected, testing the second specimen increased the sensitivity from 64 and 71 percent to 75 and 79 percent for the WHO-HKU and WHO-Hamburg RT-PCR assays, respectively. Testing more than one respiratory specimen will maximize the sensitivity of PCR assays for SARS CoV.

A global outbreak of a new emerging illness, severe acute respiratory syndrome (SARS), was associated with a novel coronavirus, SARS CoV (Lee et al., 2003; Peiris et al., 2003a; Tsang et al., 2003). By the end of April 2003, more than 1,500 patients were diagnosed with SARS in Hong Kong. Transmission within hospitals was a major contributor to disease amplification. Rapid laboratory confirmation of SARS CoV infection was important for managing patient care and for preventing nosocomial transmission. While serological testing was reliable as a retrospective diagnostic method, diagnosis of the infection in the early phase of the illness was important for patient care. The identification of the etiological agent and its partial gene sequence data made it possible to develop molecular diagnostic methods for SARS CoV (Drosten et al., 2003; Peiris et al., 2003b). The protocols were made available through the WHO website (http://www.who.int/csr/sars/primers/en). This study evaluates two of the first-generation reverse transcription (RT)-PCR assays that were used during this outbreak.

## Materials and Methods

### Patients and Specimen Collection

Specimens were available for 163 patients who presented with clinically suspected SARS according to the WHO definition (WHO, 2003) and who were admitted to three acute regional hospitals in Hong Kong between 26 February and 17 April 2003. For each patient, paired acute- and convalescent-phase serum samples and at least one respiratory specimen were collected for study. A total of 303 specimens (124 nasopharyngeal aspirate specimens, 65 throat swab specimens, 95 urine specimens, and 19 stool specimens) were available for study. Respiratory specimens were collected between days 1 and 5 after admission, whereas urine and stool specimens were collected between days 5 and 10. The acute-phase sera were collected in the first week of illness, and the convalescent-phase sera were collected 21 days after the onset of clinical symptoms. Nasopharyngeal aspirate specimens were assessed by rapid direct immunofluorescent antigen detection for influenza virus A and B, para-influenza virus types 1, 2, and 3, respiratory syncytial virus (RSV), and adenovirus as described previously (Chan et al., 2002). Paired serum samples were assayed for increasing titer against CoV. Nasopharyngeal aspirate and stool specimens from patients suffering from unrelated diseases were collected as controls.

### Extraction of CoV RNA

Nasopharyngeal aspirate and throat swab specimens were suspended in viral transport medium. Urine specimens were transported in sterile containers. Stool specimens were mixed in viral transport medium (diluted 1:10) and microcentrifuged at $10,000 \times g$ for 1 min, and supernatant was collected. Viral RNA was extracted from 140 μl samples using a Qiagen viral RNA mini kit (Qiagen, Hilden, Germany). The initial processing of specimens was performed under biohazard level 2 containment conditions. After lysis of the sample by the lysing buffer, the mixture was applied to a spin column as described by the manufacturer. The extracted RNA was eluted in a total volume of 50 μl of RNase-free water before RT-PCR amplification.

### RT-PCR Amplification

The RT-PCR protocols of two WHO SARS network laboratories (Table 4-1) were evaluated in this study. The WHO SARS network laboratory at the University of Hong Kong (WHO-HKU) used a single RT step to synthesize cDNA, followed by subsequent PCR amplification with specific primers in another reaction tube (Peiris et al., 2003a). The WHO SARS network laboratory at the Bernhard-Nocht Institute in Hamburg, Germany (WHO-Hamburg) used a single

**TABLE 4-1** RT-PCR Protocols for Rapid Diagnosis of CoV Associated with SARS[a]

| Characteristic or component of protocol | WHO-HKU — RT | WHO-HKU — PCR | RT-PVR | Second PCR |
|---|---|---|---|---|
| **Primer sequences**<br>Sense<br>Antisense | | TACACACCTTCAGCGTTG<br>CACGAACGTTGACGAAT | ATGAATTACCAAGTCAATGGTTAC<br>CATAACCAGTCGGTACAGCTAC | GAAGCTATTCGTCACG<br>CTGTAGAAAATCCTAGCTGGAG |
| **Reagent formulation** | Superscript II RTA (Invitrogen)<br>(i) 4 µl of 5x first-strand buffer<br>(ii) 10 mM DTT<br>(iii) 500 µMdNTP<br>(iv) 0.15 µg of random primer<br>(v) 200 U of Superscript II<br>(vi) 12 µl of RNA extract<br>(vii) Make up total volume of 20 µl | AmpliTaq Gold (Roche)<br>(i) 5 µl of 10x reaction buffer<br>(ii) 200 µM dIU<br>(iii) 2.5 µM MgSO4<br>(iv) 250 nM (each) primer<br>(v) 2 U of AmpliTaq Gold<br>(vi) 2 µl of RT product<br>(vii) Make up total volume of 50 µl | Superscript II RT-PCR (Invitrogen)<br>(i) 10µl of 2x reaction buffer<br>(ii) 2.45 mM MgSO4<br>(iii) 500 µM (each) primer<br>(iv) 0.4 µl of RTA-Taq mixture<br>(v) 2 µl of RNA extract<br>(vi) Make up total volume of 20 µl | AmpliTaq Gold (Roche)<br>(i) 5 µl of 10x reaction buffer<br>(ii) 200 µM dNTP<br>(iii) 2.5 µM MgSo4<br>(iv) 200 nM (each) primer<br>(v) 2 U of AmpliTaq Gold<br>(vi) 1 µl of RT-PCR product<br>(vii) Make up total volume of 50 µl |
| **Thermal cycling profile** | (i) 25°C, 10 min<br>(ii) 42°C, 50 min<br>(iii) 94°C, 3 min | (i) 94°C, 10 min<br>(ii) 40 cycles<br>(a) 94°C, 30 s<br>(b) 50°C, 40 s<br>(c) 72°C, 15 s<br>(iii) 72°C, 10 min | (i) 45°C, 30 min<br>(ii) 95°C, 3 min<br>(iii) 10 cycles<br>(a) 95°C, 10 s<br>(b) 60°C, 10 s (decrease by 1°C/cycle)<br>(c) 72°C, 30 s<br>(iv) 40 cycles<br>(a) 95°C, 10 s<br>(b) 56°C, 10 s (decrease by 1°C/cycle)<br>(c) 72°C, 30 | (i) 95°C, 5 min<br>(ii) 10 cycles<br>(a) 95°C, 10 s<br>(b) 60°C, 10 s (decrease by 1°C/cycle)<br>(c) 72°C, 20 s<br>(iii) 20 cycles<br>(a) 95°C, 10 s<br>(b) 56°C, 10 s<br>(c) 72°C, 20 s |
| **Expected PCR product size (bp)** | | 182 | 189 | 108 |

[a]The RT-PCR protocols of two WHO SARS network laboratories. WHO-HKU (Peiris et al., 2003a) and WHO-Hamburg (Drosten et al., 2003) are also available online (http://www/who.int/est/sars/primers/en). Abbreviations: RTA, reverse transcriptase; DDT, dithiothreitol; dNTP, deoxynucleoside triphosphate.

RT-PCR step, followed by transfer of the initial PCR products to the nested PCR amplification mixture (Drosten et al., 2003). Positive and negative controls were included in each run, and all precautions to prevent cross-contamination were observed. For nested PCR, RT-PCR amplicon tubes were spun (in pulses) before the tubes were opened using separate Eppendorf tube openers for transferring RT-PCR products to the nested PCR mix. Negative control was incorporated for every five nested PCRs to monitor cross-contamination. Amplified products were electrophoresed through a 2 percent agarose gel in Tris-borate buffer. Target bands were visualized by staining with ethidium bromide.

*CoV Immunoglobulin G Serology*

Smears of CoV-infected Vero cells were prepared, fixed in acetone for 10 min, and stored at −80°C before use (Peiris et al., 2003a). Each batch of SARS CoV-infected cell smears with 60 to 70 percent infected cells was prepared and tested with a high-titer, positive-control serum sample from a confirmed SARS patient as a standard to assess sensitivity and batch-to-batch variations. Serial twofold dilutions starting with a 1:10 dilution of each patient serum sample were added to the smears and incubated for 30 min at 37°C. After two 5-min washes in phosphate-buffered saline, fluorescein isothiocyanate-conjugated goat anti-human immunoglobulin G (INOVA Diagnostics, Inc., San Diego, California) was added to the smears, and the smears were incubated for 30 min at 37°C. Acute- and convalescent-phase serum samples from each patient were assayed for SARS CoV antibodies in the same experiment to minimize experimental variations. The titer was determined as the highest dilution of serum exhibiting fluorescence of the infected cells. A weakly positive patient serum sample was included as a control in each run. A sample was scored as a positive result if the fluorescent intensity was equal to or higher than that of the positive control.

*Determination of the End Points of the RT-PCR Assays*

A 96-well microtiter plate containing 0.1 ml of confluent Vero cells was used to determine the 50 percent tissue culture infective dose ($TCID_{50}$) of SARS CoV under biohazard level 3 containment conditions. Tenfold serial dilutions of a cell-adapted SARS CoV strain from $10^{-1}$ to $10^{-8}$ were prepared. One hundred microliters of each dilution were added to each well of four replicate wells and incubated at 37°C for 2 to 3 days to observe cytopathic effect. $TCID_{50}$s were determined by the Kärber method (Ballew, 1992). For the same serial dilutions of virus, 100-µl samples were subjected to RNA extraction, and the end points of the two RT-PCR assays were determined.

## Results

Of 303 specimens from clinically suspected SARS cases (see Table 4-2), 145 were positive by one or both PCR assays and more than 87 percent of PCR-positive samples were identified by both PCR assays. Common respiratory viral pathogens, including influenza virus A and B, parainfluenza virus types 1, 2, and 3, RSV, and adenovirus, were not detected in the 124 nasopharyngeal aspirate specimens. The end point for both WHO-HKU and WHO-Hamburg RT-PCR methods was determined to be 0.1 TCID50. The acute-phase serum samples from all patients were seronegative for SARS CoV. Eighty-six patients were confirmed to have SARS CoV infections on the basis of seroconversion. Using seroconversion as the gold standard for SARS diagnosis, the sensitivities of the WHO-HKU and WHO-Hamburg RT-PCR assays were found to be 61 and 68 percent (nasopharyngeal aspirate specimens), 65 and 72 percent (throat swab specimens), 50 and 54 percent (urine specimens), and 58 and 63 percent (stool specimens). A specificity of 100 percent was exhibited by both RT-PCR assays, as none of the seronegative patient samples and control samples gave a positive PCR result. Among the 163 patients, two or more respiratory specimens (nasopharyngeal aspirate or throat swab specimens) were available from 41 patients. Of the 41 patients, 28 were subsequently confirmed to have SARS CoV on the basis of seroconversion. In these 28 patients, the numbers of first specimens positive for WHO-HKU and WHO-Hamburg RT-PCR were 18 and 20, respectively, but testing a second specimen increased the overall sensitivity from 64 and 71 percent to 75 and 79 percent, respectively.

## Discussion

In Hong Kong, SARS is a serious respiratory illness that led to significant morbidity and mortality (Donnelly et al., 2003). The diagnosis depends mainly on the clinical findings of an atypical pneumonia not attributed to another cause and a history of exposure to a suspect or probable case of SARS or to the respiratory secretions and other bodily fluids of individuals with SARS. Definitive diagnosis of this novel CoV relies on classic tissue culture isolation, followed by electron microscopy studies to identify the virus on cell culture, which is technically very demanding. Serological testing for increasing titer against SARS-associated CoV was shown to be highly sensitive and specific (Peiris et al., 2003a) but was not suitable for rapid laboratory diagnosis. The rapid isolation and characterization of the novel CoV associated with SARS allowed for the timely development of diagnostic tests (Marra et al., 2003; Rota et al., 2003). RT-PCR protocols of two WHO SARS network laboratories were evaluated for rapid diagnosis of SARS-associated CoV in Hong Kong. The end point for the novel CoV by both RT-PCR assays was similar to the previous finding for human CoV (Vabret et al., 2001), yet sufficient diagnostic sensitivity was not achieved, despite attaining a

**TABLE 4-2** Performance of RT-PCR Assays for Rapid Detection of CoV Associated with SARS

| Specimens (no.) | No. of specimens tested | Seroconversion[a] | No. of specimens positive by RT-PCR assay | | |
| --- | --- | --- | --- | --- | --- |
| | | | WHO-HKU | WHO-Hamburg | Both WHO-HKU and WHO-Hamburg |
| Clinically suspected SARS | | | | | |
| Nasopharygneal aspirate specimens (124) | 72 | + | 44 | 49 | 43 |
| | 52 | − | 0 | 0 | 0 |
| Throat swab specimens (65) | 54 | + | 35 | 39 | 33 |
| Urine specimens (19) | 78 | + | 39 | 42 | 39 |
| Stool specimens | 19 | + | 11 | 12 | 11 |
| Controls | | | | | |
| Nasopharygneal aspirate specimens | 22[b] | ND | 0 | 0 | 0 |
| Stool specimen | 21[c] | ND | 0 | 0 | 0 |

[a] A fourfold rise of more in antibody titer against CoV was considered seroconversion (+). ND, not done.

[b] Samples positive for other viral pathogens included nine samples positive for influenza virus A, one sample positive for influenza virus B, six samples positive for adenovirus, and six samples positive for RSV by immunoflourescence (Chan et al., 2002).

[c] No intestinal pathogens detected.

specificity of 100 percent. A recent study using real-time RT-PCR revealed that the viral load in nasopharyngeal aspirate specimens peaked in the second week of the illness (Peiris et al., 2003b). Results indicated a more sensitive RT-PCR assay is essential for rapid diagnosis of SARS CoV during the early stage of disease. Due to the nature of respiratory specimens with inconsistent pathogen loads at various sample times, testing of multiple specimens has been shown to increase the sensitivity of laboratory diagnosis for *Mycobacterium tuberculosis* (Nelson et al., 1998). Testing a second respiratory specimen by RT-PCR increased the sensitivity of diagnosis for SARS CoV.

The examination of more than one respiratory specimen is necessary to maximize the sensitivity of RT-PCR assays for SARS CoV. As molecular characterization of this novel CoV is ongoing, targeting genomic segments of the virus for diagnostic application is still unclear. Amplification of a second genome region may further increase test specificity. In this study, the high specificity and concordance of both RT-PCR assays verified that the amplified genomic segments for both protocols are suitable for diagnostic application. Incorporation of internal probe hybridization will probably increase the sensitivity of the WHO-HKU RT-PCR assay. In this global outbreak of SARS, prompt communication and exchange of information among the WHO collaborating laboratories facilitate development of rapid diagnostic assays with shortened turnaround time. The availability of the protocols on the WHO website was helpful to diagnostic laboratories. The collaborative approach can be invaluable in our efforts to understand and control emerging pathogens in the future.

## Acknowledgments

We thank Christian Drosten of the Bernhard-Nocht Institute (Hamburg, Germany) and TIB-MOLBIOL (Hamburg, Germany) for providing DNA primers used in the WHO-Hamburg RT-PCR protocol. We also thank the staff of the Department of Microbiology, Queen Mary Hospital, The University of Hong Kong for their technical assistance.

## NOVEL BIOSENSOR FOR INFECTIOUS DISEASE DIAGNOSTICS

*Rangarajan Sampath and David J. Ecker*
Ibis Therapeutics, a division of Isis Pharmaceuticals

We describe a novel approach for surveillance of emerging infectious diseases that can be used for rapid and broad identification of infectious disease causative agents. The premise of our technology is that we can provide rapid, sensitive, and cost-effective detection of a broad range of "normal" pathogenic organisms and simultaneously also diagnose disease caused by a biological weapon or an unexpected emerging infectious organism. This broad-function technology may be the only practical way to rapidly diagnose diseases caused by a bioterrorist attack or emerging infectious diseases that otherwise might be missed or mistaken for a more common infection.

According to a recent review (Taylor et al., 2001), more than 1,400 organisms are infectious to humans. These numbers do not include numerous strain variants of each organism, bioengineered versions, or pathogens that infect plants or animals. Paradoxically, most of the new technology being developed for detection of infectious agents incorporates a version of quantitative PCR, which is based on the use of highly specific primers and probes designed to selectively detect specific pathogenic organisms. This approach requires assumptions about the type and strain of bacteria or virus. Experience has shown that it is very difficult to anticipate where the next emerging infectious agent might come from, as was the case with the outbreak of SARS early in 2003. An alternative to single-agent tests is to do broad-range consensus priming of a gene target conserved across groups of organisms (Kroes et al., 1999; Oberste et al., 2000, 2001, 2003). The drawback of this approach for unknown agent detection and epidemiology is that analysis of the PCR products requires the cloning and sequencing of hundreds to thousands of colonies per sample, which is impractical to perform rapidly or on a large number of samples. New approaches to the parallel detection of multiple infectious agents include multiplexed PCR methods (Brito et al., 2003; Fout et al., 2003) and microarray strategies (Wang et al., 2002, 2003; Wilson et al., 2002). Microarray strategies are promising because undiscovered organisms might be detected by hybridization to probes on the array that were designed to bind conserved regions of previously known families of bacteria and viruses.

Here we present an alternative, a universal pathogen-sensing approach for high-throughput detection of infectious organisms that is capable of identifying previously undiscovered organisms (see Figure 4-1).

Our strategy is based on the principle that, despite the enormous diversity of microbes, all forms of life on earth share sets of essential common features in the biomolecules encoded in their genomes. Bacteria, for example, have highly conserved sequences in a variety of locations on their genomes. Most notable is the universally conserved region of the ribosome, but there are also conserved elements in other noncoding RNAs, including RNAse P and the signal recognition particle, among others. There are also conserved motifs in essential protein-encoding genes, in bacteria as well as viruses. Use of such broad-range priming targets across the broadest possible grouping of organisms for PCR, followed by electrospray ionization mass spectrometry for accurate mass measurement, enables us to determine the base composition (numbers of A, G, C, and T nucleotides) of the PCR amplicons. The measured base compositions from strategically selected locations of the genome are used as a signature to identify and distinguish the organisms present in the original sample. An important feature of the primer design strategy used in our approach is the positioning of propynylated

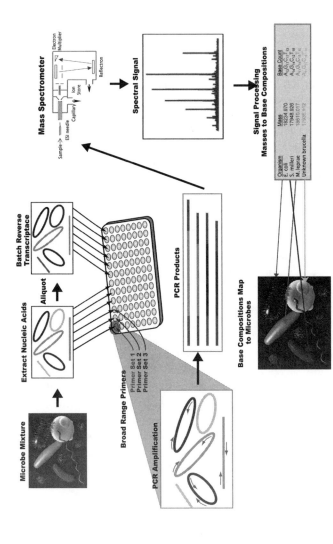

**FIGURE 4-1** Overview of the universal pathogen sensor for the detection of a diverse mixture of microbial organisms present in a sample. Genomic DNA, or cDNA obtained by batch reverse-transcription of RNA, from each sample are amplified using broad range PCR primers to generate a complex mixture of PCR products. This mixture of DNA is directly sprayed into a mass spectrometer that essentially weighs each intact nucleic acid strand in the mixture at the same time, This measurement is done at high mass accuracy, which enables us to calculate the exact number of A's, C's, G's, and T's that make up the DNA in our sample. This count serves as a base-composition fingerprint that can be mapped back to specific organisms. Examination of multiple base-count fingerprints for each organism generated by multiple pairs of broad-range primers to conserved sites distributed across the microbial genome (not shown) allows discrimination of microbial species and subspecies with great accuracy.

nucleotides (5-propynyl deoxy-cytidine and deoxy-thymidine) at highly conserved sequence positions that enables priming of short consensus regions and significantly increases the extent to which broad groups of organisms can be amplified (Barnes and Turner, 2001a,b; Wagner et al., 1993). Furthermore, we use multiple target sites spread across different parts of the genome to add further resolution and lower the risk of missed detections.

A key to the development of a practical broad priming technology is the ability to characterize signals produced by infectious organisms in the milieu of the background that might have an excess of harmless organisms. While cloning and exhaustively sequencing many colonies can solve this, this cannot be done in a rapid diagnostic device. Our strategic breakthrough was the use of mass spectrometry to analyze the products of broad-range PCR. Mass spectrometry is remarkably sensitive and can measure the weight and determine the base composition from small quantities of nucleic acids in a complex mixture with a throughput of about a sample per minute. The ability to detect and determine the base composition of a large number of PCR amplicons in a mixed sample enables analysis and identification of broad-range PCR products essentially instantaneously. In contrast to cloning and sequencing, the information product of the mass spectrometer is base composition. While the base composition of a gene fragment is not as information rich as the sequence, a base-composition signature can be thought of as a unique index of a specific gene in a specific organism. Our detection algorithm searches a database to link each sequence for a particular organism to a composition signature so that the presence of the organism can be inferred from the presence of the signature.

During the SARS epidemic outbreak in early 2003, we demonstrated that the above-described paradigm of identification of microbial nucleic acid signatures by mass spectrometry could be adapted to identify the SARS virus. In the absence of a SARS genome sequence at the onset of the epidemic, pairs of broad primers that were designed to broadly target all other known coronaviruses were used to test clinical isolates obtained from the Centers for Disease Control and Prevention (CDC). We showed that the SARS virus potentially could be identified directly from a patient sample, obviating the need for time-consuming viral culture. We further showed that this method could distinguish between SARS and other known coronaviruses, including the human coronaviruses 229E and OC43. While direct comparisons of sensitivity, using actual patient samples, have yet to be conducted between this and other methods employed to detect SARS, we did show, using titred SARS virus spiked into human serum, that we could obtain PCR sensitivities of <1 PFU, which is consistent with our previous experience. The details of the above study will be published elsewhere (Sampath et al., under preparation).

One of the limitations of our approach is that base compositions, like sequences, vary slightly from isolate to isolate within species. We have shown that it is possible to manage this diversity by building probability "clouds" around the composition constraints for each species. This permits identification of organisms in a fashion similar to sequence analysis, albeit with somewhat lower resolution. It is counterintuitive that base composition has sufficient resolving power to distinguish organisms (one might suspect that sequences from different organisms will degenerate to similar overlapping compositions). A rigorous mathematical analysis has shown, however, that base composition retains more than sufficient information to solve the problem, provided the target sequences are strategically selected. It is important to note that, in contrast to probe-based techniques, mass spectrometry determination of base composition does not require prior knowledge of the composition in order to make the measurement, only to interpret the results. In this regard, our strategy is like DNA sequencing and phylogenetic analysis, but at lower resolution. However, the resolution provided by this analysis is more than sufficient for most rapid diagnostic applications such as identification of any organism, or to classify organisms into known phylogenetic groupings (Sampath et al., under preparation).

We envision developing applications where human clinical samples can be analyzed for diagnostically relevant levels of disease-causing agents and biological weapons simultaneously. We envision that the technology will be used in reference labs, hospitals, and the laboratory response network (LRN) laboratories of the public health system in a coordinated fashion with the ability to report the results via a computer network to a common data-monitoring center in real time. Clonal propagation of specific infectious agents, as occurs in the epidemic outbreak of infectious disease, can be tracked with base composition signatures, analogous to the pulse field gel electrophoresis fingerprinting patterns used in tracking the spread of specific food pathogens in the CDC Pulse Net system (Swaminathan et al., 2001). Effectively, our technology provides a digital barcode in the form of a series of base composition signatures, the combination of which is unique for each organism. This capability enables real-time infectious disease monitoring across broad geographic locations, which may be essential in a simultaneous outbreak or attack in different cities.

## Acknowledgments

This methodology described is being developed jointly by Ibis and Science Applications International Corporation (SAIC) under a Defense Advanced Research Projects Agency (DARPA) sponsored program known as TIGER. A detailed description of the technology will be published separately. More than 25 key participants who contributed significantly to the development and implementation of various aspects of the technology are not listed individually by name.

## *IN VITRO* ANTIVIRAL ACTIVITY OF HUMAN RHINOVIRUS 3C PROTEASE INHIBITORS AGAINST THE SARS CORONAVIRUS

*David A. Matthews,[1] Amy K. Patick,[1] Robert O. Baker,[2] Mary A. Brothers,[1] Peter S. Dragovich,[1] Chris J. Hartmann,[2] Theodore O. Johnson,[1] Eric M. Mucker,[2] Siegfried H. Reich,[1] Paul A. Rejto,[1] Peter W. Rose,[1] Susan H. Zwiers,[2] and John W. Huggins[2,3]*

The construction of a homology model of the 3C-like (3CL) protease derived from the SARS coronavirus (SCoV) is described. This model is used to qualitatively evaluate the potential for several Michael acceptor-containing human rhinovirus 3C protease inhibitors to also disrupt the function of the SCoV 3CL enzyme. The antiviral activity of three such compounds (AG7088, AG7404, and AG7122) determined against SCoV in cell culture is reported (see Figure 4-2). The former two molecules fail to inhibit in vitro replication of SCoV up to the highest concentrations tested (100 µg/mL) while AG7122 exhibits measurable antiviral activity against SCoV that is distinguishable from cytotoxicity ($EC_{50}$ = 14.1 µg/mL, $CC_{50}$ >100 µg/mL).

Severe acute respiratory syndrome (SARS) is a potentially serious global health concern and the disease has been responsible for considerable negative economic impact in affected regions (Poutanen et al., 2003; Tsang et al., 2003). A newly discovered coronavirus (SCoV) has been strongly implicated as the causative agent of SARS by independent research conducted at several laboratories around the world (Drosten et al., 2003; Fouchier et al., 2003; Ksiazek et al., 2003; Lee et al., 2003; Peiris et al., 2003a). Recently, sequencing and analysis of the SARS virus genome has led to the identification of gene products that may be critical for viral replication (Marra et al., 2003; Rota et al., 2003). In particular, such analysis suggests that the SARS pathogen, like other known coronaviruses (Ziebuhr et al., 2000), encodes a critical enzyme that is required for C-proximal processing of two overlapping polyproteins produced by cellular translation of the viral RNA. This coronavirus enzyme has been termed a "3C-like" (3CL) protease due to numerous similarities with the well-known picornavirus 3C proteases including substrate preferences, particularly the requirement of a $P_1$ glutamine residue, and the use of cysteine as an active site nucleophile during catalysis (Hegyi and Ziebuhr, 2002; Ziebuhr et al., 2000). In addition, the coronavirus 3CL and picornavirus 3C proteins share a similar polypeptide fold, as evidenced by comparison of the crystal structure of the 3CL protease derived from porcine transmissible gastroenteritis coronavirus (Anand et al., 2002) with

[1]Pfizer Global Research and Development.
[2]Viral Therapeutics Branch, Virology Division, USAMRIID.
[3]We thank Drs. Catherine Laughlin, Christopher Tseng, and Jack Secrist (NIAID/NIH) for facilitating the in vitro evaluation of Pfizer compounds against SCoV.

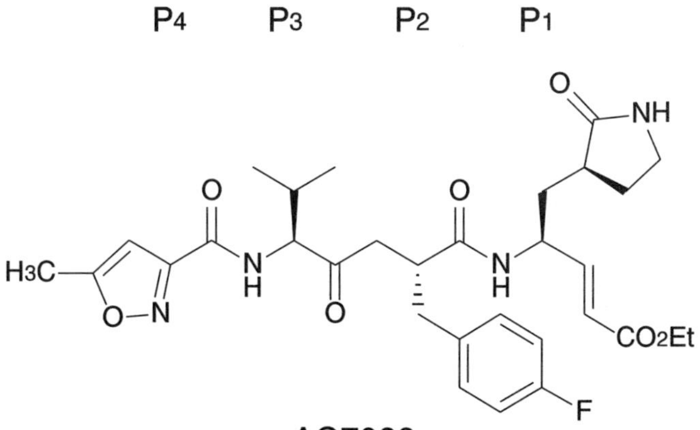


AG7088

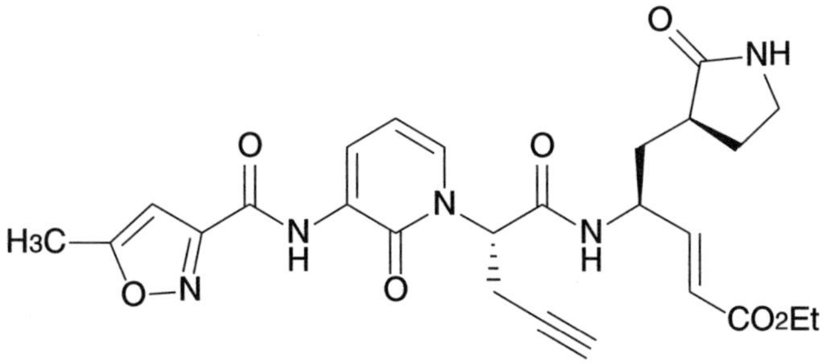

AG7404

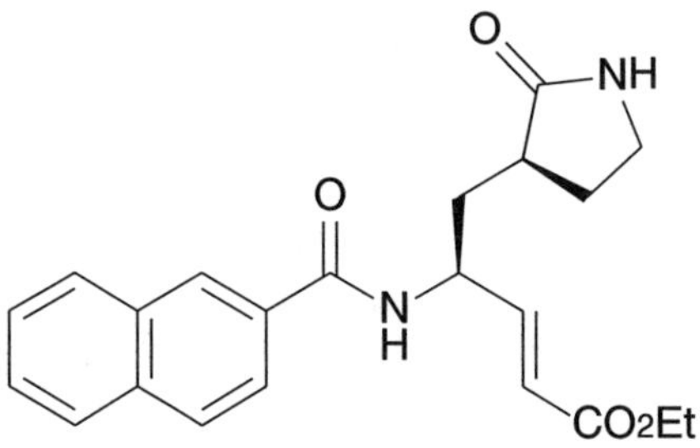

AG7122

**FIGURE 4-2** Compounds tested in cell culture for antiviral activity against SCoV.

those of corresponding picornaviral 3C enzymes (e.g., human rhinovirus 3C protease [HRV 3CP]) (Matthews et al., 1999).

The structural and functional homologies noted above between the coronavirus 3CL and picornavirus 3C enzymes were apparent (Anand et al., 2002) before the relationship between SARS and its causative agent was disclosed. Coincident with the announcement that a new coronavirus causes SARS and prior to publication of the SARS virus genome, we initiated a computational study to explore whether Michael acceptor-containing HRV 3CP inhibitors (discovered during our previous efforts to identify antirhinoviral therapeutic agents [Matthews et al., 1999]) might also bind to coronavirus 3CL proteases. The availability of the SCoV genetic sequence (Fouchier et al., 2003; Marra et al., 2003; Rota et al., 2003) enabled us to further extend these studies using a proprietary homology model of the SARS 3CL enzyme. Recently, Anand et al. (2002) disclosed an independent computational evaluation of several known picornaviral 3C protease inhibitors against SARS 3CL and reported that, although such molecules were not necessarily optimized, they could serve as starting points for the design of new SARS antiviral agents. In this communication, we report an alternate computational assessment of the potential for several Pfizer compounds to inhibit SARS 3CL along with their experimentally determined antiviral activities against SCoV in cell culture.

Our homology model for SARS 3CL protease was created using the atomic coordinates of TGEV 3CL protease (PDB accession code 1LVO) as a template. BLAST was employed to identify the 3CL protease from the genomic RNA sequence of SARS (AY274119). Minor adjustment to the BLAST output resulted in an alignment with high percent identity and few gaps (see Figure 4-3), and this alignment was used to create a homology model with the MODELLER package in Insight2000 (Sali and Blundell, 1993). Twelve residues with high structural conservation (see Table 4-3) were identified by visual inspection of the human rhinovirus 3C (1CQQ) and TGEV 3CL protease (1LVO) structures, as well as the SARS 3CL protease homology model. The structures were superimposed in a common reference frame by minimizing the root mean square distance (r.m.s.d.) between the backbone atoms of these residues, with r.m.s.d. < 0.6 Å (Drosten et al., 2003; Fouchier et al., 2003; Ksiazek et al., 2003; Peiris et al., 2003a).

Putative Michael acceptor-containing SARS 3CL protease inhibitors from the Pfizer chemical archive were computationally evaluated by first creating three-dimensional structures of the compounds using CORINA version 2.6 (Sadowski and Gasteiger, 1993), then employing a constrained docking approach using AGDOCK (Gehlhaar et al., 1999) to determine their binding mode to the model. The geometry of the reaction product as observed in the co-crystal structure of one such Pfizer compound (AG7088) with human rhinovirus 3C protease (Matthews et al., 1999) (PDB accession code 1CQQ) was used as a template to model the covalent binding of Michael acceptors with the active site cysteine of SARS 3CL protease (see Figure 4-4). The Michael acceptor portions of the in-

```
1LVO (1)     SGLRKMAQPSGLVEPCIVRVSYGNNVLNGLWLGDEVICPRHVIAS-DTTRVI
SARS (1)     SGFRKMAFPSGKVEGCMVQVTCGTTTLNGLWLDDTVYCPRHVICTAEDMLNP

1LVO (52)    NYENEMSSVRLHNFSVSKNNVFLGVVSARYKGVNLVLKVNQVNPNTPEHKFK
SARS (53)    NYEDLLIRKSNHSFLVQAGNVQLRVIGHSMQNCLLRLKVDTSNPKTPKYKFV

1LVO (104)   SIKAGESFNILACYEGCPGSVYGVNMRSQGTIKGSFIAGTCGSVGYVLENGI
SARS (105)   RIQPGQTFSVLACYNGSPSGVYQCAMRPNHTIKGSFLNGSCGSVGFNIDYDC

1LVO (156)   LYFVYMHHLELGNGSHVGSNFEGEMYGGYEDQPSMQLEGTNVMSSDNVVAFL
SARS (157)   VSFCYMHHMELPTGVHAGTDLEGKFYGPFVDRQTAQAAGTDTTITLNVLAWL

1LVO (208)   YAALINGERWFVTNTSMSLESYNTWAKTNSFTELSS--TDAFSMLAAKTGQS
SARS (209)   YAAVINGDRWFLNRFTTTLNDFNLVAMKYNYEPLTQDHVDILGPLSAQTGIA

1LVO (258)   VEKLLDSIVR-LNKGFGGRTILSYGSLCDEFTPTEVIRQMYGV---
SARS (261)   VLDMCAALKELLQNGMNGRTILGSTILEDEFTPFDVVRQCSGVTFQ
```

**FIGURE 4-3**  Sequence alignment between the TGEV 3CL protease (PDB accession code 1LVO) and SARS 3CL protease used to create the homology model.

hibitors were forced onto the template structure and then constrained during docking. The resulting protein-ligand interactions were qualitatively evaluated by visual inspection. The outcome of computationally docking AG7088 into the SARS 3CL homology model is also depicted (see Figure 4-4).

Of the Michael acceptor-containing HRV 3CP inhibitors examined, only two have been the subject of human clinical trials: AG7088 (rupintrivir) (Matthews et al., 1999; Patick et al., 1999) as an intranasally administered agent and AG7404 (Dragovich et al., 2003) as an orally delivered compound. Unfortunately, our computational evaluation detected relatively poor complementarity between the compounds' $P_3$ and $P_4$ substituents and SARS 3CL that resulted in numerous

**TABLE 4-3**  Residues Employed for the Superposition of Human Rhinovirus (HRV) 3C Protease and TGEV 3CL Protease Structures Along with Corresponding SARS 3CL Amino Acids

| HRV (1CQQ) | TGEV (1LVO) | SARS |
|---|---|---|
| PRO-38 | PRO-39 | PRO-39 |
| THR-39 | ARG-40 | ARG-40 |
| HIS-40 | HIS-41 | HIS-41 |
| LYS-143 | ILE-140 | LEU-141 |
| SER-144 | ALA-141 | ASN-142 |
| GLY-145 | GLY-142 | GLY-143 |
| TYR-146 | THR-143 | SER-144 |
| CYS-147 | CYS-144 | CYS-145 |
| ILE-160 | MET-161 | MET-162 |
| HIS-161 | HIS-162 | HIS-163 |
| VAL-162 | HIS-163 | HIS-164 |
| GLY-163 | LEU-164 | MET-165 |

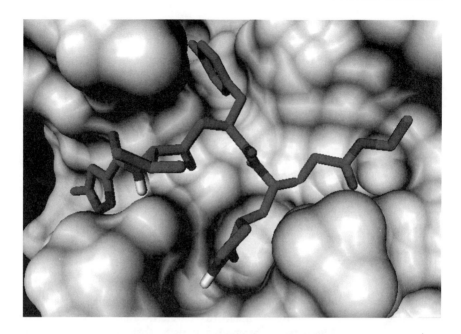

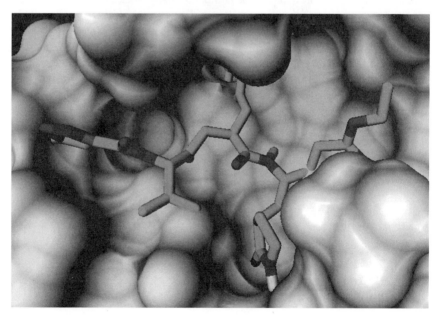

**FIGURE 4-4** Top: Co-crystal structure of AG7088 with HRV 3C protease (Connolly surface shown). Bottom: AG7088 docked into the SCoV 3CL protease homology model (Connolly surface shown).

structural clashes and several unsatisfied hydrogen bonds.[4]  These findings are in partial contrast with those reported by Anand et al. which suggest "easy accommodation" of the AG7088 $P_4$ substituent by SARS 3CL (Anand et al., 2003).  Our evaluation also indicated that a truncated compound related to AG7088 which lacks both $P_3$ and $P_4$ substituents (AG7122) interacted more favorably with the SARS 3CL protein (Johnson et al., 2002).  In order to help define the accuracy of our modeling efforts, the potential for all three molecules (AG7088, AG7404, and AG7122) to inhibit the SARS virus in cell culture was evaluated.

Stocks of tested compounds were made by dissolving them in DMSO to a concentration of 20 mg/mL.  Compounds were then diluted to 400 mg/mL in cell culture medium [high glucose Dulbeco's Modified Eagle Medium (DMEM) supplemented with 1% fetal calf serum, 10 U/mL penicillin-streptomycin, and 12.5 ng/mL fungizone], serially diluted threefold in medium, and 50 µL added to 96-well microtiter plates of confluent Vero 76 cells already containing 100 µL medium.  At each compound concentration, three wells were infected with $2 \times 10^2$ pfu/well (MOI = 0.001) of SCoV (strain 200300592) in 50 µL medium, while three were left uninfected for cytotoxicity determination (50 µl medium added to each well).  The plates were incubated at 37°C in a 5 percent $CO_2$ atmosphere, examined daily, and were stained once virus-infected, untreated cells showed maximum cytopathic effect (about 3 days).  Neutral red was added to the medium to give a final concentration of 0.22 mg/mL, and cells were returned to the incubator for 90 minutes.  The medium containing neutral red was removed, the wells were rinsed twice with buffered saline solution, and plates were decontaminated by soaking in 10 percent buffered formalin followed by a water wash.  Retained stain was solubilized by adding 100 µL of a 50 percent ethanol, 50% 0.01 M ammonium phosphate ($NH_4H_2PO_4$) (pH 3.5) solution.  The plates were incubated for 15 minutes at room temperature and the optical density (OD) of the wells at a wavelength of 450 nm was measured on a plate reader.  The data were graphed and analyzed using the four parameter-logit curve fit option of the computer program SoftMax Pro (Molecular Devices, Menlo Park, CA) to determine the 50 percent inhibitory ($EC_{50}$) and cytotoxic ($CC_{50}$) compound concentrations.

As shown in Table 4-4, both AG7088 and AG7404 failed to inhibit in vitro replication of SCoV up to the highest concentrations tested (100 mg/mL).  In contrast, AG7122 exhibited moderate but measurable inhibition of SCoV that was distinguishable from cytotoxicity (see Figure 4-5, Table 4-4).  Although these antiviral data parallel our qualitative computational evaluation of the three molecules against the SARS 3CL protease, other factors such as differing cell permeability properties may also influence the results.  We are therefore uncertain whether the poor complementarity noted in silico is responsible for the lack of

---

[4]The nomenclature used for describing the individual amino acid residues of a peptide substrate ($P_2$, $P_1$, $P_{1'}$, $P_{2'}$, etc.) and the corresponding enzyme subsites ($S_2$, $S_1$, $S_{1'}$, $S_{2'}$, etc.) is described in Schechter I, Berger A. 1967. *Biochem. Biophys. Res. Commun.* 27:157.

**TABLE 4-4**  In Vitro Antiviral Activity (EC50) and Cytotoxicity (CC50) of Pfizer Compounds Determined Against SCoV in Cell Culture

| Compound | Antiviral Activity (μg/ml) | Cytotoxicity (μg/ml) |
|----------|----------------------------|----------------------|
| AG7088 | >100 | >100 |
| AG7404 | >100 | >100 |
| AG7122 | 14.1 | >100 |

observed activity of AG7088 and AG7404 against SCoV in cell culture. While this inactivity is disappointing, the antiviral effects displayed by AG7122 encouragingly suggest that proper optimization of such Michael acceptor-containing protease inhibitors may lead to agents with improved anti-SCoV properties.[5]

Since the majority of the Michael acceptors contained in the Pfizer chemical archive are optimized against HRV 3CP, we do not anticipate that their exhaustive screening against SCoV will afford ideal therapeutic agents. However, we

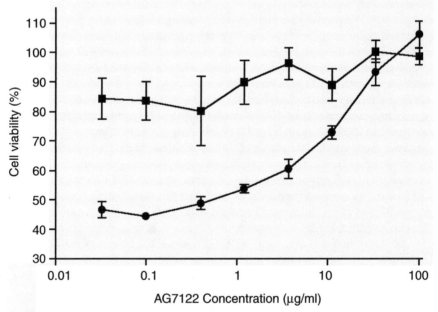

**FIGURE 4-5**  Antiviral activity of AG7122 against SCoV in Vero 76 cells. Cells were treated with the indicated compound concentrations and infected with virus (circles) or left uninfected (squares). Cell viability was measured by neutral red uptake, and is expressed as a percentage of the value in uninfected, untreated wells. Data shown are the mean of three replicate wells. Bars indicate the standard error of the mean.

---

[5]The mechanism of action by which AG7122 exerts its anti-SCoV effects has not yet been rigorously determined.

are still continuing such in vitro evaluation and have identified several additional Pfizer compounds that display improved antiviral activity ($EC_{50}$ = 1-2 µg/mL, $CC_{50}$ >100 µg/mL) relative to that exhibited by AG7122. We are currently using these molecules to help refine our SARS 3CL computational model and will report the progress of our endeavors in due course.[6]

## SARS: CLEARING THE AIR

*Jerome J. Schentag, Pharm. D.,*[7,8,9] *Charles Akers, Ph.D.,*[8]
*Pamela Campagna,*[8] *and Paul Chirayath*[8]

The integrated technologies incorporated into the FailSafe Mobile Containment Systems have a wide range of applications, including homeland security, bioterrorism, disaster management, airborne infection control, sick-building syndrome, and facility environmental service applications. The specific objective of this overview is to focus on the use of FailSafe Mobile Containment Systems for isolation precautions in a medical environment. FailSafe has not used these devices directly in an outbreak of severe acute respiratory syndrome (SARS), and thus actual clinical experience will not be reported here. Given that a major component of the spread of SARS occurs via aerosolized droplets, the systems described for clearing the air may be applicable to the containment of this new viral pathogen in hospitals and health care systems.

The guidelines for isolation precautions for hospitals and health care facilities are outlined by the Centers for Disease Control and Prevention (2004) and American Institute of Architechts (2001). These guidelines outline the precautions that infection control personnel should take to mitigate the spread of infection within facilities and protect the health care worker. Precautions must be taken to prevent the spread of infection from direct contact with contaminated surfaces (contact contamination), from large droplets of infectious material that fall out of the air, or from small droplets that can be carried by the air stream throughout the hospital (airborne contamination).

The guidelines for the creation of an isolation room are based on the principle that the isolation room is maintained under negative pressure to minimize the ability of any airborne contamination from entering the hospital. To validate the design recommendations, the precautions listed in Box 4-1 must be taken.

---

[6]The in vitro anti-SARS activity of glycyrrhizin ($EC_{50}$ = 300 µg/mL) was recently disclosed: Cinatl J, Morgenstern B, Bauer G, Chandra P, Rabenau H, Doerr HW. 2003. *Lancet* 361:2045. The precise mechanism responsible for this molecule's antiviral activity remains to be determined.

[7]University at Buffalo School of Pharmacy, Department of Pharmaceutical Sciences and Pharmacy.

[8]FailSafe Air Safety Systems Corporation.

[9]It should be noted that the author serves as a paid consultant to the FailSafe Air Safety Systems Corporation and has been involved in the development of these technologies.

---

**BOX 4-1**
**Considerations for Effective Isolation Rooms**

| | |
|---|---|
| Air flow: | Air from the hospital is to flow into the isolation room. |
| Air changes per hour (ACH) | There shall be greater than 12 ACH within the isolation room. It is preferred to pump the air from the isolation room to the outdoors. The air pump output vent must be further than 50 feet from any building air inlet vent. To augment the ACH guideline, or if outdoor venting is not possible, room air may be recirculated if the airborne particulates are filtered using an approved HEPA filter. |
| Air pressure (differential) | To ensure a negative room pressure, there should be greater than 0.01 inches of water column. It is recommended that a continuous monitor of differential air pressure be used in conjunction with an audiovisual alarm. |

---

### Failsafe Air Safety Systems Approach

FailSafe Air Safety Systems (FASS) manufactures two medical isolation units the Model 77 and the Model 07 (see Figure 4-6)—that provide personalized isolation and infection control. These medical units employ a patented air safety process that was developed in response to the lack of market availability of portable containment systems. Both the Transport Isolation Unit and the Portable Isolation Unit are equivalent in technology to an isolation room, but have the ability to bring isolation to an infected patient.

The Model 77 can be moved to an area and set up in minutes. The main components are a prefilter; an industrial, high-capacity, micro-fiberglass HEPA filter; ultraviolet lamp(s); and a high-volume blower.

The Model 07 provides isolation on wheels. At 27 inches wide, a single attendant can handle and move the unit throughout hallways and corridors. The main components are a prefilter; an industrial, high-capacity, micro-fiberglass HEPA filter; ultraviolet lamp(s); and a high-volume blower. These units are also battery powered to provide for isolation during transport.

Both of the Medical Isolation Units can be rolled to the location of a suspected infected patient, where aerosols containing SARS viruses are drawn into the system while clean air is filtered and recirculated into the air. The flexibility of the FASS Medical Isolation Units allows for a wide variety of applications:

• Immediate isolation of patients with SARS, tuberculosis, or unknown respiratory infection.

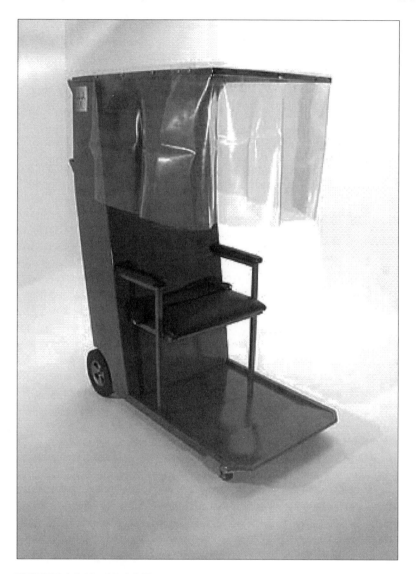

**FIGURE 4-6** The Model 07.

- Coverage during bronchoscopy or other aerosol-generating procedures.
- Removal of toxic smoke or fumes.

The FASS Medical Isolation Units offer the following benefits:

- Minimal set-up time to respond immediately to an emergency situation.

- Dual-use flexibility to provide isolation containment (negative pressure enclosure) at any place at any time.
- A system that does not alter the infrastructure within the enclosed protective area.
- A cost-effective solution to emergency isolation.
- Clean air for extended use.

## FASS Applications

The FASS Medical Isolation Units are fume hoods on wheels that combine the proven HEPA filter capacity of 99.97 percent capture at 0.1 microns with ultraviolet light. This toxic microbial capture and containment system builds on years of proven studies specifically involving *Bacillus anthracis* (anthrax) and smallpox, and can readily be applied to infection control of SARS-related incidents. These units are approved by the Food and Drug Administration (FDA) and satisfy CDC guidelines for isolation. They are the only FDA-approved portable isolation units currently on the market.

### SARS Response: Deployment Considerations

FailSafe Medical Isolation Units can be deployed in several ways as a response to a suspected SARS incident:

1. Immediate isolation and evacuation of a suspected SARS patient.
2. Transport of infected patients through crowded population (e.g., airports, train stations).
3. Transport to hospital or triage area.
4. Transport within hospital (from emergency room to SARS isolation floor).

Emergency workers can provide isolation and unrelated medical treatment to suspected SARS patients within the confines of the Medical Isolation Units while protecting caregivers and the healthy population. Bedridden patients showing symptoms of SARS can be quarantined immediately without having to be moved to another room or facility.

## System Description

Both of these FASS Isolation Units combine HEPA filtration with UVGI irradiation. The units consist of a mobile platform that allows the patient to sit in a mobile chair or a bed that is surrounded by a plastic curtain. The outside air is drawn under the curtain, across the patient, and then up into the air-purifying system that consists of a HEPA filter and a UVGI lamp, thereby reducing infectious aerosols such as tuberculosis and SARS.

The FailSafe Mobile Containment System is a patented process (U.S. Patent No. 6,162,118 [18 December 2000] entitled "Portable Isolation Device and Method") that integrates the technologies of filtration, ultraviolet germicidal irradiation, and ozone oxidation. The FailSafe process primary technology is based on high-efficiency filtration using a glass fiber HEPA filtration media that collects and traps particles greater than 0.1 micron with an efficiency greater than 99.97 percent. The filtration will collect most biological pathogens, including fungi, bacteria, and encapsulated viruses. To ensure that the pathogens collected and trapped on the HEPA filter are neutralized, the HEPA filter media surface face is illuminated with ultraviolet germicidal irradiation. Another advantage of illuminating both faces of the HEPA filter is that viruses smaller than 0.1 micron will be neutralized by irradiation.

FailSafe Mobile Containment Systems (NOT the medical Model 77 or 07 units) also incorporate ozone generation capability as a third technology. Ozone is generated with the use of ultraviolet (UV) lamps that will convert atmospheric oxygen into ozone. At concentrations below NIOSH limits, the ozone will chemically react with volatile organic compounds or odor. The FailSafe Mobile Containment Systems also have the capability of generating very high ozone levels that can be used for neutralizing pathogens on surfaces such as walls, ceilings, and floors.

## Setup and Operation

The Medical Isolation Units for health care are designed with operational simplicity to make it a "turnkey" operation and to allow health providers to focus on the individual patient and the biological contamination itself. The units are designed for easy use with three switches, and the controls are simple, as follows:

1. Power up the system. Check to see that the system is working properly and that the operation light is on. Turn the FASS system ON and select the appropriate fan speed to begin air scrubbing, treatment, and capture.
2. Identify suspected infected patient.
3. Place patient in Model 07 chair, or encompass sickbed under Model 77 unit. Place plastic curtains around patient.

### Preliminary Efficacy Testing

**Laboratory testing: FDA 510k application.** The HEPA filtration and UVGI irradiation components used in the FASS units are incorporated in Model 07 and Model 77 to protect medical personnel transporting TB and other infectious patients. Preliminary laboratory testing was performed on these units by an independent laboratory for FDA Class II certification.

## Discussion of Biological Efficacy

*Filtration*

**HEPA filters.** The safety and health protection offered by HEPA (High-Efficiency Particulate Air) filtered fume hoods has long been established by the FDA, CDC, Environmental Protection Agency (EPA), NIOSH, ASTM, and JCAHO. HEPA Filtration is the "Best Available Control Technology" at 99.99 percent at 0.3-micron efficiency level and is "Generally Accepted Control Technology" at 99.97 percent at 0.1-micron efficiency level. The added feature of the new 0.1-micron advanced filters is the "gel" seal and micro fiberglass construction that allows combining these filters with UV light disinfection. HEPA filters combined with charcoal and prefilters are the highest approved filters available for NIOSH-certified respirators. There are no adverse safety, health, or environmental aspects to HEPA filters.    HEPA filters are now the primary filtration media for electronic clean room assembly, hospital surgery rooms, bioengineering, pharmaceutical processes, and any applications where maximum reduction or removal of submicron particulates is required. Air from HEPA filters is free of 99.99 percent of all particles larger than 0.3 microns (including bacterial, fungal, and other opportunistic microbiological organisms) according to the size exclusion as described in Table 4-5.

Generally, HEPA filters belong to the "interception" family of filters and are variously referred to as "absolute" or "super interception." Such filters have a deep bed of randomly positioned fibers in which the total bed depth is very large in comparison to the average fiber diameter and effective pore or free-path cross-sectional area. Even though the media may be only 1/16 thick, this is an enormous distance compared to the 0.3- to 1.0-micron fiber diameter. The passage through which air must flow is not straight, but full of twists and turns.   As particulates impact on the fibers, they adhere. Thus the pore size becomes increasingly smaller, resulting in the filter efficacy increasing. New HEPA filters, used by FailSafe in Models 77 and 07, provide efficiency down to 0.1-micron particles at a removal efficiency of 99.97 percent.

HEPA filter bed media manufactured from glass fibers are reflective to ultraviolet irradiation, allowing the UVGI irradiation to partially penetrate the filter bed.   The result of the combination of UVGI with ozone generation and the HEPA

**TABLE 4-5** Relative Size of Fungus, Bacteria, and Viruses

| Microbe | Size Range (diameter–micron) |
| --- | --- |
| Fungus | 0.2–80 |
| Bacteria | 0.2–2.0 |
| Viruses | 0.02–0.3 |
| CDC guideline cutoff | 0.3 |
| FASS unit cutoff | 0.1 |

filter is that the bacteria, fungi, and viruses that are trapped in the filter media will be exposed to sufficient irradiation and ozone concentration to disinfect the filter. The advantage of this antimicrobial treatment combination is that the air stream is inhibited from becoming recontaminated from any growth on the filter media resulting in particle breakthrough.

*Ultraviolet*

UV irradiation can cause eye damage and surface burns on unshielded human skin, eyes, and other organs. Therefore the UV lights used in the FASS units are sealed inside and not visible to the operator or other personnel.

Ultraviolet radiation, in the wavelength range of 2,250 to 3,020 angstroms as used for air/surface disinfection and sterilization, is referred to as ultraviolet germicidal irradiation or UVGI. Ultraviolet germicidal radiation was first applied to disinfect water systems in 1909. Its use in air purification was first evaluated in the laboratory in the 1920s, in an operating room in the 1930s to sterilize the air in an operating room (Sharp, 1939), and in a school ventilation system to reduce measles infection (Riley, 1972). It is also common practice to use to disinfect medical equipment.

UVGI is currently being employed to control bacteria, fungus, and algae growth on surfaces. European breweries have been using UVGI to control microbial growth on cooling coils since 1975. The use of UVGI can control microbial growth on filter surfaces that are subject to moisture or high humidity that will allow for natural fungal growth. Figure 4-7 illustrates a filter with natural fungal growth and a filter that was irradiated with UVGI at a rated intensity of 100 micro/cm at a distance of 1m from the midpoint of the filter (Kowalski and Bahnfleth, 2000). This surface disinfection protects the air stream from being recontaminated due to bacterial, fungus, or viruses that are collected by the filter media.

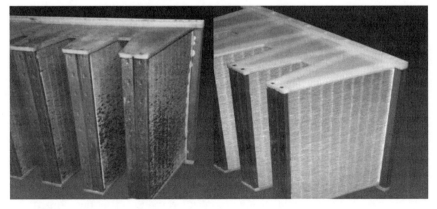

**FIGURE 4-7** (left) Microbial growth on nonirradiated filters. (right) Microbe-free UV irradiated filters (Kowalski and Bahnfleth, 2000).

*Microbial Response to Ultraviolet Radiation*

The FASS system is an integration of room recirculation to rid the air of biological threats and surface disinfection to kill the biothreat that is collected on the HEPA filters. The primary target of UV radiation is the microorganism DNA molecule with the predominant injury of strand breakage and the formation of photo-induced byproducts such as thymine diamers. This damaged DNA cannot be used for cell reproduction or for proper mRNA templates that is required for the formation of all cellular toxic products. Viruses are especially susceptible to UVGI, more so than bacteria, and are also difficult to filter because of their size. However, viruses are more susceptible to ultraviolet radiation at wavelengths slightly above the normal UVGI broadband wavelength of 253.7 nm.

Microorganisms, when exposed to UVGI irradiation, will be killed or decreased in population at a rate according to a first order equation:

$$S(t) = e^{-klt}$$

where k = standard decay-rate constant, $cm^2$/microW-s
   I = Intensity of UVGI irradiation, $microW/cm^2$
   t = time of exposure (sec)

The rate constant [k] is unique to each microorganism and defines its sensitivity of each microorganism to UVGI intensity.

The dose of ultraviolet radiation that an airborne microbe receives depends on the amount of time the microbe is being irradiated and the UV intensity. The upper limit of kill rate is obtained by mixing the air within the UVGI exposure chamber. This mixed airflow will have an average velocity that will determine the exposure time required for all microbes in the air stream. If the air is not mixed, then the flow will be partial laminar resulting in the microbes receiving different dosages of UV radiation. Microbes nearest the UV lamp will get the highest dosages and those near the wall of the chamber will have significantly less exposure to the UV radiation. Laboratory experiments can be used to determine the upper limit of Kill Rate Constant (mixed air) and lower limit of Kill Rate Constant (unmixed air).

## Ozone

Ozone, an allotropic form of oxygen, possesses unique properties when it oxidizes or interacts with chemical and biological systems. Ozone, best known for its protective role in the earth's ecological environment and its interaction with industrial pollutants, has bactericidal, virucidal, and fungicidal actions that have been used in water treatment, odor control, and medicinal applications. Ozone [$O_3$], a powerful oxidant reacting with organic molecules containing double or triple bonds, yields many complex byproducts. It is this property of ozone that has been applied as a disinfectant and sterilant against bacteria, viruses, and fungi.

Although the inhibitory and lethal effects of ozone on pathogenic organisms have been observed since the latter part of the 19th century, the mechanisms for these actions have not yet been satisfactorily highlighted. The most often cited explanation for ozone's bactericidal effects centers on disruption of envelope integrity through peroxidation of phospholipids. There is also evidence for interaction with proteins (Mudd et al., 1969). In one study (Ishizaki et al., 1987) exploring the effect of ozone on *E. coli,* investigators found cell membrane penetration with ozone, subsequent reaction with cytoplasmic substances, and conversion of the closed circular plasmid DNA to open circular DNA. It is notable that higher organisms have enzymatic mechanisms to stabilize disrupted DNA and RNA, which could provide a partial explanation for why, in clinical treatment, ozone appears to be toxic to infecting organisms and not to the patient (Cech, 1986).

Ozone possesses fungicidal effects, although the mechanism is poorly understood. In one study, *Candida utilis* cell growth inhibition with ozone was greatly dependent on phases of their growth, budding cells exhibiting the most sensitivity to its presence (Matus et al., 1981). Interestingly, low doses of ozone stimulated the growth and development of *Monilia fructagen* and *Phytophtora infestans*, while higher doses were inhibitory (Matus et al., 1982). Thus, high concentrations of ozone are required for effective antimicrobial activity.

Viruses have been studied during their interaction with ozone (Roy et al., 1981). After 30 seconds of exposure to ozone, 99 percent of the viruses were inactivated and demonstrated damage to their envelope proteins, which could result in failure of attachment to normal cells and breakage of the single-stranded RNA.

The Occupational Safety and Health Administration (OSHA) has set Public Health Air Standards of 0.1 ppm for 8 hours or 0.3 ppm for 15 minutes as the limit of the amount of ozone to which people can be safely exposed. Air cleaners based on ozone must not generate ozone levels above the Public Health Standards, which are far below any antimicrobial activity or effective odor control. Low ozone concentrations, below the EPA-acceptable indoor limit, have been used as air cleaners, but their effectiveness has been questioned by many studies (Dyas et al., 1983; Foard et al., 1997). At high ozone concentration, ozone has been used to decontaminate unoccupied spaces of some chemical and biological contaminants and odors such as smoke.

## Air Flow

The Center for Disease Control and Prevention's guidelines for air flow into an isolation room state that there shall be greater than 12 air changes per hour (ACH). However, a higher ACH means more efficiency in removing any airborne infectious materials. There are two settings on the air flow volumes. The number of ACH obtained is a function of room volume, as illustrated in Table 4-6, which is color coded based on obtaining 12 ACH as the minimal level required for meeting CDC guidelines for isolation precautions.

**TABLE 4-6** ACH as a Function of Isolation Room Volume and FASS Capabilities (calculated on a 10 percent reduction in air flow capability)

| Room Size L × W × H | Room Volume (cu ft) | FASS 700 (ACH) | FASS 1000 (ACH) | FASS 2000 (ACH) |
|---|---|---|---|---|
| 9' × 12' × 8' | 864 | 43.8 | 62.5 | 125.0 |
| 12' × 12' × 8' | 1,152 | 32.8 | 46.9 | 93.8 |
| 15' × 12' × 8' | 1,440 | 26.3 | 37.5 | 75.0 |
| 15' × 20' × 8' | 2,400 | 15.8 | 22.5 | 45.0 |
| 20' × 20' × 8' | 3,200 | 11.8 | 16.9 | 33.8 |
| 20' × 30' × 8' | 4,800 | 7.9 | 11.3 | 22.5 |
| 30' × 30' × 8' | 7,200 | 5.3 | 7.5 | 15.0 |

## Summary

The described FASS Medical Isolation Units are available in the United States, Canada, and Asia from FailSafe Air Safety Systems Corporation of Tonawanda, NY. They may offer the best opportunity to increase the numbers of isolation rooms in hospitals and especially in emergency rooms. By doing this, they provide a cost-effective solution to the challenge of new viral pathogen outbreaks. It must be emphasized that these units will only control respiratory transmissions, and are not a substitute for contact precautions or for treatment of the infection itself. Traditional measures still must be instituted to deal with surface contamination. For cleanup of biological contamination, the FASS Mobile Containment Systems also generate ozone to eradicate pathogens from surfaces. These units should be used in conjunction with the Models 77 and 07 for additional remediation of the hospital or emergency room environment.

## REFERENCES

American Institute of Architects. 2001. Guidelines for Design and Construction of Hospital and Health Care Facilities, AIA.

Anand K, Palm GJ, Mesters JR, Siddell SG, Ziebuhr J, Hilgenfeld R. 2002. Structure of coronavirus main proteinase reveals combination of a chymotrypsin fold with an extra alpha-helical domain. *EMBO Journal* 21(13):3213-24.

Anand K, Ziebuhr J, Wadhwani P, Mesters JR, Hilgenfeld R. 2003. Coronavirus main proteinase (3clpro) structure: basis for design of anti-SARS drugs. *Science* 300(5626):1763-7.

Ballew HC. 1992. Neutralization. In: Specter S, Lancz G, eds. *Clinical Virology Manual.* New York: Elsevier. Pp. 229-41.

Barnes TW 3rd, Turner DH. 2001a. C5-(1-Propynyl)-2'-deoxy-pyrimidines enhance mismatch penalties of DNA:RNA duplex formation. *Biochemistry* 40(42):12738-45.

Barnes TW 3rd, Turner DH. 2001b. Long-range cooperativity due to C5-propynylation of oligopyrimidines enhances specific recognition by uridine of ribo-adenosine over ribo-guanosine. *Journal of the American Chemical Society* 123(37):9186-7.

Brito DA, Ramirez M, de Lencastre H. 2003. Serotyping streptococcus pneumoniae by multiplex PCR. *Journal of Clinical Microbiology* 41(6):2378-84.

Centers for Disease Control and Prevention. 1994. Guidelines for preventing the transmission of mycobacterium tuberculosis in health-care facilities, 1994. *Morbidity & Mortality Weekly Report Recommendations & Reports* 43(RR-13):1-132.

Cech T. 1986. RNA as an enzyme. *Scientific American* 255(5):64-76.

Chan KH, Maldeis N, Pope W, Yup A, Ozinskas A, Gill J, Seto WH, Shortridge KF, Peiris JSM. 2002. Evaluation of the directigen FluA+B test for rapid diagnosis of influenza virus type A and B infections. *Journal of Clinical Microbiology* 40(5):1675-80.

Donnelly CA, Ghani AC, Leung GM, Hedley AJ, Fraser C, Riley S, Abu-Raddad LJ, Ho LM, Thach TQ, Chau P, Chan KP, Lam TH, Tse LY, Tsang T, Liu SH, Kong JH, Lau EM, Ferguson NM, Anderson RM. 2003. Epidemiological determinants of spread of causal agent of severe acute respiratory syndrome in Hong Kong. [Erratum Appears in *Lancet*. May 24, 2003. 361(9371):1832]. *Lancet* 361(9371):1761-6.

Dragovich PS, Prins TJ, Zhou R, Johnson TO, Hua Y, Luu HT, Sakata SK, Brown EL, Maldonado FC, Tuntland T, Lee CA, Fuhrman SA, Zalman LS, Patick AK, Matthews DA, Wu EY, Guo M, Borer BC, Nayyar NK, Moran T, Chen L, Rejto PA, Rose PW, Guzman MC, Dovalsantos EZ, Lee S, McGee K, Mohajeri M, Liese A, Tao J, Kosa MB, Liu B, Batugo MR, Gleeson JP, Wu ZP, Liu J, Meador JW 3rd, Ferre RA. 2003. Structure-based design, synthesis, and biological evaluation of irreversible human rhinovirus 3c protease inhibitors. 8. Pharmacological optimization of orally bioavailable 2-pyridone-containing peptidomimetics. *Journal of Medicinal Chemistry* 46(21):4572-85.

Drosten C, Gunther S, Preiser W, van der Werf S, Brodt HR, Becker S, Rabenau H, Panning M, Kolesnikova L, Fouchier RA, Berger A, Burguiere AM, Cinatl J, Eickmann M, Escriou N, Grywna K, Kramme S, Manuguerra JC, Muller S, Rickerts V, Sturmer M, Vieth S, Klenk HD, Osterhaus AD, Schmitz H, Doerr HW. 2003. Identification of a novel coronavirus in patients with severe acute respiratory syndrome. *New England Journal of Medicine* 348(20):1967-76.

Dyas A, Boughton BJ, Das BC. 1983. Ozone killing action against bacterial and fungal species: microbiological testing of a domestic ozone generator. *Journal of Clinical Pathology* 36:1102-4.

Foard K, van Osdell D, Steiber R. 1997. Investigation of gas-phase ozone as a potential biocide. *Applied Occupational Environmental Hygiene* 12:535-42.

Fouchier RA, Kuiken T, Schutten M, van Amerongen G, van Doornum GJ, van den Hoogen BG, Peiris M, Lim W, Stohr K, Osterhaus AD. 2003. Aetiology: Koch's postulates fulfilled for Sars virus. *Nature* 423(6937):240.

Fout GS, Martinson BC, Moyer MW, Dahling DR. 2003. A multiplex reverse transcription-Pcr method for detection of human enteric viruses in groundwater. *Applied & Environmental Microbiology* 69(6):3158-64.

Gehlhaar DK, Bouzida D, Rejto PA. 1999. Rational drug design: novel methodology and practical applications. Parrill L, Rami Reddy M, eds. Washington, DC: American Chemical Society, Pp. 292-311. ACS symposium series 719.

Hegyi A, Ziebuhr J. 2002. Conservation of substrate specificities among coronavirus main proteases. *Journal of General Virology* 83(Pt 3):595-9.

Ishizaki K, Sawadaishi D, Miura K, Shinriki N. 1987. Effect of ozone on plasmid DNA of *E. coli* in situ. *Water Research* 21(7):823-8.

Johnson TO, Hua Y, Luu HT, Brown EL, Chan F, Chu SS, Dragovich PS, Eastman BW, Ferre RA, Fuhrman SA, Hendrickson TF, Maldonado FC, Matthews DA, Meador JM, Patick AK, Reich SR, Skalitzky DJ, Worland ST, Yang M, Zalman LS. 2002. Structure-based design of a parallel synthetic array directed toward the discovery of irreversible inhibitors of human rhinovirus 3C protease. *Journal of Medicinal Chemistry* 45:2016-23.

Kowalski WJ, Bahnfleth WP. 2000. UVGI design basics for air and surface disinfection. *HPAC Engineering* 72(January):100-10.

Kroes I, Lepp PW, Relman DA. 1999. Bacterial diversity within the human subgingival crevice. *Proceedings of the National Academy of Sciences of the United States of America* 96(25):14547-52.

Ksiazek TG, Erdman D, Goldsmith CS, Zaki SR, Peret T, Emery S, Tong S, Urbani C, Comer JA, Lim W, Rollin PE, Dowell SF, Ling AE, Humphrey CD, Shieh WJ, Guarner J, Paddock CD, Rota P, Fields B, DeRisi J, Yang JY, Cox N, Hughes JM, LeDuc JW, Bellini WJ, Anderson LJ, SARS Working Group. 2003. A novel coronavirus associated with severe acute respiratory syndrome. *New England Journal of Medicine* 348(20):1953-66.

Lee N, Hui D, Wu A, Chan P, Cameron P, Joynt GM, Ahuja A, Yung MY, Leung CB, To KF, Lui SF, Szeto CC, Chung S, Sung JJ. 2003. A major outbreak of severe acute respiratory syndrome in Hong Kong. *New England Journal of Medicine* 348(20):1986-94.

Marra MA, Jones SJ, Astell CR, Holt RA, Brooks-Wilson A, Butterfield YS, Khattra J, Asano JK, Barber SA, Chan SY, Cloutier A, Coughlin SM, Freeman D, Girn N, Griffith OL, Leach SR, Mayo M, McDonald H, Montgomery SB, Pandoh PK, Petrescu AS, Robertson AG, Schein JE, Siddiqui A, Smailus DE, Stott JM, Yang GS, Plummer F, Andonov A, Artsob H, Bastien N, Bernard K, Booth TF, Bowness D, Czub M, Drebot M, Fernando L, Flick R, Garbutt M, Gray M, Grolla A, Jones S, Feldmann H, Meyers A, Kabani A, Li Y, Normand S, Stroher U, Tipples GA, Tyler S, Vogrig R, Ward D, Watson B, Brunham RC, Krajden M, Petric M, Skowronski DM, Upton C, Roper RL. 2003. The genome sequence of the SARS-associated coronavirus. *Science* 300(5624):1399-404.

Matthews DA, Dragovich PS, Webber SE, Fuhrman SA, Patick AK, Zalman LS, Hendrickson TF, Love RA, Prins TJ, Marakovits JT, Zhou R, Tikhe J, Ford CE, Meador JW, Ferre RA, Brown EL, Binford SL, Brothers MA, DeLisle DM, Worland ST. 1999. Structure-assisted design of mechanism-based irreversible inhibitors of human rhinovirus 3c protease with potent antiviral activity against multiple rhinovirus serotypes. *Proceedings of the National Academy of Sciences of the United States of America* 96(20):11000-7.

Matus V, Lyskova T, Sergienko I, Kustova A, Grigortsevich T, Konev V. 1982. Fungi: growth and sporulation after a single treatment of spores with ozone. *Mikol Fitopatot* 16(5):420-23.

Matus V, Nikava A, Prakopava Z, Konyew S. 1981. Effect of ozone on the survivability of Candida utilis cells. *Vyestsi AkadNauuk Bssr Syer Biyal Navuk* 0(3):49-52.

Mudd JB, Leavitt R, Ongun A, McManus T. 1969. Reaction of ozone with amino acids and proteins. *Atmospheric Environment* 3:669-82.

Nelson SM, Deike MA, Cartwright CP. 1998. Value of examining multiple sputum specimens in the diagnosis of pulmonary tuberculosis. *Journal of Clinical Microbiology* 36(2):467-9.

Oberste M, Schnurr D, Maher K, al-Busaidy S, Pallansch M. 2001. Molecular identification of new picornaviruses and characterization of a proposed enterovirus 73 serotype. *Journal of General Virology* 82(Pt 2):409-16.

Oberste MS, Maher K, Flemister MR, Marchetti G, Kilpatrick DR, Pallansch MA. 2000. Comparison of classic and molecular approaches for the identification of untypeable enteroviruses. *Journal of Clinical Microbiology* 38(3):1170-4.

Oberste MS, Nix WA, Kilpatrick DR, Flemister MR, Pallansch MA. 2003. Molecular epidemiology and type-specific detection of echovirus 11 isolates from the Americas, Europe, Africa, Australia, Southern Asia and the Middle East. *Virus Research* 91(2):241-8.

Patick AK, Binford SL, Brothers MA, Jackson RL, Ford CE, Diem MD, Maldonado F, Dragovich PS, Zhou R, Prins TJ, Fuhrman SA, Meador JW, Zalman LS, Matthews DA, Worland ST. 1999. In vitro antiviral activity of AG7088, a potent inhibitor of human rhinovirus 3C protease. *Antimicrobial Agents & Chemotherapy* 43(10):2444-50.

Peiris JS, Lai ST, Poon LL, Guan Y, Yam LY, Lim W, Nicholls J, Yee WK, Yan WW, Cheung MT, Cheng VC, Chan KH, Tsang DN, Yung RW, Ng TK, Yuen KY, SARS study group. 2003a. Coronavirus as a possible cause of severe acute respiratory syndrome. *Lancet* 361(9366):1319-25.

Peiris JS, Chu CM, Cheng VC, Chan KS, Hung IF, Poon LL, Law KI, Tang BS, Hon TY, Chan CS, Chan KH, Ng JS, Zheng BJ, Ng WL, Lai RW, Guan Y, Yuen KY, HKU/UCH SARS Study Group. 2003b. Clinical progression and viral load in a community outbreak of coronavirus-associated SARS pneumonia: a prospective study. *Lancet* 361(9371):1767-72.

Poutanen SM, Low DE, Henry B, Finkelstein S, Rose D, Green K, Tellier R, Draker R, Adachi D, Ayers M, Chan AK, Skowronski DM, Salit I, Simor AE, Slutsky AS, Doyle PW, Krajden M, Petric M, Brunham RC, McGeer AJ, National Microbiology Laboratory Canada, Canadian Severe Acute Respiratory Syndrome Study Team. 2003. Identification of severe acute respiratory syndrome in Canada. *New England Journal of Medicine* 348(20):1995-2005.

Riley RL. 1972. *Airborne Infections.* New York: Macmillan.

Rota PA, Oberste MS, Monroe SS, Nix WA, Campagnoli R, Icenogle JP, Penaranda S, Bankamp B, Maher K, Chen MH, Tong S, Tamin A, Lowe L, Frace M, DeRisi JL, Chen Q, Wang D, Erdman DD, Peret TC, Burns C, Ksiazek TG, Rollin PE, Sanchez A, Liffick S, Holloway B, Limor J, McCaustland K, Olsen-Rasmussen M, Fouchier R, Gunther S, Osterhaus AD, Drosten C, Pallansch MA, Anderson LJ, Bellini WJ. 2003. Characterization of a novel coronavirus associated with severe acute respiratory syndrome. *Science* 300(5624):1394-9.

Roy D, Wong PK, Engelbrecht RS, Chian ES. 1981. Mechanism of enteroviral inactivation by ozone. *Applied Environmental Microbiology* 41:718-23.

Sadowski A, Gasteiger J. 1993. From atoms and bonds to three-dimensional atomic coordinates: automatic model builders. *Chemical Reviews* 93:2567-81.

Sali A, Blundell TL. 1993. Comparative protein modelling by satisfaction of spatial restraints. *Journal of Molecular Biology* 234(3):779-815.

Sharp G. 1939. The lethal action of short ultraviolet rays on several common pathogenic bacteria. *Journal of Bacteriology* 37:447-59.

Swaminathan B, Barrett TJ, Hunter SB, Tauxe RV, CDC PulseNet Task Force. 2001. Pulsenet: the molecular subtyping network for foodborne bacterial disease surveillance, United States. *Emerging Infectious Diseases* 7(3):382-9.

Taylor LH, Latham SM, Woolhouse ME. 2001. Risk factors for human disease emergence. *Philosophical Transactions of the Royal Society of London—Series B: Biological Sciences* 356(1411):983-9.

Tsang KW, Ho PL, Ooi GC, Yee WK, Wang T, Chan-Yeung M, Lam WK, Seto WH, Yam LY, Cheung TM, Wong PC, Lam B, Ip MS, Chan J, Yuen KY, Lai KN. 2003. A cluster of cases of severe acute respiratory syndrome in Hong Kong. *New England Journal of Medicine* 348(20):1977-85.

Vabret A, Mouthon F, Mourez T, Gouarin S, Petitjean J, Freymuth F. 2001. Direct diagnosis of human respiratory coronaviruses 229e and Oc43 by the polymerase chain reaction. *Journal of Virological Methods* 97(1-2):59-66.

Wagner RW, Matteucci MD, Lewis JG, Gutierrez AJ, Moulds C, Froehler BC. 1993. Antisense gene inhibition by oligonucleotides containing C-5 propyne pyrimidines. *Science* 260(5113):1510-3.

Wang D, Coscoy L, Zylberberg M, Avila PC, Boushey HA, Ganem D, DeRisi JL. Microarray-based detection and genotyping of viral pathogens. *Proceedings of the National Academy of Sciences of the United States of America* 99(24):15687-92.

Wang D, Urisman A, Liu YT, Springer M, Ksiazek TG, Erdman DD, Mardis ER, Hickenbotham M, Magrini V, Eldred J, Latreille JP, Wilson RK, Ganem D, DeRisi JL. 2003. Viral discovery and sequence recovery using DNA microarrays. *PLOS Biology* 1(2):257.

Wilson KH, Wilson WJ, Radosevich JL, DeSantis TZ, Viswanathan VS, Kuczmarski TA, Andersen GL. 2002. High-density microarray of small-subunit ribosomal DNA probes. *Applied & Environmental Microbiology* 68(5):2535-41.

WHO. 2003. Severe acute respiratory syndrome (SARS). *Weekly Epidemiological Record* 78(12):81-3.

Ziebuhr J, Snijder EJ, Gorbalenya AE. 2000. Virus-encoded proteinases and proteolytic processing in the Nidovirales. *Journal of General Virology* 81(Pt 4):853-79.

# 5

# Preparing for the Next Disease Outbreak

## OVERVIEW

Although it is possible that the future will bring a more contagious, deadly form of SARS, it is certain to bring influenza and other infectious diseases, some of which may be introduced intentionally. Recognizing that it would be impossible to address the vast array of potential microbial threats individually, public health policy makers are formulating strategies to evaluate and respond to outbreaks of all kinds. Lessons learned from the recent SARS epidemic regarding surveillance and containment were described in earlier chapters; this chapter will discuss additional strategic issues, including anticipating the confluent threats of SARS and influenza, understanding the epidemiological factors that are likely to shape future epidemics, and ensuring that public health institutions and legal frameworks are appropriately designed for responding to any new outbreaks.

Like SARS and influenza, many of the microbial pathogens to come are likely to be viral zoonoses. The paper by Richard Webby and Robert Webster in this chapter argues that the trends that ushered SARS into the human population are in fact similar to those seen over a century of influenza outbreaks. As with SARS, livestock and poultry markets provide a breeding ground for influenza outbreaks, and laboratory sources appear to have sparked at least one epidemic. Although recent severe outbreaks of avian influenza have not featured viral transmission between humans, it may be only a matter of time until a highly contagious flu, such as the strain that is estimated to have caused over 20 million and perhaps as many as 40 million deaths in 1918–1919, confronts the world.

In the case of influenza, in which the virus can be anticipated to some extent, vaccines and antiviral therapies can play a significant role in containing an epidemic. **However, strategic actions recommended against influenza that could also inform efforts to better prepare for other viral disease outbreaks have yet to be implemented. These strategies include:[1]**

- **stockpiling of broad-spectrum antiviral drugs,**
- **advanced development of pandemic strain vaccines,**
- **the establishment of surge capacity for rapid vaccine production, and**
- **the development of models to determine the most effective means of delivering therapies during an outbreak.**

It is evident from the experience of the late 2003 influenza season that our supply and effectiveness of antiviral drugs, capabilities to accurately predict the best viral strain for annual vaccine production, and mechanisms for surge capacity production remain inadequate (Treanor, 2004). Recognition of these vulnerabilities led numerous workshop participants to call for greater scientific and financial investments to strengthen our defenses against these certain future threats.

However, most emerging infections other than influenza will represent a truly novel threat for which the world is inadequately prepared. In these cases, models based on detailed observations from previous epidemics can be used to predict demands on hospital capacity during a hypothetical epidemic and to guide the timing and nature of quarantine measures. Two papers in this chapter (Amirfar et al. and Kimball et al.) examine the modeling strategies that have been used for analyzing public health responses to epidemics as well as the particular challenges that SARS presented for international disease surveillance and alert networks. As with other public health measures, these strategies are potentially applicable not just to SARS but to any future outbreaks in which appropriate actions to protect the public's health must be taken swiftly (and possibly even before the complete clinical profile of the new disease and the etiological agent behind it are fully understood).

When containment measures such as quarantines must be put in place, establishing the trust of the public is crucial to their effectiveness. Social cohesion and compliance with SARS quarantine in Toronto, for example, have been attributed in part to a combination of clear communication and practical guidance by public health authorities. In the extreme case of mandatory quarantine, enforcement requires careful planning and a clear understanding of public health law. This is particularly true in the United States, where quarantine is likely to necessitate the coordination of federal, state, and local jurisdictions and legal authorities. As Gene Matthews' paper elaborates, additional legal considerations include: due process, which requires proper notice; legal representation; court-reviewed decisions; and remote communications to permit a quarantined person to be heard in

---

[1]Workshop presentation, Robert Webster, St. Jude Children's Research Hospital, October 1, 2003.

court, as well as practical contingencies such as the need for law enforcement officials to serve notice of quarantine.

As the world becomes more conscious of microbial threats to health, countries are increasingly recognizing the necessity of reporting outbreaks promptly and cooperating fully in international efforts to contain them. Indeed, if there is one piece of good news to be noted from last year's epidemic, it is the fact that— as David Heymann and Guenael Rodier observe in this chapter—an array of diagnostic and surveillance tools, coordinated strategies of containment, and international collaboration among scientists and public health authorities were in this case able to control the outbreak of SARS, even in the absence of curative drugs or vaccines. Nevertheless, last year's experiences further reinforce the lessons that HIV/AIDS, influenza, Ebola, malaria, and a host of other persistent and emerging infectious diseases have already made clear—that the health of any one nation cannot be isolated from the health of its neighbors, and that public health challenges in any locality have the potential to reverberate swiftly around the globe. Karen Monaghan's paper for the National Intelligence Council, which concludes this chapter, summarizes the continuing threat that SARS may still pose, as well as the challenges that lie ahead for attempting to contain any further deadly outbreaks of SARS or other infectious diseases in the future.

## ARE WE READY FOR PANDEMIC INFLUENZA?

*Richard J. Webby and Robert G. Webster*[2]
Division of Virology, Department of Infectious Diseases,
St. Jude Children's Research Hospital
Reprinted with permission from Webby and Webster, 2003. Copyright 2003 AAAS.

During the past year, the public has become keenly aware of the threat of emerging infectious diseases with the global spread of severe acute respiratory syndrome (SARS), the continuing threat of bioterrorism, the proliferation of West Nile virus, and the discovery of human cases of monkeypox in the United States. At the same time, an old foe has again raised its head, reminding us that our worst nightmare may not be a new one. In 2003, highly pathogenic strains of avian influenza virus, including the H5N1 and H7N7 subtypes, again crossed from birds to humans and caused fatal disease. Direct avian-to-human influenza transmission was unknown before 1997. Have we responded to these threats by better preparing for emerging disease agents, or are we continuing to act only as crises arise? Here we consider progress to date in preparedness for an influenza pan-

---

[2]We thank W. Shea for helpful advice, S. Naron for editorial assistance, and A. Blevins for illustrations. Influenza research at St. Jude Children's Research Hospital is supported by Public Health Service grant AI95357 and Cancer Center Support (CORE) grant CA–21765 from the National Institutes of Health and by the American Lebanese Syrian Associated Charities (ALSAC).

demic and review what remains to be done. We conclude by prioritizing the remaining needs and exploring the reasons for our current lack of preparedness for an influenza pandemic.

In February 2003, during a family visit to mainland China, a young girl from Hong Kong died of an unidentified respiratory illness. After returning to Hong Kong, both her father and brother were hospitalized with severe respiratory disease, which proved fatal to the father. When H5N1 (avian) influenza virus was isolated from both patients, the World Health Organization (WHO) went to pandemic alert status (WHO, 2003a). At about the same time, there were rumors of rampant influenza-like disease in China. Influenza experts feared that H5N1 influenza virus had acquired the ominous capacity to pass from human to human. That outbreak is now known to have been SARS, caused by a novel coronavirus.

In March 2003, another alarming situation arose on the other side of the world. A highly pathogenic H7N7 avian influenza outbreak had recently erupted in the poultry industry of the Netherlands (Koopmans et al., 2003), and workers involved in the slaughter of infected flocks contracted viral conjunctivitis. The H7N7 virus isolated from these patients had several disquieting features: Not only could it replicate in the human conjunctiva, but there was also evidence of human-to-human spread. Nearby herds of swine (which are often implicated in the adaptation of influenza viruses to humans) also showed serologic evidence of exposure (Koopmans et al., 2003). When a veterinarian died of respiratory infection (Abbott, 2003; Koopmans et al., 2003; Sheldon, 2003; van Kolfschooten, 2003), WHO again acknowledged the presence of a severe threat (WHO, 2003b).

Luckily, the worst-case scenarios did not come about in either of the 2003 avian influenza virus scares. However, the year's events eliminated any remaining doubts that global advance planning for pandemic influenza is necessary. They also highlighted how far, as a scientific community, we have come since the 1997 event: We are now much better equipped with technologies and reagents to rapidly identify and respond to pandemic influenza threats. On the other hand, the legislative and infrastructure changes needed to translate these advances into real public health benefits are alarmingly slow.

## The Role of WHO in Influenza Surveillance and Control

In 2001, WHO initiated the development of a Global Agenda for Influenza Surveillance and Control. Its four main objectives are to strengthen influenza surveillance, improve knowledge of the disease burden, increase vaccine use, and accelerate pandemic preparedness (Stohr, 2003). In May 2002, this document was adopted after proposals and public comment were invited. The document advocates the development of methods and reagents that can be used to rapidly identify all influenza virus subtypes, thereby allowing integrated influenza surveillance in humans and in other animals. WHO, with its global influenza network of more than 100 laboratories and its distinguished record of planning for yearly interpandemic influenza, is ideally situated to play a broader role in facilitating international cooperation for the rapid exchange of viruses, reagents, and information. Influenza continually evolves at the human–lower animal interface and thus can be unpredictable. As an example, within a brief period, the H7N7 virus events occurred in European poultry and humans, H5N1 viruses infected Asian poultry and humans, and novel, rapidly spreading reassortant viruses were isolated in swine in the United States (Olsen, 2002; Zhou et al., 1999). Therefore, the capacity to simultaneously manage multiple potential pandemic situations is important. The WHO global agenda document will help to prioritize areas of influenza research and facilitate national pandemic preparedness plans.

### Prioritization of Viral Subtypes for Surveillance and Control

Influenza experts agree that another influenza pandemic is inevitable and may be imminent (Figure 5-1). A major challenge in controlling influenza is the sheer magnitude of the animal reservoirs. It is not logistically possible to prepare reagents and vaccines against all strains of influenza encountered in animal reservoirs, and therefore, virus subtypes must be prioritized for pandemic vaccine and reagent preparation. Preliminary findings have identified the H2, H5, H6, H7, and H9 subtypes of influenza A as those most likely to be transmitted to humans. (Influenza viruses are typed according to their hemagglutinin [H] and neuraminidase [N] surface glycoproteins.) The influenza A subtypes currently circulating in humans, H1 and H3, continue to experience antigenic drift. That is, their antigenic surface glycoproteins are continually modified, allowing them to escape the population's immunity to the previous strain and thus to continue causing annual outbreaks. Although these continual modifications may lead to an increase in virulence, the mildness of the past three influenza seasons suggests that the dominance of the H1N1 and H3N2 viruses is waning as their ability to cause serious disease becomes increasingly attenuated. H2 influenza viruses are included in the high-risk category because they were the causative agent of the 1957 "Asian flu" pandemic and were the only influenza A subtype circulating in humans between 1957 and 1968. Counterparts of the 1957 H2N2 pandemic virus continue to circulate in wild and domestic duck reservoirs. Under the right conditions (which are still not completely understood), H2N2 viruses could again be transmitted to and spread among humans, none of whom under the age of 30 years now has immunity to this virus. Seroarchaeology data from the late 19th and early 20th centuries indicate that only the H1, H2, and H3 influenza virus subtypes have been successfully transmitted among humans. It is possible, but unlikely, that they are the only subtypes able to do so.

Not only are the H1, H2, and H3 influenza viruses of concern, but the H5 subtype has threatened to emerge as a human pandemic pathogen since 1997, when it killed 6 of 18 infected humans. Before that event, the receptor specificity of avian influenza viruses was thought to prevent their direct transmission to hu-

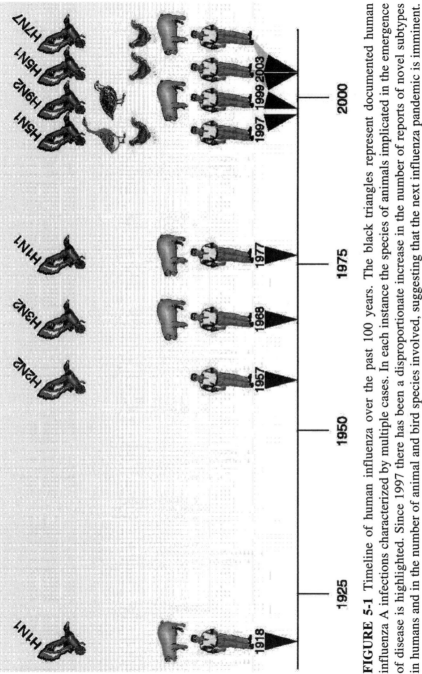

**FIGURE 5-1** Timeline of human influenza over the past 100 years. The black triangles represent documented human influenza A infections characterized by multiple cases. In each instance the species of animals implicated in the emergence of disease is highlighted. Since 1997 there has been a disproportionate increase in the number of reports of novel subtypes in humans and in the number of animal and bird species involved, suggesting that the next influenza pandemic is imminent.

mans. Transmission from aquatic birds to humans was hypothesized to require infection of an intermediate host, such as the pig, that has both human-specific ($\alpha$-6 sialic acid) and avian-specific 2-3 sialic acid) receptors on its respiratory epithelium. The 1997 H5N1 event demonstrated that domestic poultry species may also act as intermediate hosts. H5N1 viruses continue to emerge and evolve despite heroic measures taken to break their evolutionary cycle in the live poultry markets of Hong Kong: the elimination of live ducks and geese (the original source), the elimination of quail (the source of the internal genes of H5N1/97), and the institution of monthly "clean days," when all 1,000-plus retail markets are emptied and cleaned.

Two things have become clear. Live poultry markets are potential breeding grounds for influenza and other emerging disease agents, and there is an Asian source of H5N1 influenza viruses outside of Hong Kong SAR. Between 1997 and 2003, H5N1 virus was isolated from duck meat imported from China into Korea (Tumpey et al., 2002) and Japan (ProMED-mail, 2003). These observations suggest that ducks and possibly other avian species in mainland China are a reservoir of H5N1, although there have been no official reports of H5N1 virus in China.

At the beginning of the SARS outbreak, China missed an opportunity to show the world its considerable intellectual and scientific potential (Enserink, 2003a). In the case of H5N1 influenza, a pandemic in waiting, it remains to be seen whether China will show leadership in proactively addressing the problem. Concerted national and international efforts are required to deal effectively with the threat.

The third virus subtype on the most wanted list is H7. The H7 and H5 viruses have a unique ability to evolve into a form highly virulent to chickens and turkeys by acquiring additional amino acids at the hemagglutinin (HA) cleavage site (HA cleavage is required for viral infectivity) (Steinhauer, 1999). The highly pathogenic H7N7 influenza viruses that were lethal to poultry infected the eyes of more than 80 humans and killed one person (Enserink, 2003b). In the case of this outbreak, the Netherlands' policy of openness was important in reducing the potential threat and should serve as a model. When the virus was first detected at the end of February 2003, the European Community and international community, via the Office International des Epizooties, were notified so that surrounding countries, including Belgium and Germany, could immediately respond if the disease was detected. Culling of all poultry on infected farms and quarantine of surrounding farms succeeded in eradicating the virus once the etiologic agent was identified. After human infection was observed, an anti-influenza drug was given as prophylaxis, and vaccination with the current human influenza vaccine was done to reduce the likelihood that the avian virus would reassort with human H1N1 and H3N2 strains.

The remaining two viral subtypes on the priority list, H6 and H9, do not share the virulent phenotypes of the H5 and H7 viruses, but still pose a considerable threat. Both of these influenza viruses have spread from a wild aquatic bird reservoir to domestic poultry over the past 10 years. H9N2 viruses have also been detected in humans and in pigs (Peiris et al., 1999, 2001) and have acquired human-like receptor specificity (Matrosovich et al., 2001). Neither of these viruses was able to infect chickens before the mid-1980s. Now, for unknown reasons, H9 viruses are endemic in chickens in Eurasia and H6 viruses are becoming endemic in both Eurasia and the Americas. These facts highlight the continuing adaptation of influenza viruses in the aquatic bird reservoirs to domestic chickens.

## The Challenge of Developing Candidate Vaccines

If the next influenza pandemic were to begin tomorrow, inactivated vaccines would offer the only immediate means of mass prophylaxis, yet their supply is limited by inadequate production capabilities and suboptimal utilization of adjuvants (Fedson, 2003; IOM, 2003). The stocks of antiviral drugs are too low to cope with an epidemic and would be quickly depleted (IOM, 2003). Tissue culture–based and live attenuated vaccines are now licensed in some countries, and could supplement the supply of inactivated vaccine. Further development of these options is urgently needed to provide alternative substrates in the face of a pandemic.

Since the 1970s, influenza vaccines have been made by exploiting the tendency of the segmented influenza genome to reassort (Wood and Williams, 1998). This natural process has been used to produce vaccine strains that simultaneously contain gene segments that allow them to grow well in eggs and gene segments that produce the desired antigenicity. Natural reassortment is allowed to occur in embryonated chicken eggs, and reassortants with the desired characteristics are selected. These recombinant vaccine strains contain the hemagglutinin and neuraminidase genes of the target virus (encoding glycoproteins that induce neutralizing antibodies); their remaining six gene segments come from A/Puerto Rico/8/34 (H1N1), which replicates well in eggs and is safe for use in humans (Kilbourne, 1969). These "6+2" reassortants are then grown in large quantities in embryonated chicken eggs, inactivated, disrupted into subunits, and formulated for use as vaccines. Although this process creates an effective and safe influenza vaccine, it is too time-consuming and too dependent on a steady supply of eggs to be reliable in the face of a pandemic emergency. Even during interpandemic periods, 6 months is required to organize sufficient fertile chicken eggs for annual vaccine manufacture (Gerdil, 2003), and the preparation of the desired "6+2" recombinant vaccine strain can be a time-consuming process. Influenza vaccine preparation is seasonal and is a remarkable achievement, in that an essentially new vaccine is made every year. However, two of the viruses of greatest concern, those of the highly pathogenic H5 and H7 subtypes, cannot be successfully grown in eggs. Their unique ability to accumulate multiple basic amino acids at the site of hemagglutinin cleavage increases their ability to spread systemically in an infected host and cause significant disease (Steinhauer, 1999). This feature also renders H5 and H7 viruses rapidly lethal to chicken embryos.

The most promising means of expediting the response to pandemic influenza is the use of plasmid-based reverse genetic systems to construct influenza virions and vaccines. These systems also offer a successful alternative means of producing H5 and H7 vaccine seed strains. Because viable viruses can be generated from individually cloned cDNA copies of each of the eight viral RNA segments, reassortment can be prospectively defined and directed, and the extra amino acids at the HA cleavage site (which are associated with high virulence) can be removed to allow rapid generation of a vaccine seed strain in eggs. Plasmids encoding the internal genes of the base vaccine are already available. A vaccine seed strain can be created by cloning the appropriate hemagglutinin and neuraminidase genes from the target virus, altering its HA connecting peptide if necessary, and transfecting an appropriate cell line (see Figure 5-2). This technology has been shown to be effective for the production of reassortants carrying several different surface glycoprotein combinations, including those considered to have a high pandemic potential (Hoffman et al., 2002; Liu et al., 2003; Schickli et al., 2003; Subbarao et al., 2003). The next step is to take these plasmid-derived influenza vaccines through clinical trials to address crucial questions such as number and quantity of doses and the role of adjuvants. Most of the vaccines derived after the 1997 H5N1 episode by various alternative strategies induced a disappointing immune response (Wood, 2001). The optimal pandemic vaccination regimens can be anticipated only by collecting the necessary data and experience through clinical trials of vaccines against different subtypes of influenza virus.

Although they are well suited to the manufacture of inactivated influenza vaccines, reverse genetic systems introduce new variables. One of the most limiting of these is the need to use cell lines. There are surprisingly few suitable accredited cell lines and cell banks available, and many of those are the property of pharmaceutical companies. The practical options are very few, in view of the technical and regulatory restrictions. Perhaps the only cell line that meets all criteria for international use at this time is the African green monkey kidney cell line, Vero. However, although Vero cell lines are in widespread laboratory use, only those that are derived from WHO-approved sources and have a detailed history are acceptable for manufacture of human pharmaceuticals. A second new variable is the use of a genetically modified virus seed strain. Because the traditional vaccine strains are made by natural reassortment, they have escaped being labeled "genetically modified." This difference, although largely semantic, may affect the acceptance of the new vaccines. Before many of these traits can be tested, the virus must be amplified, inactivated, purified, and formulated for vaccine use (Gerdil, 2003).

In preparing for a pandemic threat, collaboration between government, industry, and academia is needed to overcome the obstacles and guarantee the most rapid production of a vaccine candidate. The recent SARS episode has shown that international collaboration in the face of a truly global threat is indeed possible.

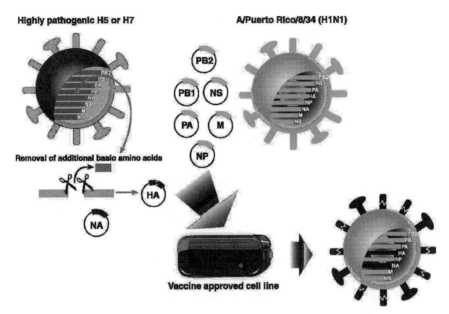

**FIGURE 5-2** Proposed method of influenza vaccine seed virus production using the eight-plasmid reverse genetics system (Hoffman et al., 2002). The hemagglutinin (HA) and neuraminidase (NA) genes from the target strain are cloned into the bacterial plasmid vector pHW2000 in a process that allows for the alteration of the HA cleavage site when necessary (see text for explanation). These two plasmids, along with six others containing the remaining influenza A gene segments derived from the master vaccine strain A/Puerto Rico/8/34 (H1N1), are then introduced into a suitable cell line (e.g., Vero). After expression of positive- and negative-sense RNA and viral proteins from these plasmids, a productive replication cycle is initiated and viable virus particles are produced.

## The Safety Testing of Candidate Pandemic Vaccines and Liability Issues

Unfortunately, there are only a few facilities available to carry out safety testing under the high-level biocontainment conditions required for handling highly pathogenic influenza viruses. Overcoming the technical hurdles to efficient vaccine production is only the start of a long, expensive process. Manufacturing scale-up presents its own problems, not least because plant workers will have no immunity to the pathogens they will be handling. Of prime importance is vaccine safety testing, but the need for safety testing will have to be balanced against the need for rapid mass production of a vaccine. In response to the 2003 H5N1 scare in Hong Kong, WHO has created an Interim Biosafety Risk Assessment (WHO Global Influenza Programme, in press) guideline for the safety testing of pandemic vaccines, particularly the H5 and H7 subtypes, signifying a substantial advance in preparedness for the production of a pandemic influenza vaccine.

A major risk for all vaccine manufacturers is the occurrence of adverse reactions in a percentage of recipients. These reactions may be attributable to the vaccine, to the host, or (most likely) to a unique combination of the vaccine and the host genetic factors. Guillain-Barré syndrome in human beings first became apparent during the U.S. swine influenza vaccination program (Roscelli et al., 1991; Safranek et al., 1991). The inevitability of adverse reactions underscores the product liability dilemma inherent in any vaccine program. The risk of devastating financial liability, and the unavailability or high cost of liability insurance, are increasingly discouraging vaccine manufacture, especially for universal use.

Legislative measures can be taken to reduce the impact of liability exposure. For example, the U.S. Congress passed the National Childhood Injury Compensation Act of 1986 (the "Vaccine Act"), which created a no-fault compensation program funded by an excise tax on vaccines. Plaintiffs need only establish that their injuries were caused by the vaccine. Claimants who are not satisfied with the administrative decision may still elect to sue the manufacturer, but the legal arguments available to the claimant are limited. Although the Vaccine Act represents progress in achieving a balance between consumer and manufacturer concerns, it would not apply to vaccines given to the general population, such as those for influenza or smallpox. Congress again attempted to address these concerns in a provision of the Homeland Security Act of 2002, and an Institute of Medicine panel is currently wrestling with the problem as well; however, drug manufacturers remain hesitant. The bottom line is that unless the government authorities of every country implement mechanisms that equitably limit vaccine liability, no prospective vaccine for H5N1, H7N7, or any other threatening influenza virus is likely to be produced for universal human use. It is hoped that governments will rise to the occasion after a crisis emerges, but logic suggests that the issue should be addressed now.

## Antiviral Drugs

A global influenza strategy would call for the stockpiling of influenza antiviral drugs for use in the event of a pandemic until vaccines can be prepared. "But," as noted by Albert Osterhaus (Abbott, 2003b), "no country has yet started to stockpile antiviral drugs." The potential value of antivirals was demonstrated in the recent H7N7 outbreak in poultry and humans. Further, because epidemiological modeling has suggested that it is more infectious than SARS (Ferguson et al., 2003; Lipsitch et al., 2003; Riley et al., 2003), influenza is unlikely to be controllable by SARS-like quarantine measures. The estimated US$ 10 billion cost of SARS and the societal disruption it caused in China and Toronto make a compelling case for stockpiling of antiviral drugs.

Pandemic influenza has already threatened twice in 2003. The events associated with these outbreaks show that we are in a much better position to rapidly respond to an influenza threat than we were in 1997; however, much remains to be accomplished. Overall, our state of preparedness is far from optimal.

## Priorities to Ensure Pandemic Preparedness

To conclude, let us revisit our concern that the next influenza pandemic alert may involve a virus that has acquired the capacity to spread from human to human. What are our most urgent needs?

1. A sufficiently large supply of anti-influenza drugs to reduce the severity and spread of infection. Specific efficacious drugs are available, but no country has yet invested in stockpiling.

2. A vaccine matching the subtype of the emerging pandemic influenza strain that has been tested in clinical trials and for which manufacturers are prepared to "scale up" production. Such a vaccine would probably not match the emerging strain antigenically and would not prevent infection, but it could reduce the severity of illness until a matching vaccine is produced. Such vaccines have been discussed for 20 years. None is available, but specific plans to produce such a vaccine are currently being formulated.

3. The preparation, testing (safety and clinical trials), and availability of a vaccine derived by reverse genetics. The scientific technology is in place to achieve this goal, but manufacturing, intellectual property, and liability issues remain unresolved. In the event of a pandemic, reverse genetics would be the most rapid means by which to produce an antigenically matched vaccine. To be truly prepared, such a vaccine needs to be produced and tested now to identify and resolve the issues, rather than doing so in direct response to an emergency.

4. An improvement in the global influenza vaccine manufacturing capacity. Without the use of adjuvants, the current capacity is inadequate and could not be quickly augmented. The country best prepared to meet this need is Canada; in Ontario, influenza vaccination is recommended and available at no charge to people of all ages during the influenza season (Schabas, 2001). This progressive strategy during interpandemic years will ensure the vaccine-manufacturing capacity of that region.

The conclusion of this analysis is inescapable: The world will be in deep trouble if the impending influenza pandemic strikes this week, this month, or even this year. It is now time to progress from talking about pandemic vaccines to taking action. Our hope is that the "Ontario experiment" will inspire other regions of the world to similarly promote the expansion of manufacturing capacity for influenza vaccines.

Although reverse genetics offers great advantages for the rapid preparation of influenza vaccine strains and for understanding pathogenesis (Hatta et al., 2001), the reverse side of this benefit is its potential for the development of bioterrorism agents (Krug, 2003). Regardless of human endeavors, nature's ongoing experiments with H5N1 influenza in Asia and H7N7 in Europe may be the greatest bioterror threat of all. The time for talking is truly over. We must be prepared.

## MODELING A RESPONSE STRATEGY

*Sam Amirfar, M.D., Mary Koshy, M.P.A., and Nathaniel Hupert, M.D., M.P.H.*
Department of Public Health, Weill Medical College of Cornell University

Containment of the 2002–2003 severe acute respiratory syndrome (SARS) epidemic posed unprecedented challenges to health care delivery and public health systems worldwide. In addition to the human costs of infection in medical workers, efforts to contain the spread of the virus led to widespread disruptions in the provision of routine medical care. Response strategies for potential recurrences of SARS will need to address treatment of infected individuals, quarantine of potential victims, and health system action plans that lead to containment of the outbreak without undue impact on the delivery of care for the wider populace. Since the outbreak of SARS, several computational models have been developed to investigate the transmission dynamics of the SARS coronavirus. Although these studies have identified certain parameters (e.g., maximum allowable delay in quarantining new cases) that may lead to more efficient management of new outbreaks, further research is needed to better define the practical steps required for such optimized response strategies. This chapter summarizes the current state of theoretical modeling for SARS and proposes a research agenda to improve forecasting of resource requirements at the hospital, health system, and regional levels for containment of future outbreaks.

Eight models of SARS transmission and control were published in the English and Chinese scientific literature in 2003 (Chen, 2003; Chowell et al., 2003; Lin et al., 2003; Lipsitch et al., 2003; Lloyd-Smith et al., 2003; Riley et al., 2003; Shi, 2003; Wang and Zhao, 2003). Seven of these utilize the standard SEIR (susceptible, exposed, infectious, recovered) dynamic mathematical model of disease transmission or variations on that model accounting for the use of quarantine (Table 5-1) (Chen, 2003; Chowell et al., 2003; Lipsitch et al., 2003; Lloyd-Smith et al., 2003; Riley et al., 2003; Shi, 2003; Wang and Zhao, 2003). SEIR models can provide estimates of critical parameters for a disease outbreak, such as the basic reproductive number $R_0$ (that is, the number of new cases for every existing case) or maximal lag time for isolation of new cases (Dye and Gay, 2003).

Five of these studies consider outbreak response variables that reflect both public health activity (e.g., time to isolation of each new case) and hospital-based measures (e.g., efficacy of isolation and reduction in transmission rate of virus) (Chowell et al., 2003; Lipsitch et al., 2003; Lloyd-Smith et al., 2003; Riley et al., 2003; Shi, 2003). For example, Chowell and colleagues predicted that containment of the Canadian outbreak would require a time-to-isolation of 3 to 6 days and a 50 to 90 percent reduction in person-to-person transmission from identified cases (Chowell et al., 2003). In a similar fashion, most of these papers provide model-derived threshold values, but do not focus on the practical steps needed to attain them. Only one paper, by Lloyd-Smith and colleagues (2003), went into

**TABLE 5-1** SARS Dynamic Transmission Models

| Authors | Disease Model Type[a] | Data Sources | Key Parameter | Threshold Values |
|---|---|---|---|---|
| Chen et al. | SIR, deterministic | Hong Kong, Beijing | In-hospital transmission | N/A |
| Wang and Zhao | SIR, deterministic | Hong Kong, Beijing | N/A | N/A |
| Chowell et al. | SEIJR, deterministic | Toronto, Hong Kong, Singapore | $R_0$=1.2<br>a. Time to diagnosis<br>b. Isolation effectiveness | a. 3-6 days to diagnosis<br>b. 50-90% effectiveness of quarantine in stopping population-based spread |
| Riley et al. | SEIR, stochastic/deterministic | Hong Kong | $R_0$=2.7<br>a. Time to isolation<br>b. Infection control<br>c. Population contact rate | a. 50% reduction in hospital infection and population contact rate<br>b. Complete cessation of pop ulation movement between r egions |
| Lipsitch et al. | SEI(QR, stochastic/deterministic | Singapore | $R_0$=1.2<br>a. "Public health interventions"<br>b. Population contact rate | Variable based on other modeled factors |
| Lloyd-Smith et al. | SEIR, deterministic with Monte Carlo simulation and heterogeneous stochastic effects | Hong Kong, Singapore | a. Time to isolation<br>b. Isolation effectiveness (hospital-based contact precaution and case management measures)<br>c. HCW-community contact | If $R_0$~3, then need:<br>a. < 3 days to isolation of new cases<br>b. 80% reduction in transmission |
| Shi | SIR, stochastic Monte Carlo | Vietnam | $R_0$=1.8<br>Days to strict isolation | ≤7 days to strict is olation of new cases |

[a]S = susceptible, E = exposed, I = infective, J = diagnosed, Q = quarantined, R = recovered.

sufficient detail about methods of disease containment to provide practical guidance for public health and hospital managers in attaining these goals. For example, these authors found that efforts to interrupt health care worker-to-patient transmission would yield greater improvements in epidemic containment than reductions in population-based transmission. This finding provided the basis for a practical recommendation to initiate hospital-wide campaigns to increase contact precautions and strict case management of infected individuals. Additionally, this report alone—among the eight model-based papers—acknowledges that containment efforts would be carried out in an environment of limited hospital resources, where scarcity of items such as gowns, gloves, and masks would require prioritization of population-wide and hospital-based strategies.

These eight reports provide the beginnings of an evidence base on which to design effective response strategies for future SARS outbreaks. In parallel with these efforts, a number of researchers have developed prediction models for medical outcomes of SARS patients (Table 5-2) (Booth et al., 2003; Chan et al., 2003; Donnelly et al., 2003; Han et al., 2003; He et al., 2003). The current challenge is to use these findings from both theoretical modeling and patient care to assist health planners in practical ways. For example, hospital administrators may benefit from guidance on determining when in the course of an epidemic it is better to cease all admissions, isolate a specific ward, or simply isolate a number of patients in individual rooms. More complex response models may begin to weigh the relative benefits of drastic steps such as shuttering entire hospitals in order to contain the spread of SARS in light of the potential harms that may accrue to affected communities through the loss of routine medical care capacity. Such cost-benefit studies will highlight the difficult choices faced by health planners and hospital administrators in the real-world setting of financial and resource constraints. Finally, with the prospect of a SARS vaccine on the horizon, new models will be needed to quantify optimal pre- and post-detection vaccination rates for disease containment given the significant resource requirements of any mass vaccination campaign. Recent efforts to model mass antibiotic prophylaxis strategies for bioterrorism response may provide insight into the methods and data requirements for this type of logistical modeling as well as techniques (e.g., Internet-based platforms) for wide dissemination of modeling tools (Hupert and Cuomo, 2003; Hupert et al., 2002).

Publication of data on resources consumed in isolating and treating SARS patients as well as quarantine of potentially infected individuals will assist modelers in developing realistic forecasting models capable of leading public health and hospital planners through "what if" scenarios that may require difficult trade-offs of personnel, materials, and patient care arrangements. The more accurate the data underlying these models, the better they can serve planners and their communities. The goal of such efforts should be to give every decision maker the ability to understand, in relevant terms and for their particular institution or community, not just the knowledge that containment of SARS would require isolation

**TABLE 5-2** Prediction Models for Medical Outcomes of SARS Patients

| Authors | Model Type | Predictor Variable(s) | Outcomes of Interest |
| --- | --- | --- | --- |
| Booth et al. | Multivariable regression | Diabetes, comorbidity | Death, intensive care admission |
| Chan et al. | Multivariable regression | Age, diabetes, heart disease | Death |
| Han et al. | Correlation | Radiology information technology systems use | Infection rate |
| He et al. | Multivariable regression | Age, hypoxia, thrombocytopenia, hypernatremia, renal failure | Death |
| Donnelly et al. | Gamma distribution | Age, infection to onset, onset to admission | Death |

of new cases within a certain number of days, but also an estimate of how to go about achieving that containment goal (i.e., how many staff, rooms, media campaigns, and other factors). Planning models that focus on critical resources in this manner can provide guidance for live exercises and may influence future investments in both infrastructure (e.g., installation of negative pressure isolation rooms) and disposable medical equipment (e.g., gowns and masks).

## REPORTING, SURVEILLANCE, AND INFORMATION EXCHANGE: THE SARS IMPERATIVE FOR INNOVATION

*Ann Marie Kimball,*[3] *Bill Lober,*[4] *John Kobayashi,*[5] *Yuzo Arima,*[6] *Louis Fox,*[7] *Jacqueline Brown,*[8] *and Nedra Floyd Pautler*[9]
Asia Pacific Economic Cooperation, Emerging Infections Network (EINET)

The emergence and widespread transmission of severe acute respiratory syndrome (SARS) in the winter of 2003 severely tested national, regional, and global reporting and surveillance systems for emergent infectious diseases. It presented a three-pronged challenge: (1) alerting responsible authorities; (2) rapidly describing the geographically diverse outbreaks in a consistent and useful fashion; and (3) providing guidance for prevention and control strategies based on experience in varied locations. Given the persistent emergence of new infections in recent years in the Asia Pacific—accompanied by the continued increase in population size and the greater range and volume of trade and travel in the region— this scenario must be considered a harbinger for the future. The gaps brought to light in this experience should be used to guide the rapid deployment of laboratory and communications systems in the region. In this article, the informatics components of the response to SARS are described and characterized. Prospective areas for applications of new technologies are discussed.

### Hypothesis

The SARS experience represents a precursor to future scenario planning for the Asia Pacific. Descriptive data suggest both successes and gaps in timeliness,

[3]Director, APEC/EINET, Professor, Departments of Epidemiology and Health Services, School of Public Health, University of Washington.

[4]Research Associate Professor, Department of Biomedical and Health Informatics, School of Medicine, University of Washington.

[5]Clinical Associate Professor, School of Public Health, University of Washington, Consultant, Japan Field Epidemiology Training Program, Government of Japan.

[6]Research Associate, Epidemiology, School of Public Health, University of Washington.

[7]Vice Provost, Educational Partnerships and Learning Technologies, University of Washington.

[8]Director, Technology Outreach Computing and Communications, University of Washington.

[9]Information Manager, APEC Emerging Infections Network.

laboratory diagnostic tools, and useful, practical transparent communications among sectors within nations, and between nations partnered in trade and travel. This report will focus on gaps in the latter two areas: practical transparent communications among sectors and between nations.

## Methods

We conducted a focused and systematic review of the 2003 SARS epidemic based on (1) our EINET experience operating an electronic, multisectoral communications network in the region, in collaboration with (2) a literature review for the identification of potential applications of informatics technology based on the 2003 experience (including response management, collaboration, capacity development, tabletops/training, and other factors).

## Findings/Conclusions

SARS presented the confluence of three urgent requirements of the global public health informatics response: (1) expansion of knowledge about the disease in a rapid, systematic manner, particularly in microbiology and epidemiology through collaborative discovery; (2) communication of appropriate aspects of that knowledge base to guide implementation of isolation, quarantine, and prevention measures by public health workers and other policy makers; and (3) mitigation of adverse societal response through broader social communication. However, with concurrent outbreaks in numerous locations, each of these requirements rapidly increased in complexity. Working relationships in the Asia Pacific public health community have been formed in the course of the outbreak response that can be reinforced in the present "inter SARS" period. Specific computing and telecommunications tools can be expanded to assist more fully in the public health response. We propose the use of a virtual tabletop (scenario) tool to proactively implement improved communications and collaboration strategies in the region.

## Background

The SARS outbreaks of 2003 have been described in numerous scientific reports (CDC, 2003a). In fact, the unprecedented volume and speed of scientific discovery and the dissemination of that knowledge has been the subject of a report (Drazen and Campion, 2003). This report focuses on (1) how informatics and telecommunications strategies assisted in the timeliness of this effort; and (2) what technologies or strategies could be tested and applied in the current "inter SARS" period to assure public health readiness for the future.

The factors related to the emergence of new infectious diseases have been described for more than a decade (IOM, 1992, 2003). The role of anthropogenic factors of emergence related to microbial pathogens in humans, while generally understood to be important, has become the object of systematic biomedical and interdisciplinary research. The overlay of globalization in manufacturing, commerce, travel, and trade on an uneven public health and sanitary infrastructure has put some populations at risk of new infections. These risks become reality in epidemics that increasingly challenge our ability to respond effectively.

The Asia Pacific has witnessed the emergence of numerous new human pathogens, including Nipah virus, enterovirus 71, *E. coli* 0157H:7, and *Cyclospora Cayetanensis*. The reemergence of "old" pathogens such as cholera and multidrug-resistant tuberculosis has also affected the region. This may reflect the pace of change that countries bordering the Pacific Ocean have experienced in their demographics, migration, and rapid shifts in economic activity. In addition, these nations are among the most trade dependent in the world. The Asia Pacific dwarfs other regions of the globe in the volume and dollar value of trade and travel revenues.

Asia has had sustained growth of Internet connectivity over the past decade, despite economic crises in the region (Kimball et al., 1999). In a recent report, the International Telecommunications Union (ITU, 2003) noted that the number of broadband subscribers rose 72 percent in 2002, with Korea (21 subscribers per 100 inhabitants), Hong Kong (15 per 100), and Canada (11 per 100) showing the highest rates of broadband use. In Korea, "Disweb," an electronic surveillance system, has been in place since 1999 using web-based reporting over the Internet. Many other economies are increasingly integrating Internet-based reporting into their disease alert and surveillance systems.

While numerous electronic disease surveillance and alert networks are operating in the region, the Asia Pacific Emerging Infections Network (APEC-EINET) is unique in that it includes membership from trade and commerce (see Figure 5-3) as well as health. Now in its eighth year of operation, the network spans the entire Asia Pacific community. The network consists of a user group of more than 500 in 19 of the 21 APEC economies. Providing a biweekly bulletin and enriched website, the APEC-EINET is supported by APEC, the U.S. government, and the University of Washington.

## Methods

Of the 1,150 articles entered into the Medline index with "SARS" in their text, 60 include the word "information" and 2 include "information technology" (Eysenbach, 2003). The 60 information-related articles were scanned for discussion on informatics or information technology employed during the outbreak by scientists or public health workers. In addition, informal discussions were held in person and through electronic communications with World Health Organization/Geneva (WHO/Geneva) and regional academic institutions and public health organizations to augment the information available for review in this report. Because the SARS experience is still being understood, the data obtained through personal communications may be incomplete.

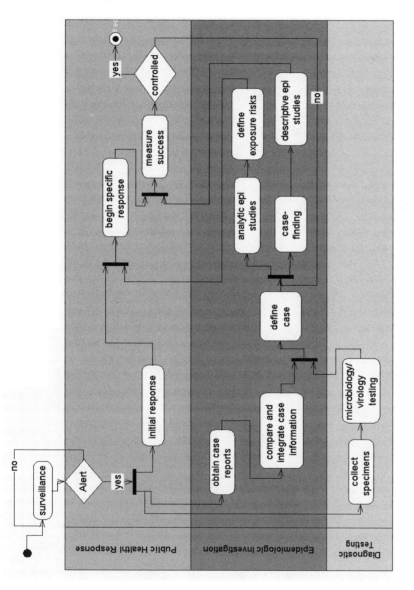

**FIGURE 5-3** Integrated process for public health disease response.

After compiling this information, we segregated our conclusions into the informatics domains of (1) generation of new biomedical knowledge about the SARS agent; and (2) generation of new knowledge about the epidemiology of SARS disease prevention for purposes of predicting and monitoring success in control. We provide our assessment based on this analysis of the need for specific new communications and collaboration strategies.

## Results

If the basic systems model of an outbreak alert, investigation, and response resembles the work model in Figure 5-4, then numerous frontiers for information technology application and evaluation exist. This diagram integrates business processes and the information flow that supports these processes in the course of work done to investigate and respond to an outbreak (Kitch and Yashoff, 2002). The focus of international information technology application during SARS centered on three aspects, which are shown in the figure: alert, diagnosis (biomedical discovery), and epidemiologic investigation.

*Alert*

According to WHO, the earliest alerts about an unknown pneumonia in Guandong were discovered by Global Public Health Information Network

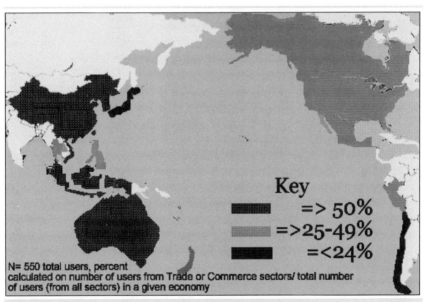

**FIGURE 5-4** Percentage of APEC EINet users from trade and commerce by economy.

(GPHIN) (Heymann et al., 2001). Essentially a webcrawler, text-mining tool, this application was developed with Canadian government funding and implemented through an agreement with WHO in 2000. The "hits" generated daily are reviewed manually in Canada, and about 200 reports are forwarded to WHO per day. However, despite such alerts, all reports from GPHIN require independent verification from reliable sources on site (Grein et al., 2000; Hsueh et al., 2003). In the absence of such confirmation, an international alert cannot be issued.

*Biomedical Discovery*

Response depends on diagnosis of what an outbreak is or is not. In the case of SARS, new scientific discovery was probably the largest beneficiary of new information technology, and this was in line with its priority in enabling effective public health response. Bioinformatics software tools were used extensively to identify the genome of SARS (Li et al., 2003), calculate the likelihood of frequencies in the annotation process (Ruan et al., 2003), and model the virus for prospective drug design among other uses. These tools, employed by teams of scientists across international boundaries, allowed bench scientists to rapidly generate new information about the SARS agent.

Interlaboratory communication was a second area in which the Internet and communications technologies added value. Stohr and colleagues report on the multicenter collaboration convened by WHO to "identify the causal agent and to develop a diagnostic test" (WHO Multicentre Collaborative Network, 2003). The 11 laboratories were located in nine countries. Countries both affected and not affected by SARS figured among the nine.

The electronic tools implemented included: (1) a secure, password-protected website where primer sequences and other information were posted for researchers; (2) electronic mail communications using the Internet; and (3) the telephone for daily teleconferences. Probably as important, the ethical framework for collaboration was established through an agreed protocol for sharing results and information. This protocol protected the work of scientists involved and fostered information sharing for advancement of the mutual collaboration. This networked activity of distributive efforts was efficient, resulting in the discovery and initial description of the coronavirus of SARS over the period of one month.

*Epidemiologic Knowledge*

Disease investigation was carried out in earnest at each of the outbreak sites. Case counts and mortality counts were reported through PROMED, WHO, EINET, and the media. However, in our experience with EINET, the need for practical guidance for the Asia Pacific outstripped the available information in the first weeks of the epidemic. We received numerous queries about hospital isolation procedures, quarantine, airport measures, treatment, and other issues. While recommendations addressing these eventually were posted by international authorities, practitioners in closely linked but unaffected economies desired more specific and detailed information in a more timely manner.

WHO has convened the Global Outbreak Alert and Response Network partners over the past 8 years to begin to address exactly the kind of crisis presented by SARS. This activity proved to be a major asset to WHO in coping with SARS. However, the secure network and website approach that was implemented was less able to cope with the volume and diversity of information required. Specifically, the need for detailed information by public health authorities in unaffected areas was not optimally met (Kimball and Pautler, 2003).

The ability to monitor the impact of interventions is important to modulating the public health response. The key epidemiologic parameter to be followed is the reproductive rate of the epidemic in progress. If this rate is above 1.0, the epidemic will continue to expand as it infects new susceptibles at a greater rate than infected individuals recover (Lipsitch et al., 2003). This rate relies on modeling, and parameters that are difficult to collect through field investigation. In retrospect, only some of the affected localities were able to collect quality data in adequate amounts to enable such modeling to be reliably applied (Donnelly et al., 2003). As noted by one group, "Limited data and inconclusive epidemiologic information place severe restrictions on efforts to model the global spread of the SARS etiological agent" (Chowell et al., 2003).

Because our own user group includes trade and commerce officials from a number of APEC economies (Figure 5-4), our network was one of the few that provided updates on the epidemic situation in the region systematically to individuals not employed in the health sector. Although we have no quantitative information to document this, anecdotally we have been told this was useful in decision-making during the epidemic period.

### Discussion: "Inter-SARS" Preparedness

SARS presented a challenge on both the research and response fronts. However, a similar challenge would be faced with any acute, severe viral respiratory infection for which diagnostic, treatment, and containment recommendations had not been well established. Influenza is an agent that could produce a similar picture and create similar chaos in the region. Thus, the overall concept of "preparedness" for such a natural disaster can serve to inform our actions in preparing for the "next wave." In fact, in the midst of SARS, this genre of concept surfaced in the literature (Augustine, 2003).

The processes to address two major domain needs of the SARS response—laboratory research and epidemic investigation—were not truly ad hoc during the outbreak period. The basic structures of the two collaborative groups—the linked laboratories and the outbreak alert and response partners (including the implementation of GPHIN)—had been created over the years prior to the outbreak. However, the implementation of emergency response was ad hoc, as was the area of epidemiologic investigation. Response encountered obstacles in communications, which can be partially addressed through preparedness exercises.

Tabletop or scenario exercises have been a centerpiece in preparation for emergency response in the United States. In Japan and Korea, exercises of alert and syndromic surveillance systems have been conducted to prepare for events such as the World Cup (Suzuki et al., 2003). The scenario "Dark Winter" convened high-level policy makers to discuss smallpox preparedness planning in the United States, and the more recent "Global Mercury" exercise carried out by the Global Health Security Action Group demonstrated the utility of this approach internationally (U.S. Department of State, 2003).

The tabletop as envisioned will: (1) bring together research universities and their public health counterparts in a collaborative process to tailor a scenario for their location in response to the threat of a travel-related, highly infectious disease; (2) create automated access to pertinent information sources at multiple sites that will add value to actual response efforts should these be needed; (3) promote international communications and collaboration using newer communications strategies among partners, thus ensuring the availability of these new tools to the public health community; and (4) create a flexible scenario for use in preparedness domestically and potentially by multiple APEC economies in training efforts. We believe the use of access node communications (see Box 5-1) for collaborative conferencing will demonstrate added value in the collaborative design process and in the debriefing on generic lessons learned in the exercises.

Beyond the virtual tabletop exercise, systematic analysis of the integrated workflow diagram suggests many other potential application sites for new information technologies. One apparent area would be the development of a software tool that could allow individual outbreak sites to assess their own data and calculate their own rate of reproduction for the outbreak they are experiencing (Chowell et al., 2003; Donnelly et al., 2003; Lipsitch et al., 2003). Such a tool could enable local public health officials to step up or step down response as success is or is not achieved. However, such a tool would rely heavily on the generation of reliable field investigation data in a timely way. The generation, compilation, and analysis of these data during the course of an outbreak remain the cornerstone of successful outbreak curtailment. Innovations in information technology need to be evaluated for their ability to support the key function of effective public health outbreak response.

Electronic networking and promoting intersectoral collaboration figure among the five strategies adopted by APEC to respond to emergent infections (Asia-Pacific Economic Corporation, 2001). The virtual tabletop will begin

---

**BOX 5-1**
**The Access Grid**

"The Access Grid™ is one example of advanced communications resources now accessible within the Asia Pacific. An ensemble of resources including multimedia large-format displays, presentation and interactive environments, and interfaces to Grid middleware and to visualization environments, access grid nodes are used to support group-to-group interactions across the Grid. The Access Grid (AG) is used for large-scale distributed meetings, collaborative work sessions, seminars, lectures, tutorials, and training. The Access Grid thus differs from desktop-to-desktop tools that focus on individual communication.

The Access Grid is now used at over 150 institutions worldwide (including institutions in Japan, Taiwan, Korea, Singapore, Canada, US, China, Hong Kong, Thailand). Each institution has one or more AG nodes, or "designed spaces," that contain the high-end audio and visual technology needed to provide a high-quality compelling user experience. The nodes are also used as a research environment for the development of distributed data and visualization corridors and for the study of issues relating to collaborative work in distributed environments" (www.accessgrid.org).

---

to leverage the sophistication already in place in communications and computing in the Asia Pacific in the service of the public good. Specifically, (1) communications technologies and middleware capacities of Asia Pacific research and education telecommunication networks are in place to be tested and adapted within the EINET community to support reporting, surveillance, and information exchange, particularly through the use of the Access Grid; and (2) a network of Pacific Rim research universities are being brought into the effort to serve as primary points of access for these advanced networks and technologies and as hubs of a broader communications network with the capacity to engage public health as well as other professionals throughout the APEC community.

## PUBLIC HEALTH LAW PREPAREDNESS

*Gene Matthews, J.D.*
Legal Advisor, Centers for Disease Control and Prevention

The Central Intelligence Agency's (CIA's) unclassified report on severe acute respiratory syndrome (SARS) sets the tone for our current status on legal preparedness for the next outbreak. "The effective application and efficacy of quarantine and isolation [during the SARS epidemic] proved a pleasant surprise to the public health community," the CIA reports. "Equally unexpected was the widespread acceptance of the need for these measures by the general public."

Another perspective on legal preparedness for an outbreak of infectious disease in the United States can be gained by considering a pair of paradoxes. The first paradox is that, in the same year (1954), the need for community-wide public health control measures was greatly reduced through the development of the Salk polio vaccine, and the U.S. Supreme Court initiated a trend toward increased procedural protections of individual liberties with its ruling that in *Brown vs. Board of Education*. Prior to 1954, the United States had regularly used community-wide quarantine in our legal system as a public health control measure. During the past 50 years, however, the judicial, legislative, and executive branches have each established ways to increase the protection of individual rights from government infringement. So, the public reaction to SARS was indeed surprising, as the CIA report says, because it marked the first true meeting in the United States of historical public health quarantine and modern civil liberties.

The second paradox could be referred to as "the paradox of the silos." As the U.S. government has evolved during the past 50 years, we have developed *more* governance, but we have partitioned various responsibilities and authorities into different jurisdictional silos. We now have a public health silo stratified at the federal, state, and local levels, and it is separated from the silos of law enforcement, emergency management, agriculture, animal control, medical services, courts, transportation, and others. Reports of the SARS outbreak in China described silos of health care in that country as well. Health care in military hospitals, for example, was totally separate from health care in hospitals run by the railway system. When this silo effect occurs in complex governments, the legal structure is limited in its ability to arch over and effectively connect all the jurisdictions that need to respond to the problem. This is the challenge we face in the "paradox of the silos."

## Quarantine and Public Health Law

The quarantine issue during the SARS outbreaks illustrates the sort of bridging of silos that has to occur in public health law. Most emergency public health measures imposed within a state are subject to state law and regulations, which can vary. Some state laws concerning quarantine are procedurally outdated, and some local laws may be very useful. The federal government also has authority concerning quarantine. The U.S. Department of Health and Human Services (HHS) has concurrent federal power to apprehend, detain, and conditionally release individuals to prevent interstate spread or international importation of certain diseases.

These federally quarantinable diseases are specified by executive order of the President. On April 4, 2003, President Bush signed an executive order adding SARS to the list of conditions that warrant quarantines; other conditions include cholera, diphtheria, infectious tuberculosis, plague, smallpox, yellow fever, and suspected viral hemorrhagic fevers (e.g., Lassa, Marburg, Ebola, Congo-Crimean, and others not yet isolated or named). Violation of quarantine authority in these cases is a criminal misdemeanor under federal law.

How would federal, state, and local laws interact to address an infectious outbreak? State and local governments have primary responsibility for isolation, quarantine and most of the emergency public health powers. The federal government has the authority to prevent interstate spread and international importation, but it can accept state and local assistance in enforcing the federal quarantine regulations. Conversely, HHS can assist state and local officials in their control of communicable diseases.

Because SARS has the potential to spread rapidly into different states, the federal quarantine authority could be applied to a single SARS case inside a state or local jurisdiction as necessary. In other words, it would not be necessary to wait for an interstate spread of SARS actually to take place before the Centers for Disease Control and Prevention (CDC), part of HHS, used this federal authority. However, any CDC action on SARS using this authority would be carefully coordinated with the appropriate state or local officials. The CDC did not use this authority during the 2003 SARS outbreak.

However, a situation may arise in which all three concurrent jurisdictions come into play. For example, if a disease outbreak occurred in a New York airport, federal, state, and local authority—all with overlapping police power—could be used. Since such activities would require coordination with the "law enforcement silo," the CDC is intensively pursuing joint training between law enforcement and public health officials.

## Lessons from Toronto

Toronto exemplifies the surprising level of public acceptance of quarantine described in the aforementioned CIA report. Dr. Barbara Yaffee and attorney Jane Speakman report that of the 13,000 persons "voluntarily" quarantined in Toronto, only 27 needed to be served with a formal quarantine order, and only one person sought to appeal (and this person later withdrew the appeal after he was told how he was exposed to SARS and could potentially transmit the disease). Few legal or public health professionals would have expected that level of public cooperation. One possible explanation is that the intense media coverage rapidly demystified the concept of quarantine. Additional analysis of this social phenomenon is urgently needed.

Toronto also exemplified social cohesion in a public health emergency; residents showed responsibility and cooperation, rather than the divisiveness and panic that some public health, media, or legal experts might have predicted. The experience seems to indicate that when the public is presented with clear communication and practical guidance in a public health emergency, they can behave quite responsibly. Interestingly, there are abundant examples in the literature of such temporary, cohesive community behavior in an emergency. Of course, it is difficult to speculate how much the Toronto (or Canadian) experience would resemble that of the United States in a similar situation. Yet despite the differences between the U.S. and Canadian legal systems, it does seem that the recent history of quarantine in Toronto will influence how the United States would handle a similar situation.

Another key lesson from Toronto, as well as from several Asian countries, is the broad range of situations encompassed under quarantine. These included "work quarantine," a concept discussed by Martin Cetron (see Chapter 1). Through "work quarantine," needed public service employees can go to work and be isolated there or at home, and continue to maintain essential services. This is an important new tool to have available to compliment "snow day" and "shelter-in-place" community emergency strategies

Finally, as CDC director Julie Gerberding said in a press conference during the SARS epidemic, the public health community must be prepared to act boldly and swiftly, yet treat individuals with dignity and fairness. That is a good description of what happened during the SARS outbreak in Toronto: People were treated fairly, they received clear messages about their situation, and quarantine proceeded smoothly.

## Practical Steps for Legal Preparedness

Some practical steps to prepare for a possible resurgence of SARS or an outbreak of another infectious disease. A more detailed treatment is available at www.cdc.gov.

• **Know the relevant legislation.** All states, and most cities and municipalities, have quarantine laws. Some of these laws have not been used on a community-wide basis in 50 or 80 years. All such laws need to be examined on a case-by-case basis to determine whether they could be applied appropriately if SARS returned.

• **Plan due process.** Be able to take the necessary steps, even if the laws are old, to give a quarantined person notice, a way to be heard, legal representation, and a final decision that a court can review. On the other hand, recognize that due process should not interfere with isolation if lives are threatened.

• **Draft documents in advance.** Examples of quarantine orders that were used in Texas, as well as orders that have been drafted in North Carolina and other areas, are available on the CDC Public Health Law website at www.phppo.cdc.gov/od/phlp. These documents are accompanied by affidavits, descriptions of due process mechanisms, and other contingent material.

- **Contact other jurisdictions.** Put law enforcement, emergency management, and health care in touch with each other. Create legal mechanisms to bridge these "silos" horizontally and vertically, and to connect federal, state, and local jurisdictions as well as geographical clusters. Personal networking is vital before an event takes place.
- **Engage the courts in advance.** Toronto judges were somewhat surprised when health agency lawyers introduced quarantine orders. If the judiciary is engaged in advance of an outbreak, it can manage due process or habeas corpus proceedings efficiently.
- **Anticipate practical problems.** In Toronto, for example, contract civil process servers refused to serve quarantine orders during the SARS epidemic. Law enforcement agents were therefore required to serve these quarantine orders.
- **Plan electronic communications for quarantined persons.** They should be able to participate in hearings via video feed, cell phone, or other mechanism, rather than risk transmitting disease in the courtroom.
- **Emphasize communication, communication, communication.** Two key reasons explain why quarantine worked so smoothly in Toronto: it was perceived as being fair and everyone was generally aware of what was happening. Communication among the "silos" is critical to success or failure of governance in a public health emergency.

## SARS: LESSONS FROM A NEW DISEASE

*David L. Heymann and Guenael Rodier*
World Health Organization

New diseases have been emerging at the unprecedented rate of one a year for the last two decades, and this trend is certain to continue. The sudden and deadly arrival of SARS on the global health stage early in 2003 was in some ways perhaps the most dramatic of all. Its rapid containment is one of the biggest success stories in public health in recent years. But how much of that success was a result of good fortune as well as good science? How narrow was the escape from an international health disaster? What tipped the scales? The international response to SARS will shape future strategies against infectious epidemics.

The day-by-day struggle to control the outbreak of severe acute respiratory syndrome (SARS) represents a major victory for public health collaboration. Key lessons emerge that will be invaluable in shaping the future of infectious disease control—and being ready for the day when the next new disease arrives without warning. First and most important is the need to report, promptly and openly, cases of any disease with the potential for international spread in a closely interconnected and highly mobile world. Second, timely global alerts can prevent imported cases from igniting big outbreaks in new areas. Third, travel recommendations, including screening measures at airports, help to contain the international spread of an emerging infection. Fourth, the world's best scientists, clinicians and public health experts, aided by electronic communications, can collaborate to generate rapidly the scientific basis for control measures. Fifth, weaknesses in health systems play a key role in permitting emerging infections to spread. Sixth, an outbreak can be contained even without a curative drug or a vaccine if existing interventions are tailored to the circumstances and backed by political commitment. Finally, risk communication about new and emerging infections is a great challenge, and it is vital to ensure that the most accurate information is successfully and unambiguously communicated to the public. WHO is applying these lessons across the Organization as it scales up its response to the HIV/AIDS emergency.

## The First Cases

On March 12, 2003, WHO alerted the world to the appearance of a severe respiratory illness of undetermined cause that was rapidly spreading among hospital staff in Hong Kong Special Administrative Region (China) and Viet Nam. Within two days, it was clear that the illness was also spreading internationally along major airline routes when hospitals in Singapore and Toronto, Canada, reported seeing patients with similar signs and symptoms. The potential for further international spread by air travel was vividly illustrated on March 15. In the early hours of the morning, the head of WHO's outbreak alert and response operations was woken by a call from health authorities in Singapore. A doctor who had treated the first cases of atypical pneumonia there had reported having similar symptoms shortly before boarding an international flight returning to Singapore from New York. Asked to intervene, WHO alerted the airline and health authorities in Germany, where the flight was scheduled for a stopover. The doctor and his wife disembarked in Frankfurt and were immediately hospitalized in isolation, becoming the first two cases in Europe. Because of these events, WHO issued a second, stronger alert later in the day. It set out a case definition, provided advice to international travellers should they develop similar symptoms, and gave the new disease its name: severe acute respiratory syndrome (SARS). The global outbreak of SARS became the focus of intense international concern, and it remained so for almost four months.

## Origins and International Spread

SARS is a newly identified human infection caused by a coronavirus unlike any other known human or animal virus in its family. Analysis of epidemiological information from the various outbreak sites is still under way, but the overall case fatality ratio, with the fate of most cases now known, approaches 11 percent, but with much higher rates among elderly people. Transmission occurs mainly from person to person during face-to-face exposure to infected respiratory droplets expelled during coughing or sneezing, or following contact with body fluids during certain medical interventions. Contamination of the environment, arising from fecal shedding of the virus, is thought to play a small role in disease transmission, illustrated by the almost simultaneous infection in late March of more than 300 residents of a housing estate in Hong Kong where faulty sewage disposal was identified. At present, the disease has no vaccine, no curative treatment, and no reliable point-of-care diagnostic test, though antibody tests have been developed that can reliably confirm previous infection using acute and convalescent sera. Management of SARS is supportive, and control strategies rely on standard epidemiological interventions: identification of those fitting the case definition, isolation, infection control, contact tracing, active surveillance of contacts, and evidence-based recommendations for international travellers. Though demanding and socially disruptive, particularly when large numbers of people were placed in quarantine, these standard interventions, supported by high-level political commitment, proved sufficiently powerful to contain the global outbreak less than four months after the initial alert.

The earliest cases of SARS are now thought to have emerged in mid-November 2002 in the southern Chinese province of Guangdong. Retrospective analysis of patient records, to date incomplete, has identified small clusters of cases, each traced to a different initial case, that occurred independently in at least seven municipalities, with the first case recorded on November 16, 2002, in Foshan City and the largest number of cases concentrated in Guangzhou City. Analysis has uncovered no links among the various initial cases in the clusters. Some cases with no previous known history of exposure also occurred (WHO, 2003c; Breiman et al., 2003). Early collaborative studies conducted in Guangdong have detected a virus almost identical to the SARS coronavirus in domesticated game animals — the masked palm civet cat and the raccoon dog—sold in Guangdong live markets, suggesting that these animals might play a role in transmission of the virus to humans.

The initial phase of the Guangdong outbreak, characterized by small, independent clusters and sporadic cases, was subsequently followed by a sharp rise in cases during the first week of February 2003, thought to result from amplification during care in hospitals. Cases gradually declined thereafter. Altogether, some 1,512 clinically confirmed cases occurred in the Guangdong outbreak, with health care workers in urban hospitals accounting for up to 27 percent of cases (WHO, 2003c; Chinese Center for Disease Control and Prevention, 2003). This pattern—occurrence in urban areas, with most cases concentrated in hospitals, and amplification during care—was repeated as the disease began to spread outside Guangdong Province to other areas in China and then internationally.

The first recorded case of SARS outside China occurred on February 21, 2003, when a medical doctor who had treated patients in Guangzhou City and was himself suffering from respiratory symptoms spent a single night in a hotel in Hong Kong. Through presumed contact, the mechanism of which is not fully understood, he transmitted SARS to at least 16 other guests and visitors, all linked to the same hotel floor. They carried the virus with them as they entered local hospitals or traveled on to Singapore, Toronto, and Viet Nam. An international outbreak that eventually spread to 30 countries had thus been seeded. Figure 5-5 maps the distribution of 8422 cases and 916 deaths that had occurred by August 7, 2003.

## Detection and Response

On March 15, 2003, when the second alert was made, the cause of SARS had not yet been identified. Cases were concentrated in hospital workers and did not respond to medicines known to be effective against a number of different lung infections. Many patients were rapidly progressing to severe pneumonia. The situation was alarming: no patients, including young and previously healthy health workers, had recovered. Many of the patients were in a critical condition, several required mechanical ventilatory support, and two had died. The spread to major cities around the world meant that any city with an international airport was at potential risk of imported cases. From the outset, WHO's objective was clear: to halt further international spread and interrupt human-to-human transmission through a global containment effort, and by so doing to minimize opportunities for the disease to establish endemicity (see Box 5-2).

The global response to SARS was in reality the roll out of a way of detecting and responding to outbreaks that had been developed over the preceding seven years by WHO and its partners, partly as a result of major weaknesses that came to light during the 1995 Ebola outbreak in the Democratic Republic of the Congo and during previous outbreaks of plague in India and cholera in Latin America. The SARS response depended on collaboration of the world's top public health and laboratory experts, and took advantage of up-to-date communication technologies, including the Internet and video and telephone conferencing.

Two principal partners of the WHO Global Outbreak Alert and Response Network (GOARN), an electronically interconnected network of experts and institutes formally set up in early 2000, contributed to the detection of the SARS outbreak. One was the Canadian Global Public Health Intelligence Network (GPHIN), a worldwide web-crawling computer application, used by WHO since 1997, that systematically searches for keywords in seven different languages to identify reports of what could be disease outbreaks. Throughout the outbreak, GPHIN provided the raw intelligence that helped WHO maintain up-to-date and high-quality information on indications that the disease might be spreading to new areas. The second partner was the WHO Influenza Laboratory Network of 110 laboratories in 84 countries that constantly keeps the world in general and

238

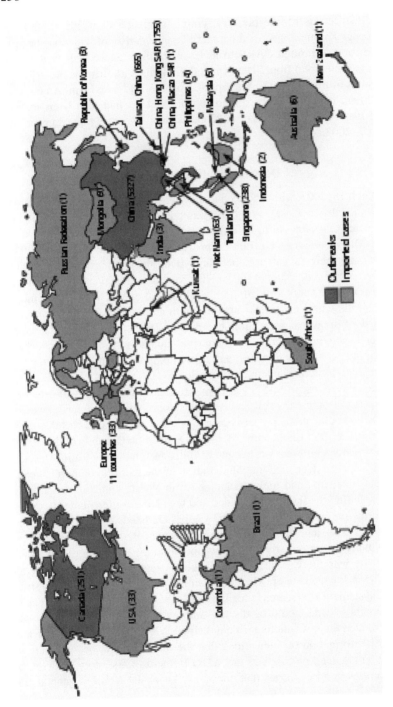

**FIGURE 5-5** Probable cases of SARS worldwide, August 7, 2003.

## BOX 5-2
## The Response to SARS in the Western Pacific Region

More than 95 percent of SARS cases occurred in the Western Pacific Region. As an immediate response, a SARS outbreak response and preparedness team—including international experts—was established in the Regional Office. The main objectives were to:

- contain and control the outbreaks,
- support the health care infrastructure in affected countries,
- provide guidance and assistance to enable vulnerable countries to prepare for the possible arrival of the virus, and
- provide the most up-to-date information to health officials and respond to public concerns.

Teams of epidemiologists and infection control experts were immediately sent to China, including Hong Kong Special Administrative Region, as well as to the Philippines, Singapore and Viet Nam and across the southern Pacific, training health care workers in infection control procedures and preparing them for the possible arrival of the disease. Practical infection control and preparedness guidelines and training tools were developed, and the first version of preparedness guidelines was issued at the beginning of April. Logistic support and supplies (personal protective equipment, including masks, collection materials for blood and respiratory samples, and internationally approved containers for shipment of samples) were sent to both affected and unaffected countries, supported by a US$ 3 million grant from the Government of Japan.

Countries were classified according to three levels of risk and three levels of capability to respond to SARS cases, in order for WHO to prioritize its support to countries. WHO worked closely with countries to ensure that enhanced surveillance was put in place to enable early detection of cases and contact tracing. Guidelines were drawn up on enhanced surveillance, hospital and community infection control, international travel, laboratory procedures and public awareness. To improve public awareness, close contact was established with national media focal points, and the web site of the Western Pacific Regional Office was regularly updated.

A regional laboratory network was established to ensure that necessary testing for SARS could be done for countries with limited laboratory capacities. National and regional reference laboratories were identified and shipping of specimens was arranged between the laboratories.

WHO's efforts were paralleled by the contribution of Member States. Viet Nam was the first to interrupt local transmission of the virus. Other countries introduced a wide range of measures, including isolation, home quarantine and comprehensive contact tracing. The willingness of governments in the Western Pacific Region to put public health considerations ahead of economic concerns about the impact of SARS was crucial to the success of the collaborative effort.

vaccine manufacturers in particular informed of which strains of influenza are circulating, so that an effective influenza vaccine can be produced each year.

On February 10, 2003, GPHIN and other partners of GOARN identified reports of an outbreak associated with health worker mortality and the closing of hospitals in Guangdong. One day later the Chinese government officially reported to WHO an outbreak of respiratory illness, beginning in mid-November, involving 300 cases and five deaths in Guangdong Province. Just over a week later, on 19 February, an outbreak of avian influenza was reported to the WHO Influenza Laboratory Network by the collaborating laboratory in Hong Kong. This outbreak first came to light when a 33-year-old man died of an unknown cause after returning from a family trip to Fujian Province, China. His 8-year-old daughter had died of a similar disease while in Fujian Province and his 9-year-old son was hospitalized in Hong Kong with the same symptoms. It was from this son that avian influenza virus was isolated and reported to the Influenza Laboratory Network. The same influenza virus had been identified in Hong Kong in 1997. Control efforts at that time required the slaughter and incineration of all chickens in the many live markets there; human-to-human transmission was never established.

This heightened level of alert led to the identification of an early SARS case in Viet Nam on February 28, 2003. At the same time as GOARN collected information about this outbreak in real time, it sent an international team of partners to work with the Viet Nam authorities to better understand the disease, and by March 12 GOARN had accumulated the initial information necessary to issue the first global alert. It was through the continued instant sharing of information by governments, public health experts, clinicians and laboratory scientists that evidence-based decisions could progressively be made, culminating in the successful containment of SARS.

Under GOARN, a virtual collaborative network of 11 leading laboratories, linked by a secure website and daily teleconferences, identified the SARS causative agent and developed early diagnostic tests. The network, in turn, served as a model for similar electronically linked groups of clinical and epidemiological experts who pooled clinical knowledge and compiled the epidemiological data needed to chart the outbreak's evolution and assess the effectiveness of control interventions.

WHO issued daily updates about the outbreaks on its website to keep the general public—especially travellers—informed and, as far as possible, to counter rumours with reliable information. Equally important, the website was used to issue a range of evidence-based technical and practical guidelines for control as knowledge and information about the disease progressed and became available through the virtual groups of experts.

As more and more evidence accumulated through real time collaboration of public health experts, a range of additional evidence-based control measures became possible. It was soon evident, for example, that people with SARS continued to travel internationally by air after March 15, and that some of them had infected passengers sitting nearby. At the same time it was also apparent that contacts of

SARS patients likewise continued to travel, becoming ill once they arrived at their destination. Recommendations were therefore made that countries with major outbreaks should screen departing passengers to make sure that they did not have fever and other signs of SARS, or known contact with SARS patients.

As the outbreak continued in Hong Kong, contact tracing there further demonstrated that transmission of SARS was occurring outside the confined environment of the health care setting, and later suggested that it was also occurring following exposure to some factor in the environment, thus creating further opportunities for exposure in the general population. Additional evidence-based guidance was therefore made for sites where contact tracing could not link all cases to a chain of transmission, on the understanding that if the disease were spreading in the wider community it would greatly increase the risk to travellers and the likelihood that cases would be exported to other countries. This guidance was aimed at international travelers, and recommended that they postpone all but essential travel to designated areas in order to minimize their risk of becoming infected. Such guidance was also needed in view of the confusion created by several different national recommendations, many of which were based on criteria other than epidemiological data.

Authorities in areas where outbreaks were occurring responded to SARS with mass public education campaigns and encouraged populations to conduct daily fever checks. Hotlines and websites answered questions. Screening measures were set up at international airports and border crossings, and procedures of infection control were reinforced in hospitals. Singapore drew on its military forces to conduct contact tracing, while Hong Kong adapted a tracing system that had been developed for use in criminal investigations and electronically mapped the location of all residences of cases. Chinese authorities opened hundreds of fever clinics throughout the country where suspected SARS cases were triaged. Heads of state and ministers of health of of countries of the Association of Southeast Asian Nations (ASEAN) and the Asia–Pacific Economic Cooperation (APEC) met and resolved to establish closer collaborative mechanisms for disease surveillance and response. Health staff everywhere worked with dedication, and many, including WHO staff member Dr. Carlo Urbani, lost their lives.

On July 5, 2003, WHO announced that Taiwan, China, where the last known probable case of SARS had been isolated 20 days earlier, had broken the chains of human-to-human transmission. A recurrence of SARS cannot, however, be ruled out. Further research on many unresolved questions is needed. In the meantime, systems are now in place to detect a re-emergence should it occur (WHO, 2003d).

## The Impact of SARS

The economic impact of the SARS outbreak has been considerable and illustrates the importance that a severe new disease can assume in a closely interdependent and highly mobile world. Apart from the direct costs of intensive medical care and control interventions, SARS caused widespread social disruption and economic losses. Schools, hospitals, and some borders were closed and thousands of people were placed in quarantine. International travel to affected areas fell sharply by 50 to 70 percent. Hotel occupancy dropped by more than 60 percent. Businesses, particularly in tourism-related areas, failed, while some large production facilities were forced to suspend operations when cases appeared among workers.

A second impact is more positive: SARS stimulated an emergency response—and a level of media attention—on a scale that has very likely changed public and political perceptions of the risks associated with emerging and epidemic-prone diseases. It also raised the profile of public health to new heights by demonstrating the severity of adverse effects that a health problem can also have on economies and social stability. The resulting high level of political commitment was decisive in the containment of SARS and has much to say about the ability of nations to achieve public health results even when drugs and vaccines are not available to cure or prevent the infection.

## Lessons Learnt

Although much about SARS—including its potential to reoccur—remains to be learnt through systematic analysis of existing data, and focused research activities in China, several important lessons are already apparent. WHO is applying these lessons across the entire Organization as it responds to the HIV/AIDS emergency.

The first and most compelling lesson concerns the need to report, promptly and openly, cases of any disease with the potential for international spread. Attempts to conceal cases of an infectious disease, for fear of social and economic consequences, must be recognized as a short-term stop-gap measure that carries a very high price: the potential for high levels of human suffering and death, loss of credibility in the eyes of the international community, escalating negative domestic economic impact, damage to the health and economies of neighboring countries, and a very real risk that outbreaks within the country's own territory will spiral out of control. Following the adoption during the World Health Assembly in May 2003 of a resolution on the International Health Regulations, WHO has been confirmed in its responsibility to take on a strong coordinating role in leading the fight against any infectious disease that threatens international public health (WHO, 2003e). In a second resolution specific to SARS, all countries are urged to report cases promptly and transparently, and to provide information requested by WHO that could help prevent international spread. It was explicitly acknowledged that across-the-board strengthening of systems for outbreak alert and response was the only rational way to defend public health security against not only SARS but also against all future infectious disease threats, including those that might be deliberately caused (WHO, 2003f).

The second lesson is closely related: timely global alerts, especially when widely supported by a responsible press and amplified by electronic communications, worked well to raise awareness and vigilance to levels that can prevent imported cases of an emerging and transmissible infection from causing significant outbreaks. The global alerts issued by WHO on March 12 and 15 provide a clear line of demarcation between areas with severe SARS outbreaks and those with none or only a few secondary cases. Following the SARS alerts, all areas experiencing imported cases, with the exception of Taiwan, China, either prevented any further transmission or kept the number of locally transmitted cases very low. Figure 5-6 shows the weekly onset of 5,910 cases. A climate of increased awareness also helps to explain the speed with which developing countries readied their health services with preparedness plans and launched SARS campaigns, often with WHO support, to guard against imported cases.

The third lesson is that travel recommendations, including screening measures at airports, appear to be effective in helping to contain the international spread of an emerging infection. Initial analysis of data on in-flight transmission of SARS has implicated four flights in the exposure of 27 probable cases, of which 22 occurred on a single flight from Hong Kong to Beijing, China, on March 15. Some of these cases may also have been exposed elsewhere because of being in the same tour group. Following the recommendation of airport screening measures on March 27, no cases associated with in-flight exposure were reported; and initial information reveals that two probable SARS cases were identified by airport screening procedures in Hong Kong and immediately hospitalized. Travel recommendations based on the epidemiological evidence also gave areas where outbreaks were occurring a benchmark for quickly containing SARS, and then regaining world confidence that the area was safe from the risk of SARS transmission. In fact, passenger movement figures provided by Hong Kong International Airport show a rapid rebound from the lowest number of passengers, 14,670 (recorded just before May 23 when the travel recommendations were removed) to 54,195 on July 12, a little over a month later.

The fourth lesson concerns international collaboration: the world's scientists, clinicians and public health experts are willing to set aside academic competition and work together for the public health good when the situation so requires. International collaboration greatly advanced understanding of the science of SARS. One month after the laboratory network was established, participating scientists collectively announced conclusive identification of the SARS virus; complete sequencing of its RNA followed shortly afterwards. The network of clinical experts provided a platform for comparison of patient management strategies to indicate to the world which treatments and strategies were effective. In addition, the epidemiology network confirmed the modes of transmission of SARS and began the long-term collaboration needed to understand clearly the clinical spectrum of disease, including its case fatality ratio, while also providing the information needed to regularly reassess and adjust the case definition.

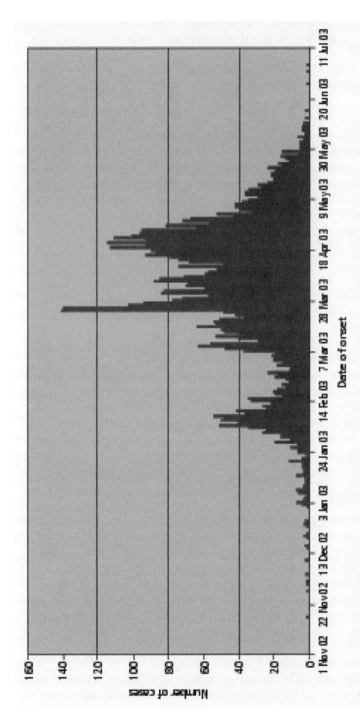

FIGURE 5-6 Probable cases of SARS worldwide, November 1, 2002, to July 11, 2003.

Lesson five is that weaknesses in health systems can permit emerging infections to amplify and spread, and can compromise patient care. The strengthening of health systems thus deserves high priority. The people at greatest risk for SARS were health workers who either became infected by close face-to-face contact with patients or by procedures that brought them into contact with respiratory secretions. Women predominate among the lower ranks of health personnel in many countries; available data reveal that infected health care workers were 2.7 times more likely to be women than men, while infection was roughly equal between the sexes in the general population. The surge of SARS patients placed an enormous burden on health services, requiring facilities for isolation, long periods of intensive and expensive care, and the use of demanding and socially disruptive measures such as mass screening, contact tracing, active surveillance of contacts and—at some outbreak sites—enforced quarantine. Even in areas with highly developed social services, the burden of coping with SARS, including the large number of hospitals with patients and the high number of health workers who became infected, often required closing some hospitals and sections of others. As a result of SARS outbreaks, many long-standing and seemingly intractable problems that have traditionally weakened health systems are being corrected in fundamental and often permanent ways. New surveillance and reporting systems, methods of data management, mechanisms for collaborative research, hospital policies, procedures for infection control, and channels for informing and educating the public are part of the initial positive legacy of SARS that will shape the capacity to respond to future outbreaks of new or re-emerging infections.

Lesson six is that in the absence of a curative drug and a preventive vaccine, existing interventions, tailored to the epidemiological data and supported by political commitment and public concern, can be effectively used to contain an outbreak. The virtual laboratory, and clinical and epidemiological collaborating networks regularly provided information that was used by WHO and its partners to update guidance for containment. Initial guidance was provided for containing outbreaks nationally—as additional evidence was obtained, guidance to limit international spread was also provided. Areas where outbreaks were occurring, and countries which considered themselves at risk of imported cases from these areas, adapted WHO guidance for their use. Some countries introduced active surveillance of suspected contacts using surveillance cameras or military personnel. Others relied on self-surveillance by contacts who voluntarily isolated themselves in their homes and regularly checked for fever. Measures introduced at airports ranged from passive screening of passengers, involving optional completion of questionnaires, to the use of interviews conducted by health workers and sophisticated infrared equipment to screen all passengers for fever and indications of possible exposure. In addition to maximizing the impact of surveillance and screening, these measures were also considered by governments to be reassuring for national citizens as well as international travelers.

The seventh lesson highlights one of the major difficulties faced during the containment activities for SARS: risk communication about new and emerging infectious diseases is a great challenge. Work along these lines is currently under way in conjunction with the risk that a biological agent might be used in an act of terrorism.

SARS will not be the last new disease to take advantage of modern global conditions. In the last two decades of the 20th century, new diseases emerged at the rate of one per year, and this trend is certain to continue (Woolhouse and Dye, 2001). Not all of these emerging infections will transmit easily from person to person as does SARS. Some will emerge, cause illness in humans and then disappear, perhaps to recur at some time in the future. Others will emerge, cause human illness and transmit for a few generations, become attenuated, and likewise disappear. And still others will emerge, become endemic, and remain important parts of our human infectious disease ecology.

The rapid containment of SARS is a success in public health, but also a warning. It is proof of the power of international collaboration supported at the highest political level. It is also proof of the effectiveness of GOARN in detecting and responding to emerging infections of international public health importance. At the same time, containment of SARS was aided by good fortune. The most severely affected areas in the SARS outbreak had well-developed health care systems. Had SARS established a foothold in countries where health systems are less well developed cases might still be occurring, with global containment much more difficult, if not impossible.

Although control measures were effective, they were extremely disruptive and consumed enormous resources resources that might not have been sustainable over time. If SARS reoccurs during an influenza season, health systems worldwide will be put under extreme pressure as they seek to isolate all those who fit the clinical case definition until diagnosis can be ascertained. Continued vigilance is vital.

## SARS: DOWN BUT STILL A THREAT

*Karen J. Monaghan*
National Intelligence Council[10]

### Scope Note

This Intelligence Community Assessment (ICA) was requested by Secretary of Health and Human Services Tommy Thompson and Ambassador Jack Chow, Deputy Assistant Secretary of State for International Health Affairs. It highlights the evolution of severe acute respiratory syndrome (SARS) and the potential im-

---

[10]Prepared under the auspices of Karen Monaghan, Acting National Intelligence Officer for Economics and Global Issues. Additional copies of this assessment can be downloaded from the NIC public website at www.odci.gov/nic or obtained from Karen Monaghan, Acting National Intelligence Officer for Economics and Global Issues, at (703) 482-4128.

plications of the disease for the United States under several scenarios; this paper does not attempt to provide a scientific assessment of the epidemiology of SARS. Even though SARS has infected and killed far fewer people than other common infectious diseases such as influenza, malaria, tuberculosis, and HIV/AIDS, it has had a disproportionately large economic and political impact because it spread in areas with broad international commercial links and received intense media attention as a mysterious new illness that seemed able to go anywhere and hit anyone.

As the first infectious disease to emerge as a new cause of human illness in the 21st century, SARS underscores the growing importance of health issues in a globalized world. The December 1999 unclassified National Intelligence Estimate, *The Global Infectious Disease Threat and Its Implications for the United States*, warned that new and reemerging diseases would pose increasing challenges to the United States and the rest of the world. The 1999 estimate highlighted several key health trends that track with the emergence of SARS:

- The forces of globalization, which are speeding the spread of infectious diseases and amplifying the impact, also are giving us better tools to protect human health.
- Major infectious disease threats to the United States and the world, like HIV/AIDS, will continue to emerge, challenging our ability to diagnose, treat, and control them.
- Infectious diseases will loom larger in global interstate relations as related embargoes and boycotts to prevent their spread create trade frictions and controversy over culpability.

In addition to coordinating the draft within the intelligence community, the National Intelligence Council asked several health experts to review the paper as part of its effort to capitalize on expertise inside and outside the government. The experts included Dr. Anthony Fauci, director of the National Institute of Allergy and Infectious Diseases at the National Institutes of Health; Dr. Steve Ostroff, deputy director, National Center for Infectious Diseases, Centers for Disease Control and Prevention (CDC); and Dr. Joshua Lederberg, professor emeritus at Rockefeller University and Nobel laureate. The NIC also shared the draft with counterparts in Canada at the Privy Council Office, Intelligence Assessment Secretariat.

## DISCUSSION

### The Global Health Challenge

The emergence of SARS illustrates the challenge of battling infectious diseases in an increasingly globalized world. SARS is the latest of more than 35 new or reemerged infectious diseases over the last 30 years. Infectious diseases have long raged through human communities, but forces of globalization—including rapid growth in international trade and travel and increasing urbanization—have amplified their spread and impact. These same forces of globalization, however, also have led to significant advances in communication, travel, and technology, which have aided in the fight against infectious diseases.

• On balance, infectious disease pathogens have the upper hand because they constantly evolve new mechanisms that can exploit weak links in human defenses.
• SARS has subsided for now, but many health experts warn that it is likely to come back when cooler weather returns to temperate areas, bringing a resurgence of respiratory infections.

*Downsides of Globalization*

Population growth and development are bringing more people into contact with non-domesticated animals, introducing new diseases more frequently into the human population. The transmission of pathogens from animals to humans is a process called zoonosis. Some researchers believe that SARS may have originated in China in animals such as wildcat species that were trapped and sold as food in exotic markets. In mid-August 2003, China lifted the ban on the sale and consumption of exotic animals imposed during the SARS epidemic.

• HIV/AIDS, monkeypox, and hantavirus are other infectious diseases believed to have originated in animals.

Modern travel and labor migration patterns played a key role in spreading SARS after it emerged in November 2002 in Guangdong Province, China (see Figure 5-7). From Guangdong, the disease made its way to Hong Kong and then to Vietnam, Singapore, and Taiwan as well as Europe and North America.

• Within China, as many as 180 million people are considered migrant labor, moving between rural areas, cities, and manufacturing centers in search of employment.
• Asia has become a major hub for business and tourist travel, putting millions of passengers within 24 hours of almost every major city in the world, providing little time to identify and isolate people infected with diseases that may take several days to show symptoms.
• More people also are migrating overseas to find jobs, and travel by workers and their families can spread diseases. For example, a Filipino nurse working in Toronto contracted SARS and transmitted it to family members on a visit to the Philippines.
In addition to spreading the disease geographically, global links also have amplified the economic and political impact of the disease. Even though SARS has killed far fewer people up to now—around 815—than those who die each

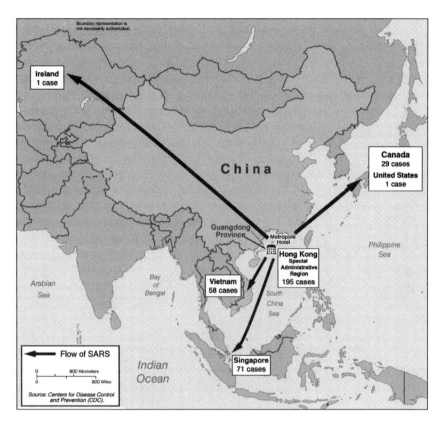

**FIGURE 5-7** Portrait of a superspreader: spread of SARS from the Metropole Hotel in Hong Kong as of March 28, 2003.

year from more common maladies such as pneumonia, influenza, malaria, and tuberculosis, as a new disease it was more disruptive and generated more attention (see Figure 5-8). The disease exhibited some characteristics of a potentially explosive epidemic in the early stages, and SARS hit countries that have extensive commercial links with other parts of the world, generating widespread economic disruptions and media attention.

• The outbreak of SARS in Asia and Canada disrupted a wide-ranging global network of businesses increasingly dependent on international trade and travel. Airlines were the highest profile economic victims, but service industries like tourism and supply chains in industries as diverse as seafood and microchips also were affected.

• Intense media attention and uncertainty about the disease fueled widespread fear, even in some areas without any cases, exacerbating economic disruptions.

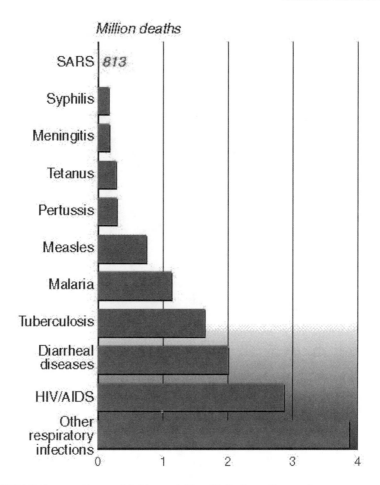

**FIGURE 5-8** Comparative worldwide mortality of infectious diseases.[a]
[a]WHO estimates of worldwide deaths in 2001 from major infectious diseases. SARS deaths occurred from November 2002 to July 2003.

• The suspicion of Asians as carriers of the disease reduced patronage of Asian businesses and communities in the United States and sparked travel bans against Asian tourist groups and conference participants worldwide.

*Benefits of Globalization*

Intense international media coverage facilitated by global communication networks increased pressure on governments to respond effectively to SARS and prompted many citizens and healthcare workers to be vigilant in taking precautions, monitoring symptoms, and seeking early treatment.

• China initially tried to cover up SARS as it did with other diseases in the past, but international media scrutiny and leaks to the press led Beijing to publicly acknowledge and respond to the disease.

• The public has been able to track the evolution of the disease more closely with everything from text messaging on cell phones to publicly and privately run websites; Singaporeans could even watch a special public service television channel devoted to SARS.

Modern communications and medical technologies provided key tools to combat SARS.

• Health workers utilized the World Health Organization's (WHO) global network of research facilities to share data and speed the identification of the virus causing SARS.

• International medical journals took the rare step of promptly publishing research on SARS on the Internet prior to hard copy publication.

• Thermal imaging equipment was acquired in numerous countries in an effort to screen large numbers of people for high fevers. Hong Kong employed software to track the spread of the disease in urban areas, and some countries employed cameras and electronic bracelets to help security officials enforce home quarantines.

## Economic and Political Fallout of SARS

Government and private sector economists have had difficulty calculating the costs of the SARS epidemic. Early on, forecasters estimated that the macroeconomic impact would be negligible but hastily cut growth estimates for several economies, including China, as the disease spread, cases mounted, and the situation appeared to be out of control (see Table 5-3). Service industries, particularly airlines and tourism, were affected immediately. SARS began to threaten the retail and manufacturing sectors, particularly in China, when business trips and trade fairs were canceled, new orders were placed on hold, and investors delayed new expansion and constructions plans.

• In late April, the World Bank cut its growth forecast for East Asia to 5.0 percent—from 5.8 percent in 2002—due in part to SARS.

• In early May, the Asian Development Bank warned that East Asia could lose $US 28 billion in income and output if the disease continued until September.

• Several investment banks shaved up to one percentage point off China's growth forecasts and cautioned that a more serious slowdown could occur if SARS were not brought under control by July.

**TABLE 5-3** Economic Impact of SARS

| Economy | Gross Domestic Product | Employment | Sectoral Impact | Stimulus Packages | Cumulative SARS cases (deaths)* |
|---|---|---|---|---|---|
| China | Early predictions of severe impact revised, forecasts suggest strong growth of 7 to 8 percent for 2003. | Major impact on jobless rate, especially among migrant workforce; unemployment nearly doubles to over 8 million. | Retail sales and restaurant sector stall, particularly in urban areas. Export and manufacturing have proven more resilient. | No comprehensive package, but some ad hoc measures for service sector, including temporary tax cuts. | 5,327(348) |
| Hong Kong | Official growth estimate cut to 1.5 percent from March-to-May earlier forecasts of 3 percent. | Unemployment hits record high 8.3 percent over period, could swell to 10 percent by year end. | Tourism and retail sector ravaged, but few signs SARS has hurt trade. Air traffic fell 80 percent in May. | A US $1.8 billion relief package, including rent reductions and tax rebates, especially for hardest hit businesses. | 1755 (298) |
| Taiwan | Official growth estimate cut to 2.7 percent from earlier forecasts of 3.7 percent. | Minimal impact as employers cut pay and grant unpaid leave but miss target of reducing unemployment to 4.5 percent in 2003. | Tourism and retail sectors hardest hit. | Emergency relief and economic stimulus packages worth $3.7 billion, and a 3-year $8.6 billion public works program. | 671 (84) |

| | | | | |
|---|---|---|---|---|
| Singapore | Private sector growth forecasts cut to I percent from earlier estimates of more than 2 percent. | Unemployment expected to rise to record high 5.5 percent; wage freezes and cuts implemented. | Hospitality and travel industries most affected; also hit retail stores and restaurants. | $US 130 million relief package targeted at SARS-affected sectors. | 206 (32) |
| Thailand | Private sector forecasts put growth as low as 4.2 percent, down one percentage point from 2002. | First quarter employment data show no impact. | Tourist arrivals were down 10 percent in the first 5 months this year; exports also suffered. | None implemented. | 9(2) |
| Canada | Growth expected to slow to 2.2 percent, down one percentage point from earlier forecasts due to SARS, mad-cow, other problems. | Unemployment increased in May to 7.8 percent; thousands of jobs lost in the hospitality sector nationwide. | Lost tourism and airport revenues amounted to $950 million, $570 million in Toronto alone. | In July, the Bank of Canada cut interest rate one-quarter to 3 percent. | 250 (38) |

*Information from VMO as of July 8, 2003.

NOTE: The chart below reflects estimates for 2003 based on second quarter data, but the delayed impact and potential for recurrence in the fall suggest that it may be premature to measure the full impact on growth.

- North Korea imposed tight border restrictions and quarantines, slowing trade flows and temporarily closing a lucrative new tourist resort.

Recent data suggest that growth in most countries plummeted in April and May but started to recover as the disease was brought under control, reports of new cases dwindled, and the WHO removed countries from its travel advisory list. Most notably, no major disruptions in trade and investment flows occurred. Moreover, most factories in China, including those in Guangdong where the disease originated, continued to operate even during the height of the epidemic. In some countries, monetary and fiscal stimulus packages also helped to cushion the blow.

Certain locales, notably Hong Kong, Beijing, and Toronto, were hurt more than others. Moreover, additional indirect costs—the so-called SARS tax—probably will be incurred by businesses consumers, governments, and nongovernment agencies.

- Collectively, the ASEAN countries—Brunei, Cambodia, Indonesia, Laos, Malaysia, Myanmar, the Philippines, Singapore, Thailand, and Vietnam—are estimated to have lost $US 25 billion to $US 30 billion, mostly in the tourism, service, aviation, and restaurant sectors.
- Although China is forecast to achieve growth of 7 to 8 percent this year, the economies of China and Hong Kong will take longer to recover because the tourism, transport, communication, food, and entertainment industries suffered substantial losses.
- Most analysts forecast that SARS would shave a minimal amount off Canada's 2003 growth but cut 1 percent off Toronto's $200 billion economy.

SARS dealt a body blow to the travel and tourism industries, already facing a slowdown from post-9/11 terrorism concerns. They will be slow to recover. Business travel has resumed more rapidly as firms catch up on a backlog of deals, but tourist travel is far below last year's levels. Hotels in Asia are cutting room rates in a bid to attract customers.

An industry trade group estimates the tourist sector in China, Hong Kong, Singapore, and Vietnam will lose up to $US 10 billion and 3 million jobs this year because of SARS.

Airlines have restored most canceled flights, but carriers will have difficulty recouping lost revenues, and some may be forced into bankruptcy. The airline industry's slow recovery will be a further drag on the aviation industry. Asian airlines were to account for one-quarter of Airbus deliveries and 30 percent of Boeing's deliveries in 2003. Several Asia-Pacific carriers asked Airbus and Boeing to postpone deliveries of new aircraft. Both manufacturers have been counting on robust growth in the Asian travel market to boost revenues.

Anecdotal evidence suggests that some export-oriented industries, particularly clothing manufacturers, temporarily shifted some orders to Bangladesh, Turkey, India, and Pakistan. Foreign electronics manufacturers, including a large Japanese electronics firm, shifted some production to plants in Philippines and Malaysia with highly specialized sectors and relatively low costs. There is no evidence to suggest that foreign manufacturers pulled out investments or permanently shifted production outside China or East Asian production plants. Some multinationals probably have begun to rethink the costs and benefits of concentrating investment in one country or region, however.

- Over the last decade, China has attracted massive amounts of foreign direct investment (FDI)—$53 billion in 2002—thanks to its reputation as a low-cost and relatively low-risk manufacturing locale with a rapidly growing domestic market.

SARS has had minimal impact on global semiconductor production, even though nearly 80 percent of production in this $US 8 billion industry is located in Asia, largely in Taiwan and China.

None of the semiconductor operations was forced to curtail production, although SARS disrupted some visits by foreign equipment suppliers and prompted the temporary closing of some Hong Kong sales and marketing offices.

*Political Impact*

SARS seriously tested the leadership skills of politicians and civil servants in every country affected. The public was quick to criticize leaders in China, Canada, Hong Kong, and Taiwan for failing to grasp the seriousness of the situation, to act quickly to contain the spread, and to accept responsibility for missteps. In some countries, public confidence in the ability of government leaders and state institutions to protect them may be permanently damaged.

- In China, SARS intensified behind-the-scenes jockeying between President Hu Jintao and his predecessor, Jiang Zemin, who initially downplayed the disease. Hu publicly acknowledged the threat of SARS, allowed greater media coverage of the crisis, and sacked one of Jiang's loyalists as Minister of Health.
- In Canada the Prime Minister, Premier of Ontario, and Mayor of Toronto drew fire from media and opposition party critics accusing them of failing to respond effectively and address public fears.

In contrast, the WHO and CDC lauded the Vietnamese government's swift action and willingness to accept outside assistance, noting these factors were key to its success in containing the spread of SARS. In Singapore, the public expressed confidence and support for the government's rigorous efforts to identify and isolate suspected SARS patients. An early April poll showed three out of four Singaporeans were confident that the government could stop SARS.

## Tracking the Downturn in SARS

Since WHO first issued a global alert about SARS in March 2003, almost 8,500 probable cases have been reported from 29 countries around the world, with most cases (over 7,000) occurring in China. At one point in May, over 180 new infections were being reported daily, mostly in China.

The number of SARS cases peaked in May and steadily declined worldwide with the WHO declaring on July 5 that all transmission chains of the disease had been broken. The decline may reflect a seasonal retreat of the disease in warmer months, which is common for respiratory illnesses in temperate climates. Nonetheless, the downturn clearly illustrates that, even in a globalized world, the old-fashioned work of identifying and isolating suspected cases, tracing and quarantining others who might be exposed, and issuing travel advisories can control an emerging disease.

• Most countries hit by SARS had not used traditional public health tools such as quarantine and isolation on such a large scale for decades, which slowed the containment.

• Governments also had to mobilize enormous resources to implement large-scale quarantine operations.

### Surveillance

The first line of defense in arresting the spread of SARS has been the success in identifying possible cases—despite the lack of a proven screening test and symptoms common to many respiratory ailments. Taking people's temperature generally has been the simplest, most cost-effective means of initial screening for possible SARS cases, followed by clinical examination for respiratory symptoms in those with fevers.[11]

• Singapore issued over a million SARS toolkits with thermometers and facemasks to every residence in the country. Residents were regularly stopped at office buildings, schools, and other public places for temperature checks.

• China mobilized local party and government officials, including 85 million family planning workers, to try to monitor citizens for symptoms. China also mobilized its large militia to provide the rural public with instructions on SARS prevention. The government distributed tens of thousands of thermometers to the provinces.

---

[11] Anecdotal evidence suggests that some people with SARS may not have classic respiratory symptoms, which makes detection more difficult.

## BOX 5-3
## SARS Basics

**Origins.** The SARS epidemic spread rapidly because people had little immunity to the newly emerged coronavirus that causes the disease. Close contact with sick individuals appears to be the primary means of virus transmission, although research indicates that SARS does not transmit as easily from person-to-person as more common diseases like the cold or flu. The disease spread most rapidly among healthcare workers and family members of infected individuals. Evidence indicates that the virus also is spread through contact with inanimate objects contaminated with virus-containing secretions. Recent detection of a related coronavirus in wildcat species in China raises concerns that SARS may continue to have an animal reservoir, which would complicate control efforts.

**Symptoms.** SARS can progress rapidly from fever and cough to serious pneumonia after an average four-to-six-day incubation period, with up to 20 percent of patients needing mechanical ventilation to survive. In some patients, progression to pneumonia may be delayed. Death may occur several weeks to months after initial symptoms.

**Diagnosis.** Accurate, rapid screening diagnostic tests for SARS are being developed but are not yet licensed in the United States. During the epidemic healthcare workers generally relied on clinical symptoms for detection. WHO defines a suspected SARS case as someone with a temperature over 38° Celsius, a cough or difficulty breathing, and one or more of the following exposures: close contact with a person who is a suspect or probable SARS case, or someone who has lived in or visited a region with SARS transmissions. A "probable case" is a suspected case with radiographic evidence of pneumonia or positive laboratory tests that may take days to weeks to complete.

**Treatment.** No proven therapy is available for severe SARS pneumonia cases. Most clinicians employ respiratory support, antibiotics, fever reduction, and hydration. Some Chinese doctors have used steroids and the antiviral drug ribavirin with varying degrees of success.

**Fatalities.** Although the overall lethality of SARS is higher than initially believed, most deaths continue to be among older patients and those with underlying health problems, such as diabetes or hepatitis B. The WHO reported in May 2003 that death rates vary substantially by age:

- Less than 1 percent in persons 24 years or younger.
- Up to 6 percent in persons 25 to 44 years old.
- Up to 15 percent in persons 44 to 64 years old.
- Greater than 55 percent in persons aged 65 or older.

*Continued*

---

**BOX 5-3 Continued**

Preliminary reports on nonfatal cases showed SARS patients required longer hospital stays—an average of three weeks for those under 60 years of age—than patients with other typical respiratory viruses, raising the economic costs of the SARS outbreak. Moreover, preliminary evidence suggests that some people who survive SARS could suffer long-term respiratory damage that increases health complications and costs.

---

- After WHO confirmed that SARS could be transmitted on airline flights, including 22 infections traced to a single flight in March, airlines have become more stringent at keeping people who might be infected off airplanes.

Even though checks of passengers at airports were relatively effective at keeping infected people off airplanes, some lapses did occur.

- Japan installed infrared thermometers to monitor passengers at Tokyo's international airport after voluntary testing proved ineffective, but press reports indicate that the machines cannot keep up with all travelers at peak times.
- An Asian man suspected of having SARS boarded a flight to the United States in May because his flight left before lab results were received and he had no other symptoms.

*Quarantines and Isolation*[12]

As SARS spread and political and economic stakes rose, countries took tougher measures to contain it. Some countries resorted to strong steps, such as closing schools despite the low number of cases among children, probably to compensate for weaknesses in their health-care infrastructure. Open societies seemed to have trouble enforcing quarantine orders.

- Some Chinese citizens fled cities and industrial hubs in response to early government efforts to isolate suspected cases and quarantine their contacts. Subsequently, Beijing forcibly locked both patients and healthcare workers in hospitals during the peak of infections, and the government instituted fines for people violating isolation orders and employed citizens to keep outsiders out of various villages. Shanghai officials announced in late May they had quarantined nearly 29,000 people in the previous 2 months.

---

[12]Quarantine is the sequestering of those possibly exposed to an infection, while isolation is the sequestering of those individuals with known or suspected infection.

**BOX 5-4**
**The World Health Organization:**
**Playing Fairly Well with a Weak Hand**

The World Health Organization (WHO) issued an international health warning on SARS in March 2003 and travel advisories regarding particular regions hit by the disease. The WHO, in collaboration with the U.S. Centers for Disease Control and Prevention (CDC) and other organizations, worked to identify the cause of the disease, assisted local investigators, and provided guidance on control measures.

The SARS experience highlights the bureaucratic and technical limitations WHO faces in trying to identify and control the international spread of infectious diseases. Under existing international health regulations, countries are only required to report to WHO outbreaks of yellow fever, cholera, and plague. With these diseases, WHO, the United Nations, and domestic officials have the authority to intervene and prevent the movement of people and goods to avert cross-border transmission. With other diseases, WHO plays an advisory role, including issuing travel advisories and offering advice to member governments on screening procedures. Unless a country invites in WHO investigators, WHO has a limited ability to respond to outbreaks. Moreover, WHO has limited capability to investigate suspicious outbreaks before a country officially reports them.

• The World Health Assembly, the body that oversees the WHO, recommended expanding the list of reportable diseases by 2005 to include notification for public health emergencies of international concern.

• In 2000, WHO, with assistance from the Canadian Government, set up the Global Outbreak Alert and Response Network to enhance global surveillance, detection, and response to emerging infectious diseases. It uses an electronic collection system to scan worldwide news reports, websites, discussion groups, and other open source information networks for rumors or reports of disease outbreaks. These notifications trigger WHO staff to notify country representatives, who query national authorities for more information about possible disease outbreaks, bypassing official government notification channels.

• Despite these advances, the system may not have picked up early clues to the SARS outbreak. The electronic monitoring system currently only searches in English and French, although WHO plans to add search capabilities in Arabic, Chinese, Russian, and Spanish. In addition, once WHO receives notification, country cooperation is essential to validate the outbreak, something Chinese officials avoided until late in the outbreak.

**BOX 5-5**
**The World's Quick Response to SARS**

Several factors appeared to facilitate a faster international reaction to SARS in comparison to other diseases in recent decades.

*Fear and Uncertainty.* The rapid geographic spread of the mysterious illness created a sense of urgency to respond to a disease that seemed able to "go anywhere and hit anyone."

*Stronger Leadership.* The World Health Organization took a more public, activist stance in sounding the alarm and mobilizing the global response.

*Scientific Advances.* New tools and techniques allowed researchers better and faster ways to study everything from patterns of lung damage to the genetic sequence of the coronavirus.

*Heightened Awareness of BW Threat.* Concerns about the threat posed by biological weapons enhanced the ability and speed of many countries to identify new infectious diseases.

*Concern About Missing "Another" AIDS.* Some health officials acknowledge they reacted more quickly to SARS partly due to fears that the world's slow response in the 1980s to the emergence of HIV/AIDS allowed the disease to build up devastating momentum.

• Canada threatened those who violated quarantines with fines or court-ordered isolation after some people defied voluntary measures, but news reports indicate that some people violated quarantines when the SARS threat appeared to be fading.

• Singapore's strict quarantines proved particularly effective in bringing the disease under control.

Sometimes the most effective isolation and quarantine policies raised concerns about political freedom and human rights. For example, India and Thailand at one point isolated foreign visitors from countries that had SARS outbreaks, even though they did not have symptoms or known exposures.

• North Korea, which has quarantined entire areas to deal with epidemics in the past, imposed such tight restrictions for SARS that it constrained some international aid flows.

*Political Leadership*

A key variable in managing the SARS epidemic was the willingness of political leaders to raise public awareness of the disease, focus resources, and speed the government response. As noted above, Vietnamese leaders promptly acknowledged the SARS threat at an early stage in the outbreak and sought international help. In contrast, China's political leaders clearly exacerbated the situation by initially suppressing news of the disease.

## Reasons to Stay on Guard

Despite the downturn in cases, SARS has not been eradicated and remains a significant potential threat. Senior WHO officials and many other noted medical experts believe it highly likely that SARS will return. SARS, like other respiratory diseases such as influenza, may have subsided in the northern hemisphere as summer temperatures rise, only to come back in the fall.

- Most infectious diseases follow a similar epidemiological curve, emerging, peaking, and declining over time to a steady state, but the number of infections, the lethality, and length of time can vary enormously.
- Even as WHO officials removed the last of its travel advisories for SARS early this summer, officers repeatedly emphasized the risk that the disease would be back.
- Some experts caution that SARS might even lay low for several years before reappearing, as diseases such as Ebola and Marburg have done.
- The apparent reservoir of the coronavirus in animals, Beijing's decision to lift the ban on sales of exotic animals, and lack of a reliable diagnostic kit, vaccine, or antiviral drug are factors that preclude eradication.

### No Reliable Screening Tests

Diagnosis remains almost as much an art as a science as long as no proven screening test has been developed. Diagnostic kits currently under development can catch only about 70 percent of SARS cases, and their utility for widespread deployment is not yet known. SARS is difficult to detect, particularly in the early stages, even for countries with the most modern medical capabilities, raising the risk that healthcare workers will miss mild cases. Moreover, there is little prospect of a vaccine in the short-term.

Various countries have different definitions of suspected and probable cases and have changed the definitions over time.

### SARS Could Mutate

Natural mutations in the coronavirus which causes SARS could alter basic characteristics of the disease, but whether a mutation would make SARS more or less dangerous is impossible to predict. A significant increase in the transmissibility or lethality of SARS obviously would pose greater health risks and raise fears around the globe.

- Mutations could be particularly problematic if they alter the symptoms associated with SARS, making it harder to identify suspected cases.
- Researchers are studying a group of Canadians who tested positive for the SARS virus last spring but never got sick in order to see if they still might have infected others.
- Mutations also would complicate the development of a treatment or vaccine, which already probably is several years away.

### Difficult to Maintain Vigilance

The willingness of healthcare workers to serve in the face of significant infection risks has been a key variable in the battle against SARS and other emerging diseases. Most healthcare workers in countries hit by SARS toiled long hours under dangerous conditions. The rate of infection among hospital workers was much higher than among the general public, underscoring the difficulty even professionals had in maintaining stringent infection control procedures.

- At one point 20 percent of those infected in Hong Kong were nurses, and over 300 healthcare workers were infected within a 17-day period in China during April.

Some health workers refused to work in SARS wards. This problem is likely to grow in both rich and poor countries if the disease resurges.

- In Taiwan, where over 90 percent of SARS infections occurred in hospitals, over 160 health workers quit or refused to work on SARS wards. The government threatened to revoke their professional licenses.
- The Chinese government fired at least six doctors who refused to treat SARS patients and barred them from practicing for life. China also tried to encourage healthcare workers by launching public relations campaigns hailing the work of the Angels in White, and Beijing offered bonus pay and staffed SARS hospitals with Army medical staff.
- Press reports in Canada indicate that some nurses refused to work in SARS wards in Toronto despite a doubling of their wages and lobbied for an official government inquiry on the handling of the epidemic.

Shortages in trained healthcare personnel were exacerbated when many healthcare workers fell ill to SARS and were replaced by workers with less training.

- Taiwan appeared so eager to declare victory over SARS that it relaxed its standards before the disease was brought under control. Press reports suggest that some health-care workers were so fatigued from the crisis that they cut corners.
- Canadian officials acknowledge that the second outbreak in Toronto resulted from hospitals relaxing infection control regimes too quickly.

## SARS Scenarios

Faced with these uncertainties, we have constructed three scenarios to consider potential trajectories for the disease and the implications for the United States. We have not attempted to identify a most likely scenario because the future course of SARS will depend on a host of complex variables, including the scope of present infections, mutations in the virus, the vulnerability of host populations, how individuals and governments respond, and chance.

### Scenario One: SARS Simmers

SARS could resurface this fall but be limited to random outbreaks in a few countries. Rapid activation of local and international surveillance systems and isolation procedures would be key to identifying suspect cases and containing the spread. Initially, some cases might elude detection by hospital workers and airport personnel, who have relaxed screening procedures since the disease ebbed. Smaller, poorly funded transit facilities would remain vulnerable because they lacked trained staff and equipment to effectively monitor all passengers.

- In most affected countries, the small number of cases and transmission would render SARS more of a public health nuisance than a crisis.

Some countries would be tempted to hide a resurgence. China's experience demonstrated that hiding an outbreak is increasingly difficult and costly in a globalized world, but some governments still probably calculate that transparency also has drawbacks. Indeed, the economic repercussions of WHO travel advisories for SARS probably reinforce the incentives countries have to hide or underreport cases.

- The WHO had to lean on Beijing throughout the crisis to share data.
- Some countries over the past decade have not acknowledged HIV/AIDS cases in the military for security reasons, suggesting they would withhold information on other diseases that might affect readiness.

Even if new SARS outbreaks were sporadic and small-scale, economic, political, and psychological ripples would occur. China faces the biggest risks. Although foreign investors are unlikely to withdraw substantial amounts of FDI, firms with considerable exposure to China might redirect a percentage of new investment to other locations to diversify their manufacturing operations. Companies that already have temporarily shifted some production outside China probably would establish more permanent arrangements.

- Companies and governments outside China probably would attempt to exploit these concerns by more aggressively trying to turn temporary production into longer-term investments.

Multinationals also are likely to become more concerned about the "SARS tax" on their businesses, including increased healthcare expenditures for expatriate employees and expanded insurance to cover the risk to operations and personnel from infectious diseases. Some firms probably would calculate that the risks of frequent business travel outweighed the costs and switch to teleconferencing, telecommuting, and e-commerce.

- SARS has alerted companies to the potential operational disruptions caused by a contagious disease, risks that are rarely priced into business costs or considered in contingency planning.
- Whereas previous business continuity plans focused on data protection and recovery, businesses probably will begin to consider plans that involve protection of human resources, backup teams, and alternate locations for operation.

Paradoxically, keeping SARS out of the United States might become more difficult as fewer cases are seen, because health, transportation, and security workers are more likely to drop their guard in monitoring for infected people if only a few cases pop up now and then.

- The U.S. status as a major hub for international travel increases the statistical risk that lapses in surveillance abroad could facilitate the spread of SARS to American cities.
- It is difficult for many visitors to acquire visas for travel to the United States; thus they probably would be inclined to withhold information that could complicate their visit.

*Scenario Two: SARS Spreads to Poor Countries, Regions*

SARS could gain a foothold in one or more poor countries, potentially generating more infections and deaths than before but with relatively little international economic impact. Few poor countries have had SARS appear on their doorstep up to now because most have relatively few links to the affected regions, but the longer the disease persists the more likely it is that SARS will spread more widely.

- Impoverished areas of Africa, Asia, and Latin America remain at potential risk for SARS because of weak healthcare systems and vulnerable populations. Even a small number of cases in large, underdeveloped cities such as Dhaka, Kinshasa, or Lagos could generate a large number of victims in a short period.
- No evidence thus far suggests that people with malaria or HIV/AIDS are

more susceptible to becoming infected by SARS, but experience indicates that diseases are more lethal among sick and malnourished populations. Sub-Saharan Africa has the highest concentration of HIV-infected people in the world, and those with full-blown AIDS have severely deficient immune response.

Most poor countries would have trouble organizing control measures against SARS, especially if the disease gained momentum before it was identified by healthcare workers. Most countries have inadequate hospital facilities to effectively isolate large numbers of patients, and most hospitals even lack the resources to provide food and care to patients.

• Voluntary home quarantine might not be viable in crowded urban slums, where large families might share small dwellings and people might have to go out each day for food or work.
• Identifying and tracking down people who might have been exposed probably would be substantially more difficult in countries with poor infrastructure and underfunded local security services.
• Repressive countries, fearful that the disease could spark political upheaval, probably would quarantine entire towns or villages with military force or incarcerate quarantine violators. Outside countries and international organizations providing assistance are likely to split over how much to condemn or withhold aid over apparent human rights violations.

The spread of SARS into various poor countries is likely to significantly disrupt local economies while having relatively little impact on broader international markets.

• The local impact could be worse than in places like Taiwan and Canada, because people in poor countries are living closer to the margin and governments have less resources for emergencies. In countries with a much smaller pool of skilled workers, the loss of key personnel can have a relatively large effect on society—as HIV/AIDS has illustrated in Africa.
• Even poor countries like Bangladesh have at least some global trade and business links that could be disrupted if they were hit by SARS, but the more isolated the country, the smaller the global economic impact probably would be.

The spread of SARS to poor countries also would complicate international efforts to control the disease.

• Diagnosing SARS is likely to be more difficult among populations with many preexisting health problems.
• Even if SARS claimed hundreds of victims in poor countries, their gov-

ernments probably would not be inclined to devote substantial resources to the fight when other diseases—such as malaria, tuberculosis, and HIV/AIDS—were claiming many more lives.

The spread of SARS to countries with weak healthcare systems and vulnerable populations also is likely to make the disease appear more transmissible and lethal, heightening public fears in other parts of the world:

• Poor, isolated regions of Russia and China would have trouble containing an outbreak, although their governments probably could mobilize more resources to respond once infections began to climb.
• Even if SARS outbreaks were limited to poor countries, the persistence of the disease probably would fuel some unease around the world about a broader resurgence. The impact probably would marginally decrease demand for travel and increase demand for medical products.

An outbreak of SARS in poor countries would pose particular challenges for the United States and other governments and multilateral organizations providing assistance. WHO and CDC probably would come under pressure to provide money and technical assistance to compensate for weak healthcare systems. The higher the number of infected people, the more the international community would be called on to do something.

• Neighboring countries are likely to press for help with disease monitoring to prevent SARS from spreading into their countries, especially if panic began generating refugee flows.
• Repressive regimes like North Korea might accept material assistance but block outside experts from visiting, even at the risk of putting more of their own citizens at risk. North Korea in previous years has been accused of diverting NGO assistance to the military and not allowing outsiders to monitor how it is used.

*Scenario Three: SARS Resurges in Major Trade Centers*

SARS could stage a comeback this fall in the main places it hit before—such as China, Hong Kong, Taiwan, and Canada—or gain a foothold in other places with extensive international travel and trade links like the United States, Japan, Europe, India, or Brazil.

• An outbreak almost certainly would spark another wave of WHO health warnings and travel advisories; Japan already has canceled an international conference on HIV/AIDS planned for this winter due to fears it would coincide with a resurgence of SARS.

Even if the number of infected persons were not greater in a second wave, an outbreak of SARS in major trade centers again would be likely to have significant economic and political implications. The resurgence of SARS in Asia probably would cause less disruption as citizens, companies, and governments learn to live with it, as they do with other diseases, unless the transmissibility or lethality rose substantially. Nonetheless, a second wave of SARS in Asia probably would prompt some multinationals to modestly reduce their exposure to the region if they concluded that SARS posed a long-term health challenge.

• Given the size of the Asian market and low wage-rates, few companies are likely to yank existing production out of China unless SARS debilitates or kills large numbers of workers. Firms probably would divert some future investments to other regions to diversify their supply chains.
• Disruptions due to SARS are likely to persuade some companies to loosen just-in-time production chains by creating some cushion in key inventories, increasing costs but not productivity.
• Global trade and investment flows could seize up if quarantines shut down factories and shipments.

A substantial decline in China's manu-facturing sector would reverberate in Southeast Asian economies that provide critical manufactured inputs, raw materials, and energy and disrupts production chains throughout East Asia.

Bigger outbreaks in places such as Europe and the United States would affect new sets of business and government players. The level of public fear almost certainly would be higher in places that had not been affected by the first wave of SARS, driving up social disruption and economic costs.

• The economic cost of SARS probably would skyrocket if fears grew about the transmission of the disease in planes or on objects.
• Some buyers this spring demanded that Asian manufacturers irradiate their export goods after research indicated that SARS could survive for several days on inanimate objects.

Even the health systems of rich countries could be overwhelmed if the resurgence of SARS cases coincided with the annual influenza epidemic this winter. As long as no quick and reliable test to diagnose SARS exists, people with fevers and a cough could overwhelm hospitals and clinics as healthcare workers struggled to distinguish patients with SARS and isolate them from others.

• A pneumonia-like illness erupted in western Canada in mid-August, raising questions among health experts about whether a milder version of SARS had returned.
• Surges of people seeking medical care almost certainly would increase the odds of healthcare workers missing some cases.

• Some SARS patients have not displayed classic respiratory symptoms, suggesting some "silent" spreaders may not even know they have the disease, and some travelers with mild symptoms might lie about contact with infected persons to avoid quarantine.

Given the high economic and political stakes already seen in the SARS epidemic, some jurisdictions probably would try to fudge health data in an effort to avoid official health warnings or get them lifted more quickly.

• Some governments might narrow the definition of "probable" SARS cases to reduce crowding in hospitals, yet such moves could spark tensions with WHO and other countries over the accuracy of data.

### Building Better Defenses Against Disease

The emergence of SARS has sparked widespread calls for greater international surveillance and cooperation against such diseases. SARS has demonstrated to even skeptical government leaders that health matters in profound social, economic, and political ways.

---

**BOX 5-6**
**Influenza: Lurking Killer**

Influenza is an ideal virus for worldwide spread (a pandemic) and many epidemilogists argue that the world is "overdue" for a major influenza pandemic. When a new type of flu virus emerges from a reassortment of animal and human viruses to which humans have no prior immunity, a pandemic may ensue. Scientists believe the past two influenza pandemics originated in China where people live in close contact with birds and swine, the major sources of animal flu viruses. Influenza spreads even more quickly than SARS because flu can be transmitted efficiently through the air. As a result, close contact is not required for people to become infected, making it almost impossible to trace and isolate ill people who are spreading the disease.

Three major flu epidemics stand out in modern U.S. history:

• 1918-19: "Spanish Flu" caused 20-50 million deaths worldwide, including 500,000 in the United States.
• 1957-58: "Asian Flu" originated in China and spread globally, killing around 70,000 Americans.
• 1968-69: "Hong Kong Flu," a global pandemic, began in Hong Kong and ultimately claimed 34,000 U.S. lives.

- The experience with SARS probably will help countries prepare for future disease outbreaks.

This intense focus on SARS has opened a window of opportunity to pursue bilateral and international cooperation against infectious diseases. The United States and WHO may be able to develop new institutional channels to foster long-term cooperation on health issues.

- Momentum is likely to flag if SARS continues to subside and political leaders lose interest.
- Budget constraints and turf battles almost certainly will retard progress and agreements may fail to be implemented at the provincial, state and local levels if added responsibilities are not accompanied by additional funding.

## Areas of Need

Several countries already are seeking assistance from the WHO and the U.S. CDC in an effort to strengthen their health systems. Some even are moving to commit more resources.

- Both China and Taiwan have held technical discussions with US officials exploring ways to improve their health system, and Beijing publicly has committed $1.3 billion in new funds.

## Surveillance

Despite substantial progress in recent decades in building networks to monitor disease, the surveillance systems in most countries remain weak. Many surveillance systems have been built over the years to detect specific diseases, such as polio and guinea worm. The WHO also has created a global network of over 100 centers in 83 countries to track influenza. The longer-term challenge is to build networks throughout countries and regions and the means to issue warnings to national and international authorities.

- Systems focusing on specific diseases generally have been more cost effective than trying to increase surveillance for all diseases, but either approach leaves holes.
- International surveillance networks also must work out differences between countries over what health patterns are "normal" and which should set off alarm bells. The death of working-age pneumonia patients in the United States would be so unusual it would trigger closer examination, but this phenomenon probably was not considered abnormal in China in the early stage of SARS.

---

**BOX 5-7**
**Health Surveillance and Biological Weapons**

The SARS outbreak illustrates the difficulty in distinguishing the emergence of new infectious disease from the release of a BW agent. Ongoing efforts to improve global health surveillance, however, probably will aid international monitoring for detecting the possible release of biological warfare agents, especially traditional types. As baselines for natural diseases are established in the coming years, a deliberate release of traditional BW agents could be more readily recognized. Unfortunately, many developing countries probably will not acquire domestic detection capabilities, such as tools to identify genetic sequences in disease organisms. Moreover, history suggests that some countries will not support internal disease surveillance efforts for political or economic reasons, leaving significant gaps in a global surveillance system.

---

• Even if local health workers identify worrisome developments, many medical facilities in developing countries lack communications equipment and vehicles to alert national officials and transport samples or patients.

• Although rapid online journal publication aided in sharing information on the new SARS virus, outbreak responders need to share data even earlier.

*Epidemiological Expertise*

Many countries lacked trained experts to map the trajectory of SARS. Such expertise was critical to understanding the transmissibility, lethality, and scope of the disease.

• Press reports indicate that Chinese officials have had trouble processing and sharing research information within China and with outsiders, such as WHO.

*Laboratory Facilities*

Few countries have the sophisticated laboratories or trained personnel to do the hard science of cracking mysterious new illnesses. As a result, regional or mobile labs may be the most viable prospect for speeding up diagnoses and research.

• WHO reports that staff in over 90 percent of developing country laboratories are not familiar with quality assurance principles, and 60 percent of the lab equipment is inoperable or outdated.

*Equipment*

The cost of basic diagnostic and protective equipment is relatively modest yet still unaffordable for many countries. SARS highlighted a widespread shortage of ventilators to support patients with pneumonia. The lack of adequate sterilization equipment raises the risk of spreading disease when medical instruments are reused.

• The highest priority for many countries is likely to be diagnostic tests to determine which patients need to be isolated; the need for such tests would be all the more pressing if research indicates SARS can be transmitted through the blood supply.

---

**BOX 5-8**
**SARS and HIV/AIDS**

SARS has focused greater international attention on the importance of health, but the new disease probably will not lead to a significant boost in the fight against HIV/AIDS in the coming years. Indeed, many countries are likely to view spending on diseases like SARS and HIV/AIDS as a zero-sum game in the short term.

• SARS is generating international interest in improving health surveillance systems that could broaden screening for HIV/AIDS as well, but the interests will not always coincide on allocating limited resources. The small number of HIV/AIDS surveillance sites already in most countries is designed to gather health data on specific groups, such as young women, drug users, or prostitutes, rather than samples of the population at large.
• Some countries may be willing to devote more resources to improving general health and fighting HIV/AIDS within their security services. With HIV/AIDS prevalence rates running as high as 50 percent in some African militaries, a growing number of governments are working with the US on control programs. Political leaders may see it as critical and cost effective to work with outsiders for better healthcare for soldiers as well.

China's new health minister has said she plans to focus on HIV/AIDS now that SARS has subsided, according to press reports. Some AIDS activists and NGOs within China also have expressed hope that the government response to SARS will translate into more action on HIV/AIDS.

A resurgence of SARS this winter could delay activity on AIDS, and some AIDS activists in China fear the government might believe the stringent controls used to fight SARS should be used against HIV/AIDS as well.

• Many countries need more ventilators to support patients with pneumonia. In addition, negative pressure rooms to isolate infected patients are in shorter supply; even many hospitals in affluent countries are not likely to have enough rooms to handle a serious outbreak.

### Developing Countermeasures

Progress in developing diagnostic tests, treatments, and vaccines would fundamentally improve prospects for combating SARS. This will take time, however, and first-generation products often are not completely effective without further research and improvement.

• Tracking down infected and exposed persons on airline flights also could be improved significantly if airlines retained electronic records of passenger lists.

### Political Hurdles

Almost all countries will express support for improving international healthcare capabilities, but negotiations are likely to be contentious, and many players will see this as an opportunity to win concessions or score points with Washington. Some areas of possible contention are:

• *Money.* Many developing countries will say they cannot improve their surveillance systems and healthcare infrastructure without significant outside assistance, in the form of training, equipment, or grants.
• *"Rich" vs. "poor" Diseases.* Some developing countries may argue that they will work to improve surveillance for diseases like SARS if the United States and the international community do more to help them fight diseases which claim more lives in their countries, such as malaria and tuberculosis.
• *Multilateral Channels.* European countries are likely to use the focus on health issues to renew pressure on the United States to work through multilateral organizations such as the Global Fund for AIDS, Tuberculosis, and Malaria.
• *Pharmaceutical Access.* Any forum to discuss international health cooperation almost certainly will include some criticism of U.S. positions in the WTO on pharmaceutical sales. Research to develop tests, treatments, and vaccines is underway, but drug companies will have little incentive to bring such products to market without public sector support if SARS appears to fade away.
• *WHO Authority.* Some countries probably will argue for strengthening the authority of the WHO to sanction states that do not share health data or bar outside health experts from visiting. Other countries, such as China and Malaysia, are likely to resist any moves they see as infringing on sovereignty. Taiwan almost certainly will continue trying to use health issues to win recognition from WHO and other multilateral organizations.

# REFERENCES

Abbott A. 2003a. Human fatality adds fresh impetus to fight against bird flu. *Nature* 423(6935):5.

Abbott A. 2003b. *Nature* 423:5.

Asia-Pacific Economic Corporation. 2001. Infectious Diseases in the Asia Pacific Region: A Reason to Act and Acting with Reason. 22nd Industrial Science and Technology Working Group Strategy Paper. Singapore: Asia-Pacific Economic Corporation.

Augustine JJ. 2003. Developing a highly contagious disease readiness plan: the SARS experience. *Emergency Medical Services* 32(7):77-83.

Booth CM, Matukas LM, Tomlinson GA, Rachlis AR, Rose DB, Dwosh HA, Walmsley SL, Mazzulli T, Avendano M, Derkach P, Ephtimios IE, Kitai I, Mederski BD, Shadowitz SB, Gold WL, Hawryluck LA, Rea E, Chenkin JS, Cescon DW, Poutanen SM, Detsky AS. 2003. Clinical features and short-term outcomes of 144 patients with SARS in the greater Toronto area. *JAMA* 289(21):2801-9.

Breiman RF, Evans MR, Preiser W, Maguire J, Schnur A, Li A, Bekedam H, MacKenzie JS. 2003. Role of China in the quest to define and control severe acute respiratory syndrome. [Review] [16 Refs]. *Emerging Infectious Diseases* 9(9):1037-41.

CDC. 2003a. Update: severe acute respiratory syndrome—worldwide and United States, 2003. *MMWR–Morbidity & Mortality Weekly Report* 52(28):664-5.

Chan JW, Ng CK, Chan YH, Mok TY, Lee S, Chu SY, Law WL, Lee MP, Li PC. 2003. Short term outcome and risk factors for adverse clinical outcomes in adults with severe acute respiratory syndrome (SARS). *Thorax* 58(8):686-9.

Chen Q. 2003. [Application of SIR model in forecasting and analyzing for SARS]. *Beijing Da Xue Xue Bao* 35(Suppl.):75-80.

Chinese Center for Disease Control and Prevention. 2003. Overview of the epidemics and repsonses to the severe acute respiratory syndrome (SARS) in the People's Republic of China, Beijing.

Chowell G, Fenimore PW, Castillo-Garsow MA, Castillo-Chavez C. 2003. SARS outbreaks in Ontario, Hong Kong and Singapore: the role of diagnosis and isolation as a control mechanism. *Journal of Theoretical Biology* 224(1):1-8.

Department of State. 2003. Global mercury: an international bioterrorism exercise. Media Note. Available: http://www.state.gov/pa/prs/ps/2003/23878.htm.

Donnelly CA, Ghani AC, Leung GM, Hedley AJ, Fraser C, Riley S, Abu-Raddad LJ, Ho LM, Thach TQ, Chau P, Chan KP, Lam TH, Tse LY, Tsang T, Liu SH, Kong JH, Lau EM, Ferguson NM, Anderson RM. 2003. Epidemiological Determinants of Spread of Causal Agent of Severe Acute Respiratory Syndrome in Hong Kong. May 24, 2003. [Erratum Appears in *Lancet* 361(9371):1832]. *Lancet* 361(9371):1761-6.

Drazen JM, Campion EW. 2003. SARS, the Internet, and the journal. [See Comment]. *New England Journal of Medicine* 348(20):2029.

Dye C, Gay N. 2003. Epidemiology: modeling the SARS epidemic. *Science* 300(5627):1884-5.

Enserink M. 2003a. SARS in China. China's missed chance. *Science* 301(5631):294-6.

Enserink M. 2003b. Infectious diseases: Avian flu outbreak sets off alarm bells. *Science* 300(5620):718.

Eysenbach G. 2003. SARS and population health technology. *Journal of Medical Internet Research* 5(2):e14.

Fedson DS. 2003. Pandemic influenza and the global vaccine supply. *Clinical Infectious Diseases* 36(12):1552-61.

Ferguson NM, Mallett S, Jackson H, Roberts N, Ward P. 2003. A population-dynamic model for evaluating the potential spread of drug-resistant influenza virus infections during community-based use of antivirals. *Journal of Antimicrobial Chemotherapy* 51(4):977-90.

Gerdil C. 2003. The annual production cycle for influenza vaccine. *Vaccine* 21(16):1776-9.

Grein TW, Kamara K-BO, Rodier G, Plant AJ, Bovier P, Ryan MJ, Ohyama T, Heymann DL. 2000. Rumors of disease in the global village: outbreak verification. *Emerging Infectious Diseases* 6(2):97-102.

Han H, Li X, Qu W, Shen T, Xu F, Gao D. 2003. [The regression analysis of the in hospital medical staffs infection rate and the application of the isolation measures including the emergency-isolation radiology information system]. *Beijing Da Xue Xue Bao* 35(Suppl.):89-91.

Hatta M, Gao P, Halfmann P, Kawaoka Y. 2001. Molecular basis for high virulence of Hong Kong H5N1 influenza A viruses. *Science* 293(5536):1840-2.

He WQ, Chen SB, Liu XQ, Li YM, Xiao ZL, Zhong NS. 2003. Death risk factors of severe acute respiratory syndrome with acute respiratory distress syndrome. *Zhongguo Wei Zhong Bing Ji Jiu Yi Xue* 15(6):336-7.

Heymann DL, Rodier GR, WHO Operational Support Team to the Global Outbreak Alert and Response, Network. 2001. Hot spots in a wired world: who surveillance of emerging and re-emerging infectious diseases. [Review] [44 Refs]. *The Lancet Infectious Diseases* 1(5):345-53.

Hoffmann E, Krauss S, Perez D, Webby R, Webster RG. 2002. Eight-plasmid system for rapid generation of influenza virus vaccines. *Vaccine* 20(25-26):3165-70.

Hsueh PR, Hsiao CH, Yeh SH, Wang WK, Chen PJ, Wang JT, Chang SC, Kao CL, Yang PC, SARS Research Group of National Taiwan University College of Medicine and, National Taiwan University Hospital. 2003. Microbiologic characteristics, serologic responses, and clinical manifestations in severe acute respiratory syndrome, Taiwan. *Emerging Infectious Diseases* 9(9):1163-7.

Hupert N, Cuomo J. 2003. BERM: The Weill/Cornell Bioterrorism and Epidemic Outbreak Response Model. [Online] Available: http://www.ahrq.gov/research/biomodel.htm [accessed September 17, 2003].

Hupert N, Mushlin AI, Callahan MA. 2002. Modeling the public health response to bioterrorism: using discrete event simulation to design antibiotic distribution centers. *Medical Decision Making* 22(5 Suppl.):S17-S25.

IOM (Institute of Medicine). 1992. Emerging infections: microbial threats to health in the United States. Washington, DC: National Academy Press.

IOM. 2003. Microbial threats to health: emergence, detection, and response. Washington, DC: The National Academies Press.

ITU Internet Report. Birth of broadband. [Online] Available: http://www.itu.net [accessed September 17, 2003].

Kilbourne ED. 1969. Future influenza vaccines and the use of genetic recombinants. Bulletin of the World Health Organization 141(3):643-5.

Kimball AM, Horwitch CA, O'Carroll PW, Arjoso S, Kunanusont C, Lin YS, Meyer CM, Schubert LE, Dunham PL. 1999. The Asian Pacific Economic Cooperation emerging infections network. *American Journal of Preventive Medicine* 17(2):156-8.

Kimball AM, Pautler NF. 2003. Lessons of SARS, The APEC-EINET experience. [Online] Available: http://apec.org/infectious/SARS_Lessons.pdf.

Kitch P, Yasnoff WA. 2002. Assessing the value of information systems. In: Gotham I, Smith P, Birkhead S, Davisson MC. Policy issues in developing information systems for public health surveillance systems of communicable diseases. In: O'Carroll P, Yasnoff WA, Ward ME, Ripp LH, Martin EL, eds., *Public Health Informatics and Information Systems*. New York: Springer Verlag.

Koopmans M, Fouchier R, Wilbrink B, Meijer A, Natrop G, Osterhaus ADME, van Steenbergen JE, du Ry van Beest Holle M, Conyn van Spaendonck MAE, Bosman A. 2003. Update on human infections with highly pathogenic avian influenza virus A/H7N7 during an outbreak in poultry in the Netherlands. *Eurosurveillance Weekly* 7(18).

Krug RM. 2003. The potential use of influenza virus as an agent for bioterrorism. *Antiviral Research* 57(1-2):147-50.

Li L, Wang Z, Lu Y, Bao Q, Chen S, Wu N, Cheng S, Weng J, Zhang Y, Yan J, Mei L, Wang X, Zhu H, Yu Y, Zhang M, Li M, Yao J, Lu Q, Yao P, Bo X, Wo J, Wang S, Hu S. 2003. Severe acute respiratory syndrome-associated coronavirus genotype and its characterization. *Chinese Medical Journal* 116(9):1288-92.

Lin G, Jia X, Ouyang Q. 2003. [Predict SARS infection with the small world network model]. *Beijing Da Xue Xue Bao* 35(Suppl.):66-9.

Lipsitch M, Cohen T, Cooper B, Robins JM, Ma S, James L, Gopalakrishna G, Chew SK, Tan CC, Samore MH, Fisman D, Murray M. 2003. Transmission dynamics and control of severe acute respiratory syndrome. *Science* 300(5627):1966-70.

Liu M. et al. 2003. *Virology* 314:589.

Lloyd-Smith JO, Galvani AP, Getz WM. 2003. Curtailing transmission of severe acute respiratory syndrome within a community and its hospital. *Proceedings of the Royal Society of London. Series B, Biological Sciences* 270(1528):1979-89.

Matrosovich MN, Krauss S, Webster RG. 2001. H9N2 influenza A viruses from poultry in Asia have human virus-like receptor specificity. *Virology* 281(2):156-62.

Olsen CW. 2002. The emergence of novel swine influenza viruses in North America. *Virus Research* 85(2):199-210.

Pearson H, Clarke T, Abbott A, Knight J, Cyranoski D. 2003. SARS: what have we learned? *Nature* 424(6945):121-6.

Peiris JS, Guan Y, Markwell D, Ghose P, Webster RG, Shortridge KF. 2001. Cocirculation of avian H9n2 and contemporary human H3n2 influenza a viruses in pigs in Southeastern China: potential for genetic reassortment? *Journal of Virology* 75(20):9679-86.

Peiris M, Yuen KY, Leung CW, Chan KH, Ip PL, Lai RW, Orr WK, Shortridge KF. 1999. Human infection with influenza H9N2. *Lancet* 354(9182):916-7.

ProMED-Mail. May 14, 2003. Influenza H5N1, avian-China: suspected. ProMED-mail. [Online] Available: http://www.promedmail.org [accessed January 17, 2004].

Riley S, Fraser C, Donnelly CA, Ghani AC, Abu-Raddad LJ, Hedley AJ, Leung GM, Ho LM, Lam TH, Thach TQ, Chau P, Chan KP, Lo SV, Leung PY, Tsang T, Ho W, Lee KH, Lau EM, Ferguson NM, Anderson RM. 2003. Transmission dynamics of the etiological agent of SARS in Hong Kong: impact of public health interventions. *Science* 300(5627):1961-6.

Riley S, Fraser C, Donnelly CA, Ghani AC, Abu-Raddad LJ, Hedley AJ, Leung GM, Ho LM, Lam TH, Thach TQ, Chau P, Chan KP, Lo SV, Leung PY, Tsang T, Ho W, Lee KH, Lau EM, Ferguson NM, Anderson RM. 2003. Transmission dynamics of the etiological agent of SARS in Hong Kong: impact of public health interventions. [See Comment]. *Science* 300(5627):1961-6.

Roscelli JD, Bass JW, Pang L. 1991. Guillain-Barré syndrome and influenza vaccination in the U.S. Army, 1980-1988. [See Comment]. *American Journal of Epidemiology* 133(9):952-5.

Ruan YJ, Wei CL, Ee AL, Vega VB, Thoreau H, Su ST, Chia JM, Ng P, Chiu KP, Lim L, Zhang T, Peng CK, Lin EO, Lee NM, Yee SL, Ng LF, Chee RE, Stanton LW, Long PM, Liu ET. 2003. Comparative full-length genome sequence analysis of 14 SARS coronavirus isolates and common mutations associated with putative origins of infection. *Lancet* 361(9371):1779-85.

Safranek TJ, Lawrence DN, Kurland LT, Culver DH, Wiederholt WC, Hayner NS, Osterholm MT, O'Brien P, Hughes JM. 1991. Reassessment of the association between Guillain-Barré syndrome and receipt of swine influenza vaccine in 1976-1977: results of a two-state study. Expert Neurology Group. *American Journal of Epidemiology* 133(9):940-51.

Schabas RE. 2001. Mass influenza vaccination in Ontario: a sensible move. *CMAJ* 164(1):36-7.

Schickli JH, Flandorfer A, Nakaya T, Martinez-Sobrido L, Garcia-Sastre A, Palese P. 2001. Plasmid-only rescue of influenza A virus vaccine candidates. *Philosophical Transactions of the Royal Society of London. Series B, Biological Sciences* 356(1416):1965-73.

Sheldon T. 2003. Vet dies from pneumonia in avian flu case. *British Medical Journal* 326(7396):952.

Shi Y. 2003. Stochastic dynamic model of SARS spreading. *Chinese Science Bulletin* 48(13):1287-92.

Steinhauer DA. 1999. Role of hemagglutinin cleavage for the pathogenicity of influenza virus. *Virology* 258(1):1-20.

Stohr K. 2003. The global agenda on influenza surveillance and control. *Vaccine* 21(16):1744-8.

Subbarao K, Chen H, Swayne D, Mingay L, Fodor E, Brownlee G, Xu X, Lu X, Katz J, Cox N, Matsuoka Y. 2003. Evaluation of a genetically modified reassortant H5N1 influenza A virus vaccine candidate generated by plasmid-based reverse genetics. *Virology* 305(1):192-200.

Suzuki S, Ohyama T, Taniguchi K, Kimura M, Kobayashi J, Okabe N, Sano T, Kuwasaki T, Nakatani H. 2003. Web-based Japanese syndromic surveillance for FIFA World Cup 2002. Section II: Event-Based Syndromic Surveillance Systems, *Journal of Urban Health: Bulletin of the New York Academy of Medicine.* 80(2)(Suppl.) 1:i123.

Treanor J. 2004. Influenza vaccine—outmaneuvering antigenic shift and drift. *New England Journal of Medicine* 350(3):218-20.

Tumpey TM, Suarez DL, Perkins LE, Senne DA, Lee JG, Lee YJ, Mo IP, Sung HW, Swayne DE. 2002. Characterization of a highly pathogenic H5N1 avian influenza A virus isolated from duck meat. *Journal of Virology* 76(12):6344-55.

van Kolfschooten F. 2003. Dutch veterinarian becomes first victim of avian influenza. *Lancet* 361(9367):1444.

Wang D, Zhao X. 2003. [Empirical analysis and forecasting for SARS epidemic situation]. *Beijing Da Xue Xue Bao* 35(Suppl.):72-4.

Webby RJ, Webster RG. 2003. Are we ready for pandemic influenza? [Review] [37 Refs]. *Science* 302(5650):1519-22.

WHO Global Influenza Programme. In press.

Wood JM. 2001. Developing vaccines against pandemic influenza. *Philosophical Transactions of the Royal Society of London. Series B, Biological Sciences* 356(1416):1953-60.

Wood JM, Williams MS. 1998. In: Nicholson KG, Webster RG, Hay AJ, eds., *Textbook of Influenza.* Oxford, UK: Blackwell Science. Pp. 317-23.

Woolhouse MEJ, Dye CE. 2001. Population biology of emerging and re-emerging pathogens. *Philosophical Transactions of the Royal Society for Biological Sciences* (356):981-2.

WHO (World Health Organization). 2003a. Influenza A(H5N1) in Hong Kong Special Administrative Region of China. [Online] Available: http://www.who.int/csr/don/2003_2_19/en/ [accessed January 17, 2004].

WHO. 2003b. Avian influenza in the Netherlands. [Online] Available: http://www.who.int/csr/don/ 2003_04_24/en/ [accessed January 17, 2004].

WHO. 2003c. *Visit of WHO Team to Review the Outbreak of Atypical Pneumonia in Guandong Province, March 24-April 9, 2003, Final Report, April 30, 2003.*

WHO. 2003d. Alert, verification and public health management of SARS in the post-outbreak period. [Online] Available: http://www.who.int/csr/sars/postoutbreak/en/ [accessed January 15, 2004].

WHO. 2003e. Revision of the International Health Regulations. [Online] Available: http:// www.who.int/gb/EB_WHA/PDF/WHA56/ea56r28.pdf [accessed January 18, 2004].

WHO. 2003f. Severe Acute Respiratory Syndrome. [Online] Available: http://www.who. int/gb/ EB_WHA/PDF/WHA56/ea56r29.pdf [accessed January 18, 2004].

WHO Multicentre Collaborative Network for Severe, Acute Respiratory Syndrome Diagnosis. 2003. A Multicentre Collaboration to Investigate the Cause of Severe Acute Respiratory Syndrome. *Lancet* 361(9370):1730-3.

Zhou NN, Senne DA, Landgraf JS, Swenson SL, Erickson G, Rossow K, Liu L, Yoon K, Krauss S, Webster RG. 1999. Genetic reassortment of avian, swine, and human influenza A viruses in American pigs. *Journal of Virology* 73(10):8851-6.

# Appendix A

# Learning from SARS:
# Preparing for the Next Disease Outbreak

September 30-October 1, 2003
SMITHSONIAN S. DILLON RIPLEY CENTER
WASHINGTON, DC

## AGENDA

### TUESDAY, SEPTEMBER 30, 2003

8:30      Continental Breakfast
9:00      **Welcome and Opening Remarks**
         **Adel Mahmoud, M.D., Ph.D.**
         Chair, Forum on Emerging Infections
         President, Merck Vaccines

### RECAPPING THE EVENTS: EXPERIENCES FROM THE FIELD

#### Session I: The Evolution of the Outbreak

#### Moderator: Harvey Fineberg, President, Institute of Medicine

9:15-9:40      **CHINA: The Epicenter**
         **Yi Guan, M.D., Ph.D.,** *The University of Hong Kong,*
         *Queen Mary Hospital*
9:40-10:00    *Discussion*

10:00-10:25    **SARS: Lessons from Toronto**
         **Don Low, M.D., FRCPC.,** *Toronto Medical Laboratories,*
         *Mt. Sinai Hospital, Toronto*
10:25-10:45    *Discussion*

10:45-11:10     **WHO: The Global Response**
                **David Heymann, M.D.,** *World Health Organization, Geneva*
11:10-11:30     *Discussion*

11:30           BREAK

### Session II: Discussion Panel

**Moderator: Stanley Lemon, M.D.,** Vice Chair, Forum on Emerging Infections/ Dean of Medicine, The University of Texas Branch at Galveston

11:45   Discussants:     **Reporting Tools and Surveillance Networks:**
                         ***Ann-Marie Kimball, M.D., M.P.H.,***
                         School of Public Health and Community Medicine,
                         University of Washington
                         **International Coordination and Collaboration:**
                         ***Ray Arthur, Ph.D.,*** *National Center for Infectious*
                         *Diseases, Global Health, CDC (Invited)*
                         **Animal Coronaviruses—Lessons from SARS:**
                         ***Linda Saif, Ph.D.,*** *Ohio Agricultural Research*
                         *Center, Ohio State University*

12:30   Open Discussion

1:00    **Lunch**

### Session III: The Spectrum of Consequences and Responses

**Moderator: James Hughes, M.D.,** NCID, CDC

2:00-2:25   **Economic Impacts**
            **Warwick McKibbin, Ph.D.,** *Australian National University*
2:25-2:45   *Discussion*

2:45-3:10   **The Implications of SARS Epidemic for China's Public**
            **Health Infrastructure and Political System**
            **Yanzhong Huang, Ph.D.,** *Seton Hall University, Whitehead*
            *School of Diplomacy and International Relations,*
            *Center for Global Health Studies*
3:10-3:30   *Discussion*

| | |
|---|---|
| 3:30-3:55 | **Quarantine and Containment Strategies**<br>**Marty Cetron, M.D.,** *National Center for*<br>*Infectious Diseases, CDC* |
| 3:55-4:15 | *Discussion* |

| | |
|---|---|
| 4:15-4:40 | **Impacts on Health Care Systems**<br>**G. Neil Thomas, M.D.,** *Department of Community Medicine,*<br>*University of Hong Kong (Invited)* |
| 4:40-5:00 | *Discussion* |

**Session IV: Open Discussion**

| | |
|---|---|
| 5:00 | **Moderator: Joshua Lederberg, Ph.D.,** Nobel Laureate,<br>Sackler Foundation Scholar, Rockefeller University |

Open Discussion

| | |
|---|---|
| 6:00 | **Adjournment of the first day** |

**WEDNESDAY, OCTOBER 1, 2003**

| | |
|---|---|
| 8:30 | Continental Breakfast |
| 9:00 | **Opening Remarks/Summary of Day 1**<br>**Stanley Lemon, M.D.**<br>Vice Chair, Forum on Emerging Infections |

**LEARNING FROM OUR LESSONS: THE AGENDA AHEAD**

**Session V: The Research Agenda and Emerging Technologies**

**Moderator: Carole Heilman Ph.D.,** Director, Division of Microbiology and Infectious Diseases, NIAID, NIH

| | |
|---|---|
| 9:15-9:40 | **Coronavirus Research**<br>**Mark Denison, M.D.,** *Vanderbilt University* |
| 9:40-10:00 | *Discussion* |

| | |
|---|---|
| 10:00-10:25 | **TIGER Technology for Emerging Infectious**<br>**Disease Surveillance**<br>**Ranga Sampath, Ph.D.,** *Ibis Therapeutics, A Division of*<br>*Isis Pharmaceuticals* |
| 10:25-10:45 | *Discussion* |

| | |
|---|---|
| 10:45-11:20 | **Pharmaceutical Approaches to Antiviral Drug Development** |
| | **Amy Patick, Ph.D. and Peter Dragovich, Ph.D.,** *Pfizer Inc.* |
| 11:20-11:30 | *Discussion* |
| 11:30 | BREAK |
| 11:45-12:10 | **Vaccines: Can We Prevent the Unexpected?** |
| | **Alan Shaw, Ph.D.,** *Merck Research Laboratories* |
| 12:10-12:30 | *Discussion* |
| 12:30-12:50 | **SARS: Clearing the Air** |
| | **Jerome Schentag, Pharm.D.,** *State University of New York-Buffalo* |
| 12:50-1:00 | *Discussion* |
| 1:00 | LUNCH |

**Session VI: Panel Discussion—Preparing for the Next Disease Outbreak**

**Moderator: Frederick Sparling, M.D.,** Professor of Medicine, Microbiology, and Immunology, University of North Carolina

| | | |
|---|---|---|
| 2:00 | **Discussants:** | **The Quest to Define and Control SARS:** *Robert Breiman, M.D.,* Centre for Health and Population Research, Dhaka, Bangladesh |
| | | **Regulatory Laboratory Planning/Preparedness:** *Kathryn Carbone, M.D., Center for Biologics, Food and Drug Administration* |
| | | **Future Threats Assessment:** *Karen Monaghan, NIC, National Intelligence Council Report* |
| | | **Public Health Law:** *Gene Matthews, J.D., Legal Advisor to CDC* |
| | | **Modeling a Response Strategy:** *Nathaniel Hupert, M.D., M.P.H., Weill Cornell Medical College* |
| | | **Face to Face w/ Influenza:** *Robert Webster, Ph.D., St. Jude Children's Research Hospital* |
| 3:30 | Open Discussion | |
| 5:00 | Closing Remarks/Adjourn | |

# Appendix B

# Clinical Guidance on the Identification and Evaluation of Possible SARS-CoV Disease Among Persons Presenting with Community-Acquired Illness[1,2]

Version 2. Reprinted with Permission from the Centers for Disease Control and Prevention, 2003.

## INTRODUCTION

Severe acute respiratory syndrome (SARS) is a recently recognized febrile severe lower respiratory illness that is caused by infection with a novel coronavirus, SARS-associated coronavirus (SARS-CoV). During the winter of 2002 through the spring of 2003, WHO received reports of >8,000 SARS cases and nearly 800 deaths. No one knows if SARS-CoV transmission will recur, but it is important to be prepared for that possibility. Early recognition of cases and application of appropriate infection control measures will be critical in controlling future outbreaks.

Many studies have been undertaken or are underway to evaluate whether there are specific laboratory and/or clinical parameters that can distinguish

---

[1]This document provides guidance on the clinical evaluation and management of patients who present from the community with fever and/or respiratory illnesses. The material in this document supplements the information provided in *Public Health Guidance for Community-Level Preparedness and Response to Severe Acute Respiratory Syndrome (SARS)*. Available: http://www.cdc.gov/ncidod/sars/guidance/index.htm.

[2]Summary of Changes in Version 2: This updated version of the clinical guidance clarifies that, in a setting of ongoing SARS-CoV transmission in a facility or community, the presence of either fever *or lower* respiratory symptoms should prompt further evaluation for SARS-CoV disease. In addition, in accordance with the new SARS case definition, when persons have a high risk of exposure to SARS-CoV (e.g., persons previously identified through contact tracing or self-identified as close contacts of a laboratory-confirmed case of SARS-CoV disease; persons who are epidemiologically linked to a laboratory-confirmed case of SARS-CoV disease), the clinical screening criteria should be expanded to include, in addition to fever or lower respiratory symptoms, the presence of other early symptoms of SARS-CoV disease.

---

**BOX B-1**
**Key Concepts**

• The vast majority of patients with SARS-CoV disease 1) have a clear history of exposure either to a SARS patient(s) or to a setting in which SARS-CoV transmission is occurring, and 2) develop pneumonia.
• Laboratory tests are helpful but do not reliably detect infection early in the illness.

---

SARS-CoV disease from other febrile respiratory illnesses. Researchers are also working on the development of laboratory tests to improve diagnostic capabilities for SARS-CoV and other respiratory pathogens. To date, however, no specific clinical or laboratory findings can distinguish with certainty SARS-CoV disease from other respiratory illnesses rapidly enough to inform management decisions that must be made soon after the patient presents to the healthcare system. Therefore, **early clinical recognition of SARS-CoV disease still relies on a combination of clinical and epidemiologic features.**

## IDENTIFICATION OF POTENTIAL CASES OF SARS-COV DISEASE

The diagnosis of SARS-CoV disease and the implementation of control measures should be based on the risk of exposure. In the absence of any person-to-person transmission of SARS-CoV worldwide, the overall likelihood that a patient being evaluated for fever or respiratory illness has SARS-CoV disease will be exceedingly low unless there are both typical clinical findings and some accompanying epidemiologic evidence that raises the suspicion of exposure to SARS-CoV. Therefore, one approach in this setting would be to consider the diagnosis only for patients who require hospitalization for unexplained pneumonia and who have an epidemiologic history that raises the suspicion of exposure, such as recent travel to a previously SARS-affected area (or close contact with an ill person with such a travel history), employment as a healthcare worker with direct patient contact or as a worker in a laboratory that contains live SARS-CoV, or an epidemiologic link to a cluster of cases of unexplained pneumonia. Once person-to-person SARS-CoV transmission has been documented anywhere in the world, the positive predictive value of even early clinical symptoms (e.g., fever or lower respiratory symptoms in the absence of pneumonia), while still low, may be sufficiently high—when combined with an epidemiologic link to settings in which SARS-CoV has been documented— to lead clinicians to consider a diagnosis of SARS-CoV disease.

In that context, the guidance that follows should be considered in the evaluation and management of patients who present from the community with fever or lower respiratory illnesses. For more detailed guidance on infection control, see Supplement I in *Public Health Guidance for Community-Level Preparedness and Response to Severe Acute Respiratory Syndrome (SARS)*: http://www.cdc.gov/ncidod/sars/guidance/index.htm.

## GUIDELINES FOR EVALUATION OF SARS-COV DISEASE AMONG PERSONS PRESENTING WITH COMMUNITY-ACQUIRED ILLNESS (SEE FIGURES B-1 AND B-2)

The following is an approach for the evaluation of possible SARS-CoV disease among persons presenting with community-acquired illness. As part of the evaluation, in addition to identification of suggestive clinical features, clinicians should routinely incorporate into the medical history questions that may provide epidemiologic clues to identify patients with SARS-CoV disease.

### ADDITIONAL CONSIDERATIONS

In some settings, early recognition of SARS-CoV disease may require additional measures. The following guidance is provided to assist in the evaluation of patients in settings or with characteristics not detailed/outlined in Figures B-1 and B-2. These include SARS outbreaks in the surrounding community, management of patients who become ill while already in the hospital, workers from laboratories that contain live SARS-CoV, pediatric patients, the elderly, and persons with chronic underlying diseases.

### Additional Epidemiologic Risk Factors to Consider in Community Outbreak Settings

The risk factors that should trigger suspicion for SARS-CoV disease may vary depending on the level of SARS-CoV transmission occurring in the community. Specifically, as outbreaks become more widespread, the types of epidemiologic characteristics that are considered as risk factors for SARS-CoV disease should be broadened appropriately. Two examples are given below.

1. Evaluating patients in the midst of a community outbreak in which more extensive secondary transmission of SARS-CoV is occurring **in well-defined settings with all cases linked to other cases (e.g., an outbreak in a local hospital)**

- **Continue the activities for evaluation of persons with 'fever and/or lower respiratory illness' outlined in Figure B-2, but in addition:**
- **Consider the diagnosis of SARS-CoV disease** among *all* persons with radiographic evidence of pneumonia (*even if not requiring hospitalization*) if they:

  - Have had exposure to hospitals in the 10 days before onset of symptoms (e.g., patient, visitor, or staff), *or*
  - Are employed in an occupation at particular risk for SARS-CoV exposure, including a healthcare worker with *or without* direct patient contact or a worker in a clinical or research virology laboratory, *or*
  - Have close contact with a patient with documented pneumonia.

## BOX B-2
## Diagnosis of SARS-CoV Disease

In the absence of person-to-person transmission of SARS-CoV anywhere in the world, the diagnosis of SARS-CoV disease should be considered only in patients who require hospitalization for radiographically confirmed pneumonia and who have an epidemiologic history that raises the suspicion of SARS-CoV disease. The suspicion for SARS-CoV disease is raised if, within 10 days of symptom onset, the patient:

• Has a history of recent travel to mainland China, Hong Kong, or Taiwan (see Figure B-1, footnote 3) or close contact[a] with ill persons with a history of recent travel to such areas, OR
• Is employed in an occupation at particular risk for SARS-CoV exposure, including a healthcare worker with direct patient contact or a worker in a laboratory that contains live SARS-CoV, OR
• Is part of a cluster of cases of atypical pneumonia without an alternative diagnosis

Persons with such a clinical and exposure history should be evaluated according to the algorithm in **Figure B-1.**

**Once person-to-person transmission of SARS-CoV has been documented in the world, the diagnosis should still be considered** in patients who require hospitalization for pneumonia and who have the epidemiologic history described above. In addition, all patients with fever or lower respiratory symptoms (e.g., cough, shortness of breath, difficulty breathing) should be questioned about whether within 10 days of symptom onset they have had:

• Close contact with someone suspected of having SARS-CoV disease, OR
• A history of foreign travel (or close contact with an ill person with a history of travel) to a location with documented or suspected SARS-CoV, OR
• Exposure to a domestic location with documented or suspected SARS-CoV (including a laboratory that contains live SARS-CoV), or close contact with an ill person with such an exposure history.

Persons with such an exposure history should be evaluated for SARS-CoV disease according to the algorithm in **Figure B-2.**

---

[a]Close contact: A person who has cared for or lived with a person with SARS-CoV disease or had a high likelihood of direct contact with respiratory secretions and/or body fluids of a person with SARS-CoV disease. Examples of close contact include kissing or hugging, sharing eating or drinking utensils, talking within 3 feet, and direct touching. Close contact does not include activities such as walking by a person or briefly sitting across a waiting room or office.

2. Evaluating patients in the midst of a community outbreak in which transmission is widespread and epidemiologic linkages between cases are not well defined

- Since epidemiologic links to persons with SARS-CoV disease may not be identifiable at this point, SARS-CoV disease should be considered in any patient presenting with fever or lower respiratory illness, even in the absence of known epidemiologic risk factors.

### Persons with a High Risk of Exposure

For persons with a high risk of exposure to SARS-CoV (e.g., persons previously identified through contact tracing as close contacts of a laboratory-confirmed case of SARS-CoV disease; persons who are epidemiologically linked to a laboratory-confirmed case of SARS-CoV disease), symptoms that should trigger the clinical algorithm should be expanded to include the presence of any of the following: sore throat, rhinorrhea, chills, rigors, myalgia, headache, diarrhea. For more details on the clinical features of SARS-CoV disease, see Figure B-2, footnote 1.

### Management of Patients Who Acquire Illness While in the Hospital

This document focuses on the evaluation and management of patients who present from the community, although many of the same principles apply to hospitalized patients who develop nosocomial fever or lower respiratory symptoms. The diagnosis of nosocomial SARS-CoV disease may be particularly challenging, however, since many inpatients may have other reasons for developing nosocomial fever, lower respiratory symptoms, and pneumonia. Therefore, in hospitals known to have or suspected of having patients with SARS-CoV disease, clinicians and public health officials must be particularly vigilant about evaluating fever and respiratory illnesses among inpatients. Additional guidance on when to apply Figure B-2 in the evaluation of patients who develop fever and/or respiratory illness while hospitalized is provided in Supplement C, *Public Health Guidance for Community-Level Preparedness and Response to Severe Acute Respiratory Syndrome (SARS)*: http://www.cdc.gov/ncidod/sars/guidance/index.htm.

### Laboratory Workers

Breaks in technique in laboratories that contain live SARS-CoV can result in laboratory-acquired cases of SARS-CoV disease. Personnel working in laboratories that contain live SARS-CoV should report any febrile and/or lower respiratory illnesses to the supervisor, be evaluated for possible exposures, and be closely monitored for clinical features and course of illness. If laboratory workers with

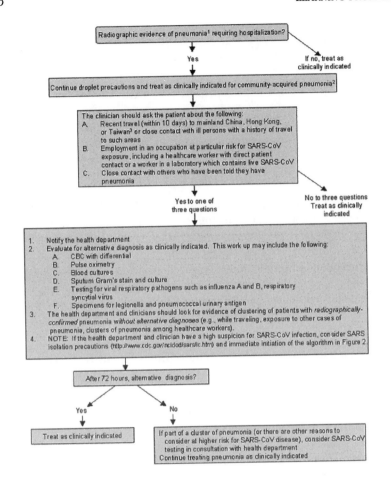

**FIGURE B-1** Algorithm for evaluation and management of patients requiring hospitalization for radiographically confirmed pneumonia, in the absence of person-to-person transmission of SARS-CoV in the world.

---

[1]Or Acute Respiratory Distress Syndrome (ARDS) of unknown etiology.

[2]Guidance for the management of community-acquired pneumonia is available from the Infectious Diseases Society of America (IDSA) and can be found at www.journals.uchicago.edu/IDSA/guidelines/.

[3]The 2003 SARS-CoV outbreak likely originated in mainland China, and neighboring areas such as Taiwan and Hong Kong are thought to be at higher risk due to the high volume of travelers from mainland China. Although less likely, SARS-CoV may also reappear from other previously affected areas. Therefore, clinicians should obtain a complete travel history. If clinicians have concerns about the possibility of SARS-CoV disease in a patient with a history of travel to other previously affected areas (e.g., while traveling abroad, had close contact with another person with pneumonia of unknown etiology or spent time in a hospital in which patients with acute respiratory disease were treated), they should contact the health department.

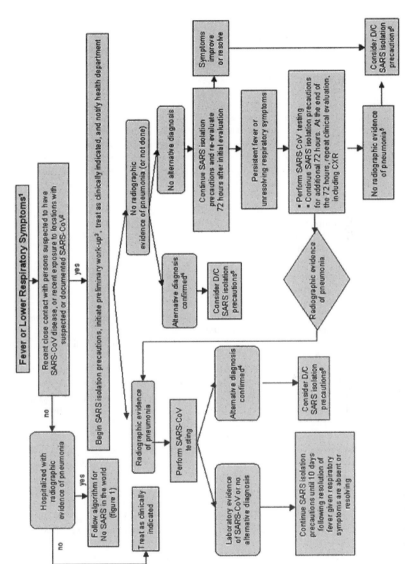

**FIGURE B-2**

**FIGURE B-2** Algorithm for management of patients with fever or lower respiratory symptoms when person-to-person transmission of SARS-CoV is occurring in the world.

[1]Clinical description of SARS-CoV disease and approach to treatment:

Clinical judgment should be used to determine when symptoms trigger initiation of the algorithm in Figure B-2. The early symptoms of SARS-CoV disease usually include fever, chills, rigors, myalgia, and headache. In some patients, myalgia and headache may precede the onset of fever by 12-24 hours. Respiratory symptoms often do not appear until 2-7 days after the onset of illness and most often include shortness of breath and/or dry cough. Diarrhea, sore throat, and rhinorrhea may also be early symptoms of SARS-CoV disease. In the absence of fever, when screening patients for potential SARS-CoV disease, respiratory symptoms that would trigger the clinical algorithm are generally defined as lower respiratory tract symptoms (e.g., cough, shortness of breath, difficulty breathing). However, when screening patients who have a high risk of exposure to SARS-CoV (e.g., persons previously identified through contact tracing or self-identified as close contacts of a laboratory-confirmed case of SARS-CoV disease; persons who are epidemiologically linked to a laboratory-confirmed case of SARS-CoV disease), symptoms that should trigger the clinical algorithm should be expanded to include any of the following: sore throat, rhinorrhea, chills, rigors, myalgia, headache, diarrhea.

Although not diagnostic, the following laboratory abnormalities have been seen in some patients with laboratory-confirmed SARS-CoV disease:

- Lymphopenia with normal or low white blood cell count
- Elevated hepatic transaminases
- Elevated creatine phosphokinase
- Elevated lactate dehydrogenase
- Elevated C-reactive protein
- Prolonged activated partial thromboplastin time

As of December 1, 2003, no specific treatment recommendations can be made for management of SARS-CoV disease. Empiric therapy for community-acquired pneumonia should include treatment for organisms associated with any community-acquired pneumonia of unclear etiology, including agents with activity against both typical and atypical respiratory pathogens. Treatment choices may be influenced by both the severity of and the circumstances surrounding the illness. Infectious disease consultation is recommended. The Infectious Diseases Society of America has guidelines for the management of community-acquired pneumonia at www.journals.uchicago.edu/IDSA/guidelines/.

[2]Exposure history for SARS-CoV, once SARS-CoV transmission is documented in the world:

In settings of no or limited local secondary transmission of SARS-CoV, patients are considered exposed to SARS-CoV if, within 10 days of symptom onset, the patient has:

- Close contact with someone suspected of having SARS-CoV disease, OR
- A history of foreign travel (or close contact with an ill person with a history of travel) to a location with documented or suspected SARS-CoV, OR
- Exposure to a domestic location with documented or suspected SARS-CoV (including a laboratory that contains live SARS-CoV), or close contact with an ill person with such an exposure history.

In settings with more extensive transmission, all patients with fever or lower respiratory symptoms should be evaluated for possible SARS-CoV disease, since the ability to determine epidemiologic links will be lost.

For up-to-date information on where recent SARS-CoV transmission is suspected or documented, see the CDC and WHO websites: www.cdc.gov/sars and www.who.int.

[3]Clinical work-up: Clinicians should work up patients as clinically indicated. Depending on symptoms and exposure history, initial diagnostic testing for patients with suspected SARS-CoV disease may include:

- Complete blood count (CBC) with differential
- Chest radiograph
- Pulse oximetry

- Blood cultures
- Sputum Gram's stain and culture
- Testing for viral respiratory pathogens, notably influenza A and B and respiratory syncytial virus
- Legionella and pneumococcal urinary antigen testing if radiographic evidence of pneumonia (adults only)

An acute serum sample and other available clinical specimens (respiratory, blood, and stool) should be saved for additional testing until a specific diagnosis is made.

SARS-CoV testing may be considered as part of the initial work-up if there is a high level of suspicion for SARS-CoV disease based on exposure history. For additional details on specialized laboratory testing options available through the health department and the Laboratory Response Network (LRN), see CDC's SARS website: www.cdc.gov/sars/.

[4]Alternative diagnosis:

An alternative diagnosis should be based only on laboratory tests with high positive-predictive value (e.g., blood culture, viral culture, Legionella urinary antigen, pleural fluid culture, transthoracic aspirate). In some settings, PCR testing for bacterial and viral pathogens can also be used to help establish alternative diagnoses. The presence of an alternative diagnosis does not necessarily rule out co-infection with SARS-CoV.

[5]Radiographic testing:

Chest CT may show evidence of an infiltrate before a chest radiograph (CXR). Therefore, a chest CT should be considered in patients with a strong epidemiologic link to a known case of SARS-CoV disease and a negative CXR 6 days after onset of symptoms. Alternatively, the patient should remain in SARS isolation, and the CXR should be repeated on day 9 after symptom onset.

[6]Discontinuation of SARS isolation precautions:

SARS isolation precautions should be discontinued only after consultation with the local public health authorities and the evaluating clinician. Factors that might be considered include the strength of the epidemiologic exposure to SARS-CoV, nature of contact with others in the residential or work setting, strength of evidence for an alternative diagnosis, and evidence for clustering of pneumonia among close contacts. Isolation precautions should be discontinued on the basis of an alternative diagnosis only when the following criteria are met:

- Absence of strong epidemiologic link to known cases of SARS-CoV disease
- Alternative diagnosis confirmed using a test with a high positive-predictive value
- Clinical manifestations entirely explained by the alternative diagnosis
- No evidence of clustering of pneumonia cases among close contacts (unless >1 case in the cluster is confirmed to have the same alternative diagnosis)
- All cases of presumed SARS-CoV disease identified in the surrounding community can be epidemiologically linked to known cases or locations in which transmission is known to have occurred.

fever and/or lower respiratory illness are found to have an exposure to SARS-CoV, they should be managed according to the guidance in Figure B-2. In addition, in an exposed laboratory worker, symptoms that should trigger the clinical algorithm in Figure B-2 should be expanded to include the presence of any of the following: sore throat, rhinorrhea, chills, rigors, myalgia, headache, diarrhea (see Figure B-2, footnote 1, for more information). Detailed information for persons who work in laboratories that contain live SARS-CoV is provided in Supplement F, *Public Health Guidance for Community-Level Preparedness and Response to Severe Acute Respiratory Syndrome (SARS)*, http://www.cdc.gov/ncidod/sars/guidance/index.htm.

### Considerations for the Pediatric Population

The document does not specifically address the evaluation and management of infants and children. Much less is known about SARS-CoV disease in pediatric patients than in adults. During the 2003 outbreaks, infants and children accounted for only a small percentage of patients and had much milder disease with better outcome. Their role in transmission is not well described but is likely much less significant than the role of adults. Taking these factors into account, the following guidance may change as more information becomes available on SARS-CoV disease in the pediatric population:

- In the absence of person-to-person SARS-CoV transmission in the world, evaluation and management for possible SARS-CoV disease should be considered only for adults, unless special circumstances make the clinician and health department consider a child to be of potentially high risk for having SARS-CoV disease.
- In the presence of person-to-person SARS-CoV transmission in the world, the evaluation algorithm established for adults can be used in children with the following caveats:
  - Both the rate of development of radiographically confirmed pneumonia and the timing of development of such radiographic changes in children are unknown.
  - The positive predictive value of rapid virus antigen detection tests (e.g., RSV) "in season" will be higher in a pediatric population.
  - Pneumococcal and legionella urinary antigen testing are not recommended for routine diagnostic use in children.

### Elderly Persons and Patients with Underlying Chronic Illnesses

Typical symptoms of SARS-CoV disease may not always be present in elderly patients and those with underlying chronic illnesses, such as renal failure. Therefore, the diagnosis should be considered for almost any change in health status, even in the absence of typical clinical features of SARS-CoV disease, when such patients have epidemiologic risk factors for SARS-CoV disease (e.g., close contact with someone suspected to have SARS-CoV disease or exposure to a location [domestic or international] with documented or suspected recent transmission of SARS-CoV).

# Appendix C

# In the Absence of SARS-CoV Transmission Worldwide: Guidance for Surveillance, Clinical and Laboratory Evaluation, and Reporting[1,2]

## BACKGROUND

Severe acute respiratory syndrome (SARS) came to global attention in February 2003, when officials in China informed the World Health Organization (WHO) about 305 cases of atypical pneumonia that had occurred in Guangdong Province. By the time the new infectious disease was declared contained in July 2003, more than 8,000 cases and 780 deaths had been reported from 29 countries worldwide. Since then, active global surveillance for SARS-associated coronavirus (SARS-CoV) disease in humans has detected no laboratory-confirmed person-to-person transmission of SARS-CoV.

No one knows if, when, or where person-to-person transmission of SARS-CoV will recur. However, the rapidity of spread of infection and the high levels

---

[1]This is an updated version of a document first issued by CDC in December 2003. The document provides guidance for surveillance, clinical and laboratory evaluation, and reporting in the setting of no known person-to-person transmission of SARS-CoV worldwide. Recommendations are derived from *Public Health Guidance for Community-Level Preparedness and Response to Severe Acute Respiratory Syndrome (SARS)*: www.cdc.gov/ncidod/sars/guidance/index.htm.

[2]Summary of Changes in Version 2: This version of the guidance document clarifies that the recommendations apply to situations in which no known person-to-person transmission of SARS-CoV is occurring in the world. Some wording has also been revised for consistency with the companion documents, Public Health Guidance for Community-Level Preparedness and Response to Severe Acute Respiratory Syndrome (SARS), and Clinical Guidance on the Identification and Evaluation of Possible SARS-CoV Disease among Persons Presenting with Community-Acquired Illness.

of morbidity and mortality associated with SARS-CoV call for careful monitoring for the recurrence of transmission and preparations for the rapid implementation of control measures. The 2003 global outbreaks demonstrated the ease with which SARS-CoV can seed and spread in human populations when cases remain undetected or when infected persons are not cared for in controlled environments that reduce the risk of transmission to others. The two laboratory-acquired infections and the recent cases in Southern China show that SARS-CoV continues to be a threat. Early detection of SARS cases and contacts, plus swift and decisive implementation of containment measures, are therefore essential to prevent transmission. Although the United States had only a limited SARS-CoV outbreak during the 2003 epidemic—with only eight laboratory-confirmed cases and no significant local spread—the U.S. population is clearly vulnerable to the more widespread, disruptive outbreaks experienced in other countries. During this period of no known person-to-person transmission of SARS-CoV in the world, healthcare and public health officials must therefore do what they can to prepare for the possibility that SARS-CoV transmission may recur.

This document provides guidance for surveillance, clinical and laboratory evaluation, and reporting in the setting of no known person-to-person transmission of SARS-CoV worldwide. Recommendations are derived from *Public Health Guidance for Community-Level Preparedness and Response to Severe Acute Respiratory Syndrome (SARS)* www.cdc.gov/ncidod/sars/guidance/index.htm. If such transmission recurs anywhere in the world, CDC will promptly review all available information and provide additional guidance via the Health Alert Network (HAN), Epi-X, and partner organizations. Current information will also be posted on CDC's SARS website: www.cdc.gov/sars.

## CLINICAL FEATURES OF SARS-COV DISEASE

The median incubation period for SARS-CoV appears to be approximately 4 to 6 days; most patients become ill within 2 to 10 days after exposure. Early clinical features of SARS-CoV disease can be similar to other viral illnesses and are not sufficiently distinct to enable diagnosis by signs and symptoms alone. The illness usually begins with systemic symptoms such as fever, headache, and myalgias. Respiratory complaints often develop 2 to 7 days after illness onset and usually include a non-productive cough and dyspnea. Upper respiratory symptoms such as rhinorrhea and sore throat may occur but are uncommon. Almost all patients with laboratory evidence of SARS-CoV disease evaluated to date developed radiographic evidence of pneumonia by day 7-10 of illness, and most (70 percent-90 percent) developed lymphopenia. The overall case-fatality rate of approximately 10 percent can increase to >50 percent in persons older than age 60.

## BOX C-1
## Key Clinical Features of SARS-CoV Disease

• Incubation period of 2-10 days
• Early systemic symptoms followed within 2-7 days by dry cough and/or shortness of breath, often without upper respiratory tract symptoms
• Development of radiographically confirmed pneumonia by day 7-10 of illness
• Lymphopenia in most cases

## SURVEILLANCE: EARLY CASE DETECTION

Potential sources of virus for a recurrence of person-to-person spread of SARS-CoV include reintroduction to humans from an animal reservoir, persistent infection in previously ill persons, or the laboratory. Since SARS-CoV currently exists in the animals in southern China—the apparent source of the 2003 outbreak—this area remains under scrutiny for SARS-CoV disease activity. Potential sources of recurrence also include other areas where SARS-CoV transmission occurred and large cities that are international travel hubs connecting to locales that might harbor persistent infections in humans. Laboratory personnel working with SARS-CoV might also become infected as a result of compromised laboratory techniques.[3] Because persons with SARS-CoV disease tended to appear in clusters (e.g., in healthcare facilities, households, and a few special settings) during the 2003 outbreaks, early signals of the reappearance of the illness in U.S. communities could include unusual clusters of unexplained pneumonia.

**In the absence of person-to-person transmission of SARS-CoV worldwide, the goal of domestic surveillance is to maximize early detection of cases of SARS-CoV disease while minimizing unnecessary laboratory testing, concerns about SARS-CoV, implementation of control measures, and social dis-**

---

[3]Persons who work in laboratories that contain live SARS-CoV should report any febrile and/or respiratory illnesses to the supervisor. They should be evaluated for possible exposures, and their clinical features and course of illness should be closely monitored, as described in Appendix F6, Supplement F, in *Public Health Guidance for Community-Level Preparedness and Response to Severe Acute Respiratory Syndrome (SARS):* www.cdc.gov/ncidod/sars/guidance/F/pdf/app6.pdf.

If laboratory workers with fever and/or lower respiratory illness are found to have an exposure to SARS-CoV, they should be managed according to the algorithm in Figure 2, Clinical Guidance on the Identification and Evaluation of Possible SARS-CoV Disease among Persons Presenting with Community-Acquired Illness (www.cdc.gov/ncidod/sars/clinicalguidance.htm). In an exposed laboratory worker, symptoms that should trigger the clinical algorithm in Figure 2 should be expanded to include the presence of any of the following: sore throat, rhinorrhea, chills, rigors, myalgia, headache, diarrhea (see Figure 2, footnote 1, for more details).

**ruption**. Early and efficient detection of SARS cases is not, however, a straightforward task. In the absence of known transmission worldwide, the overall likelihood that a person in the United States with fever and respiratory symptoms will have SARS-CoV disease is exceedingly low. Moreover, the nonspecific clinical features of early SARS-CoV disease and the current lack of diagnostic tests that can reliably detect the virus during the first few days of illness pose challenges to finding SARS-CoV-infected persons during the predictable seasonal upsurge in respiratory infections.

Nonetheless, lessons learned from the 2003 outbreaks have identified three features of SARS-CoV disease that can be used to focus surveillance activities during the period of no transmission worldwide: (1) most patients infected with SARS-CoV develop radiographic evidence of pneumonia; (2) most SARS-CoV transmission occurs when patients are seriously ill and require hospitalization; and (3) most infected patients have an identifiable exposure to a known SARS-CoV case or a suggestive cluster of SARS-like illness or a location with known SARS transmission.

Given these features, the potential sources of recurrence of SARS-CoV, and the predilection for SARS-CoV transmission to occur in healthcare settings or to be associated with geographically focused pneumonia clusters, surveillance efforts in the absence of person-to-person SARS-CoV transmission should aim to **identify patients who require hospitalization for radiographically confirmed pneumonia or acute respiratory distress syndrome without identifiable etiology AND who have one of the following risk factors in the 10 days before the onset of illness**:

- Travel to mainland China, Hong Kong, or Taiwan, or close contact[4] with an ill person with a history of recent travel to one of these areas, *OR*
- Employment in an occupation associated with a risk for SARS-CoV exposure (e.g., healthcare worker[5] with direct patient contact; worker in a laboratory that contains live SARS-CoV), *OR*
- Part of a cluster of cases of atypical pneumonia without an alternative diagnosis

Infection control practitioners and other healthcare personnel should also be alert for clusters of pneumonia among two or more healthcare workers who work in the same facility.

---

[4]Close contact: A person who has cared for or lived with a person with SARS-CoV disease or had a high likelihood of direct contact with respiratory secretions and/or body fluids of a person with SARS-CoV disease. Examples of close contact include kissing or hugging, sharing eating or drinking utensils, talking within 3 feet, and direct touching. Close contact does not include activities such as walking by a person or briefly sitting across a waiting room or office.

[5]Healthcare worker: Any employee in a healthcare facility who has close contact with patients, patient-care areas, or patient-care items.

The 2003 SARS-CoV outbreak likely originated in mainland China, and neighboring areas such as Taiwan and Hong Kong are thought to be at higher risk due to the large volume of travelers from mainland China. Although less likely, SARS-CoV may also reappear from other previously affected areas. Therefore, clinicians should obtain a complete travel history. If clinicians have concerns about the possibility of SARS-CoV disease in a patient with a history of travel to other previously affected areas (e.g., while traveling abroad, had close contact with another person with pneumonia of unknown etiology or spent time in a hospital in which patients with acute respiratory disease were treated), they should contact the health department.

In the absence of person-to-person transmission of SARS-CoV in the world, the screening of persons requiring hospitalization for radiographically confirmed pneumonia for risk factors suggesting SARS-CoV exposure should be limited to adults, unless there are special circumstances that make the clinician and public health personnel consider a child to be of potentially high risk for having SARS-CoV disease. During the 2003 global outbreaks, infants and children accounted for only a small percentage of SARS cases and had a much milder disease and better outcome than adults. Although information on SARS-CoV disease in pediatric patients is limited, the role of children in transmission is likely much less significant than the role of adults.

---

**BOX C-2**
**Case Detection**

Severe respiratory illness in the context of a documented exposure risk is the key to diagnosing SARS-CoV disease. Providers should therefore consider SARS-CoV disease in patients requiring hospitalization for:

- Radiographically confirmed pneumonia or acute respiratory distress syndrome of unknown etiology, AND
- One of the following risk factors in the 10 days before illness onset:
  - Travel to mainland China, Hong Kong, or Taiwan, or close contact with an ill person with a history of recent travel to one of these areas; OR
  - Employment in an occupation associated with a risk for SARS-CoV exposure (e.g., healthcare worker with direct patient contact; worker in a laboratory that contains live SARS-CoV); OR
  - Part of a cluster of cases of atypical pneumonia without an alternative diagnosis.

Infection control practitioners and other healthcare personnel should be alert for clusters of pneumonia among two or more healthcare workers who work in the same facility.

# INFECTION CONTROL AND CLINICAL EVALUATION

SARS-CoV disease provides a reminder of the risks of nosocomial transmission of respiratory pathogens and an opportunity to improve overall infection control in healthcare facilities. All healthcare facilities need to re-emphasize the importance of basic infection control measures for the control of SARS-CoV disease and other respiratory illnesses. Facilities should also consider adopting a "respiratory hygiene/ cough etiquette" strategy to help limit nosocomial transmission of respiratory pathogens. To contain respiratory secretions, all persons with signs and symptoms of a respiratory infection, regardless of presumed cause, should be instructed to:

- Cover the nose and mouth when coughing or sneezing.
- Use tissues to contain respiratory secretions.
- Dispose of tissues in the nearest waste receptacle after use.
- Perform hand hygiene after contact with respiratory secretions and contaminated objects and materials.

Healthcare facilities should ensure the availability of materials for adhering to respiratory hygiene/cough etiquette in waiting areas for patients and visitors:

- Provide tissues and no-touch receptacles for used tissue disposal.
- Provide conveniently located dispensers for alcohol-based hand rub.
- Provide soap and disposable towels for hand washing where sinks are available.

During periods of increased respiratory infection in the community, healthcare facilities should offer procedure or surgical masks to persons who are coughing and encourage coughing persons to sit at least 3 feet away from others in waiting areas. Healthcare workers should practice Droplet Precautions, in addition to Standard Precautions, when examining a patient with symptoms of a respiratory infection. Droplet precautions should be maintained until it is determined that they are no longer needed (see www.cdc.gov/ncidod/hip/ISOLAT/ Isolat.htm). An algorithm for patient evaluation is provided in Appendix 1.

If the clinician and health department have a high index of suspicion for SARS-CoV disease or if laboratory evidence of SARS-CoV disease is found, then the patient should be placed immediately on SARS isolation precautions, and contacts should be immediately identified, evaluated, and monitored for evidence of respiratory disease. Prompt SARS-CoV laboratory diagnostics should be arranged through the health department. Initial diagnostic evaluation to look for an alternative diagnosis in suspected SARS-CoV patients should be performed as clinically indicated, and may include:

- Chest radiograph
- Pulse oximetry

> ## BOX C-3
> ## Infection Control and Clinical Evaluation
>
> • Healthcare facilities should re-emphasize the importance of basic infection control measures for respiratory infections and consider adopting a "respiratory hygiene/cough etiquette" strategy.
> • All patients admitted to the hospital with radiographically confirmed pneumonia should be:
>   • Placed on Droplet Precautions
>   • Screened for risk factors for possible exposure to SARS-CoV
>   • Evaluated with a chest radiograph, pulse oximetry, complete blood count, and etiologic workup as indicated.
> • If there is a high index of suspicion for SARS-CoV disease (by clinicians and health department), the patient should immediately be placed on SARS isolation precautions, and all contacts of the ill patient should be identified, evaluated, and monitored. Prompt SARS-CoV laboratory diagnostics should be arranged through the health department.

• Complete blood count with differential
• Blood cultures
• Sputum Gram's stain and culture
• Testing for viral respiratory pathogens, notably influenza A and B and respiratory syncytial virus
• Specimens for *Legionella* and pneumococcal urinary antigen testing

## LABORATORY TESTING FOR SARS-COV

Laboratory testing for SARS-CoV is now available at many state public health laboratories. Available tests include antibody testing using an enzyme immunoassay (EIA) and reverse transcription polymerase chain reaction (RT-PCR) tests for respiratory, blood, and stool specimens. In the absence of person-to-person transmission of SARS-CoV, the positive predictive value of a diagnostic test is extremely low. False-positive test results may generate tremendous anxiety and concern and expend valuable public health resources. Therefore, **SARS-CoV testing should be performed judiciously, and preferably only in consultation with the local or state health department.** SARS-CoV testing should be considered if no alternative diagnosis is identified 72 hours after initiation of the clinical evaluation and the patient is thought to be at high risk for SARS-CoV disease (e.g., is part of a cluster of unexplained pneumonia cases).

Providers should immediately report all positive SARS-CoV test results to the local or state health department. Confirmatory SARS-CoV testing at an ap-

---

**BOX C-4**
**Laboratory testing for SARS-CoV**

- Perform laboratory testing judiciously and in consultation with the local or state health department.
- Providers should report all positive test results immediately to the local or state health department.
- Arrange for confirmatory testing at an appropriate test site through the local or state health department.

---

propriate confirmatory test site should be arranged through the local or state health department as outlined in Supplement F, *Public Health Guidance for Community-Level Preparedness and Response to Severe Acute Respiratory Syndrome (SARS)* www.cdc.gov/ncidod/sars/guidance/index.htm.

Guidelines for the collection and transport of specimens for SARS-CoV testing are provided in Appendix F4, Supplement F, in *Public Health Guidance for Community-Level Preparedness and Response to Severe Acute Respiratory Syndrome (SARS)* www.cdc.gov/ncidod/sars/guidance/F/pdf/app4.pdf.

CDC is working with the Association of Public Health Laboratories (APHL) and the Laboratory Response Network (LRN) to ensure that SARS RT-PCR and EIA tests meet quality control guidelines. CDC will also be distributing proficiency testing materials to participating laboratories.

## REPORTING OF POTENTIAL SARS-COV CASES

**Healthcare providers** should report to the state or local health department:

- All persons requiring hospitalization for radiographically confirmed pneumonia who report at least one of the three risk factors for exposure to SARS-CoV outlined in Section III above.
- Any clusters (two or more persons) of unexplained pneumonia, especially among healthcare workers
- Any positive SARS-CoV test result

Note: In the absence of known person-to-person transmission of SARS-CoV in the world, any **SARS-CoV-positive test result** should be phoned in to the state or local health department immediately for confirmation and implementation of urgent and appropriate isolation precautions, contact tracing, and follow-up.

**Health departments** should immediately report any SARS-CoV positive test result to CDC. Health departments should also inform CDC of other cases or clusters of pneumonia that are of particular concern by calling 770-488-7100.

---

**BOX C-5**
**Report to state or local health department:**

• All persons requiring hospitalization for radiographically confirmed pneumonia who report at least one of the three risk factors for exposure to SARS-CoV
• Any clusters of unexplained pneumonia, especially among healthcare workers
• Any positive SARS-CoV test result

---

## APPENDIX C-1

## IN THE ABSENCE OF PERSON-TO-PERSON TRANSMISSION OF SARS-COV WORLDWIDE: GUIDANCE FOR EVALUATION AND MANAGEMENT OF PATIENTS REQUIRING HOSPITALIZATION FOR RADIOGRAPHICALLY CONFIRMED PNEUMONIA

In the absence of SARS-CoV transmission in the world, a diagnosis of SARS-CoV disease should be considered only in patients who require hospitalization for radiographically confirmed pneumonia and who have an epidemiologic history that raises the suspicion for SARS-CoV disease (see Figure C-1, page 296). The suspicion for SARS-CoV disease is increased if, within 10 days of the onset of SARS-like symptoms, the patient: 1) traveled to mainland China, Hong Kong, or Taiwan, or had close contact with an ill person with a history of recent travel to one of these areas; 2) is employed in an occupation associated with a risk for SARS-CoV exposure (e.g., healthcare worker with direct patient contact; worker in a laboratory that contains live SARS-CoV); or 3) is part of a cluster of cases of atypical pneumonia without an alternative diagnosis. Persons with such a clinical and exposure history should be evaluated according to the following algorithm.

In some settings, early recognition of SARS-CoV disease may require additional measures:

• Laboratory workers—Breaks in technique in laboratories that contain live SARS-CoV could result in laboratory–acquired cases of SARS. Persons working in laboratories that contain live SARS-CoV should report any fever and/or lower respiratory illness to the supervisor. They should be evaluated for possible exposures, and their clinical features and course of illness should be closely monitored as described in Appendix F6 in Supplement F, *Public Health Guidance for Community-Level Preparedness and Response to Severe Acute Respiratory Syndrome (SARS)* www.cdc.gov/ncidod/sars/guidance/index.htm. If laboratory workers with fever and/or lower respiratory illness are found to have an exposure to SARS-CoV, they should be managed according to the algorithm in

Figure 2, *Clinical Guidance on the Identification and Evaluation of Possible SARS-CoV Disease among Persons Presenting with Community-Acquired Illness* (www.cdc.gov/ncidod/sars/clinicalguidance.htm). In an exposed laboratory worker, symptoms that should trigger the clinical algorithm in Figure 2 should be expanded to include the presence of any of the following: sore throat, rhinorrhea, chills, rigors, myalgia, headache, diarrhea (see Figure 2, footnote 1, for more details).

• Pediatric populations—Information on SARS-CoV disease in pediatric patients is limited. During the global outbreaks of 2003, infants and children accounted for only a small percentage of cases and had a much milder disease and better outcome than adults. Their role in transmission is not well described but is likely much less significant than the role of adults. Therefore, in the setting of no person-to-person SARS-CoV transmission in the world, the evaluation and management algorithm applies only to adults, unless there are special circumstances that make the clinical and health department consider a child to be of potentially high risk for having SARS-CoV disease.

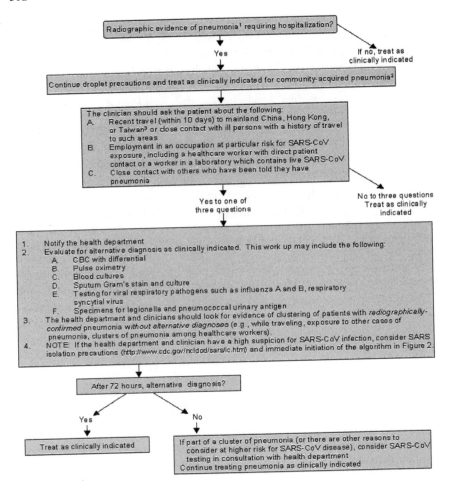

**FIGURE C-1** Evaluation and management of patients requiring hospitalization for radiographically confirmed pneumonia, in the absence of person-to-person transmission of SARS-CoV in the world

[1] Or acute respiratory distress syndrome (ARDS) of unknown etiology

[2] Guidance for the management of community-acquired pneumonia is available from the Infectious Diseases Society of America (IDSA) at: www.journals.uchicago.edu/IDSA/guidelines/.

[3] The 2003 SARS-CoV outbreak likely originated in mainland China, and neighboring areas such as Taiwan and Hong Kong are thought to be at higher risk due to the high volume of travelers from mainland China. Although less likely, SARS-CoV may also reappear from other previously affected areas. Therefore, clinicians should obtain a complete travel history. If clinicians have concerns about the possibility of SARS-CoV disease in a patient with a history of travel to other previously affected areas (e.g., while traveling abroad, had close contact with another person with pneumonia of unknown etiology or spent time in a hospital in which patients with acute respiratory disease were treated), they should contact the health department.

# Appendix D

# Selected Bibliography

## OVERVIEW

Berger A, Drosten CH, Doerr HW, Stürmer M, Preiser W. 2004. Severe acute respiratory syndrome (SARS): paradigm of an emerging viral infection. *Journal of Clinical Virology.* 29(1):13-22.

CDC. Severe acute respiratory syndrome (SARS). 2004. Web Page. Available at: http://www.cdc.gov/ncidod/sars/.

Groneberg DA, Zhang L, Welte T, Zabel P, Chung KF. 2003. Severe acute respiratory syndrome: global initiatives for disease diagnosis. *QJM.* 96(11):845-52.

Lai MM. 2003. SARS virus: the beginning of the unraveling of a new coronavirus. *Journal of Biomedical Science.* 10(6:2):664-75.

Lingappa JR, McDonald LC, Simone P, Parashar UD. 2004. Wresting SARS from uncertainty. *Emerging Infectious Diseases* [serial online]. 10(2). Available at: http://www.cdc.gov/ncidod/EID/vol10no2/03-1032.htm.

Peiris JSM, Yuen KY, Osterhaus ADME, Stöhr K. 2003. The severe acute respiratory syndrome. *New England Journal of Medicine.* 349(25):2431-2441.

SARS Expert Committee. *SARS in Hong Kong: From Experience to Action.* Hong Kong (SAR), China: Hong Kong Government; 2003. Available at: http://www.sars-expertcom.gov.hk/english/reports/reports.html.

WHO. Severe acute respiratory syndrome (SARS). 2004. Web Page. Available at: http://www.who.int/csr/sars/en/.

## ORIGIN AND SPREAD

Booth CM, Matukas LM, Tomlinson GA, Rachlis AR, Rose DB, Dwosh HA, Walmsley SL, Mazzulli T, Avendano M, Derkach P, Ephtimios IE, Kitai I, Mederski BD, Shadowitz SB, Gold WL, Hawryluck LA, Rea E, Chenkin JS, Cescon DW, Poutanen SM, Detsky AS. 2003. Clinical features and short-term outcomes of 144 patients with SARS in the greater Toronto area. *JAMA.* 289(21):2801-9. [Erratum appears in *JAMA.* 2003. 290(3):334.]

Drosten C, Gunther S, Preiser W, van der Werf S, Brodt HR, Becker S, Rabenau H, Panning M, Kolesnikova L, Fouchier RA, Berger A, Burguiere AM, Cinatl J, Eickmann M, Escriou N, Grywna K, Kramme S, Manuguerra JC, Muller S, Rickerts V, Sturmer M, Vieth S, Klenk HD, Osterhaus AD, Schmitz H, Doerr HW. 2003. Identification of a novel coronavirus in patients with severe acute respiratory syndrome. *New England Journal of Medicine.* 348(20): 1967-76.

Hsu LY, Lee CC, Green JA, Ang B, Paton NI, Lee L, Villacian JS, Lim PL, Earnest A, Leo YS. 2003. Severe acute respiratory syndrome (SARS) in Singapore: clinical features of index patient and initial contacts. *Emerging Infectious Diseases* [serial online]. 9(6). Available at: http://www.cdc.gov/ncidod/eid/vol9no6/03-0264.htm.

Ksiazek TG, Erdman D, Goldsmith CS, Zaki SR, Peret T, Emery S, Tong S, Urbani C, Comer JA, Lim W, Rollin PE, Dowell SF, Ling AE, Humphrey CD, Shieh WJ, Guarner J, Paddock CD, Rota P, Fields B, DeRisi J, Yang JY, Cox N, Hughes JM, LeDuc JW, Bellini WJ, Anderson LJ, SARS Working Group. 2003. A novel coronavirus associated with severe acute respiratory syndrome. *New England Journal of Medicine.* 348(20):1953-66.

Kuiken T, Fouchier RA, Schutten M, Rimmelzwaan GF, van Amerongen G, van Riel D, Laman JD, de Jong T, van Doornum G, Lim W, Ling AE, Chan PK, Tam JS, Zambon MC, Gopal R, Drosten C, van der Werf S, Escriou N, Manuguerra JC, Stohr K, Peiris JS, Osterhaus AD. 2003. Newly discovered coronavirus as the primary cause of severe acute respiratory syndrome. *Lancet.* 362(9380):263-70.

Lee N, Hui D, Wu A, Chan P, Cameron P, Joynt GM, Ahuja A, Yung MY, Leung CB, To KF, Lui SF, Szeto CC, Chung S, Sung JJ. 2003. A major outbreak of severe acute respiratory syndrome in Hong Kong. *New England Journal of Medicine.* 348(20):1986-94.

Liang W, Zhu Z, Guo J, Liu Z, He X, Zhou W, Chin DP, Schucat A, Beijing Joint SARS Expert Group. 2004. Severe acute respiratory syndrome, Beijing, 2003. *Emerging Infectious Diseases* [serial online]. 10(1). Available at: http://www.cdc.gov/ncidod/eid/vol10no1/03-0553.htm.

Peiris JS, Lai ST, Poon LL, Guan Y, Yam LY, Lim W, et al. 2003. Coronavirus as a possible cause of severe acute respiratory syndrome. *Lancet.* 361(9366): 1319-25.

Poutanen SM, Low DE, Henry B, Finkelstein S, Rose D, Green K, Tellier R, Draker R, Adachi D, Ayers M, Chan AK, Skowronski DM, Salit I, Simor AE, Slutsky AS, Doyle PW, Krajden M, Petric M, Brunham RC, McGeer AJ, National Microbiology Laboratory Canada, Canadian Severe Acute Respiratory Syndrome Study Team. 2003. Identification of severe acute respiratory syndrome in Canada. *New England Journal of Medicine*. 348(20):1995-2005.

Tsang KW, Ho PL, Ooi GC, Yee WK, Wang T, Chan-Yeung M, Lam WK, Seto WH, Yam LY, Cheung TM, Wong PC, Lam B, Ip MS, Chan J, Yuen KY, Lai KN. 2003. A cluster of cases of severe acute respiratory syndrome in Hong Kong. *New England Journal of Medicine*. 348(20):1977-85.

Wong RSM, Hui DS. 2004. Index patient and SARS outbreak in Hong Kong. *Emerging Infectious Diseases* [serial online]. 10(2). Available at: http://www.cdc.gov/ncidod/EID/vol10no2/03-0645.htm.

Wu W, Wang J, Liu P, Chen W, Yin S, Jiang S, Yan L, Zhan J, Chen X, Li J, Huang Z, Huang H. 2003. A hospital outbreak of severe acute respiratory syndrome in Guangzhou, China. *Chinese Medical Journal*. 116(6):811-8.

Zhao Z, Zhang F, Xu M, Huang K, Zhong W, Cai W, Yin Z, Huang S, Deng Z, Wei M, Xiong J, Hawkey PM. 2003. Description and clinical treatment of an early outbreak of severe acute respiratory syndrome (SARS) in Guangzhou, PR China. *Journal of Medical Microbiology*. 52(Pt 8):715-20.

Zhong NS, Zheng BJ, Li YM, Poon, Xie ZH, Chan KH, Li PH, Tan SY, Chang Q, Xie JP, Liu XQ, Xu J, Li DX, Yuen KY, Peiris, Guan Y. 2003. Epidemiology and cause of severe acute respiratory syndrome (SARS) in Guangdong, People's Republic of China, in February, 2003. *Lancet*. 362(9393):1353-8.

## EPIDEMIOLOGY

The Chinese SARS Molecular Epidemiology Consortium. 2004. Molecular evolution of the SARS coronavirus during the course of the SARS epidemic in China. *Science*. 303(5664)1666-9.

Choi BC, Pak AW. 2003. A simple approximate mathematical model to predict the number of severe acute respiratory syndrome cases and deaths. *Journal of Epidemiology & Community Health*. 57(10):831-5.

Chow PKH, Ooi E-E, Tan H-K, Ong K-W, Sil BK, Teo M, et al. 2004. Healthcare worker seroconversion in SARS outbreak. *Emerging Infectious Diseases* [serial online]. 10(2). Available at: http://www.cdc.gov/ncidod/EID/vol10no2/03-0397.htm.

Donnelly CA, Ghani AC, Leung GM, Hedley AJ, Fraser C, Riley S, Abu-Raddad LJ, Ho LM, Thach TQ, Chau P, Chan KP, Lam TH, Tse LY, Tsang T, Liu SH, Kong JH, Lau EM, Ferguson NM, Anderson RM. 2003. Epidemiological determinants of spread of causal agent of severe acute respiratory syndrome in Hong Kong. *Lancet.* 361(9371):1761-6. [Erratum appears in *Lancet.* 2003. 361(9371):1832.]

Flint J, Burton S, Macey JF, Deeks SL, Tam TW, King A, Bodie-Collins M, Naus M, MacDonald D, McIntyre C, Krajden M, Petric M, Halpert C, Gustafson L, Larder A. 2003. Assessment of in-flight transmission of SARS: results of contact tracing, Canada. *Canada Communicable Disease Report.* 29(12):105-10.

Goh DLM, Lee BW, Chia KS, Heng BH, Chen M, Ma S, et al. 2004. Secondary household transmission of SARS, Singapore. *Emerging Infectious Diseases* [serial online]. 10(2). Available at: http://www.cdc.gov/ncidod/EID/vol10no2/03-0676.htm.

Guan Y, Peiris JSM, Zheng B, Poon LLM, Chan KH, Zeng FY, Chan CWM, Chan MN, Chen JD, Chow KYC, Hon CC, Hui KH, Li J, Li VYY, Wang Y, Leung SW, Yuen KY, Leung FC. 2004. Molecular epidemiology of the novel coronavirus that causes severe acute respiratory syndrome. *Lancet.* 363(9403):99-104.

Ha LD, Bloom SA, Nguyen QH, Maloney SA, Le MQ, Leitmeyer KC, et al. 2004. Lack of SARS transmission among public hospital workers, Vietnam. *Emerging Infectious Diseases* [serial online]. 10(2). Available at: http://www.cdc.gov/ncidod/EID/vol10no2/03-0707.htm.

Ho AS, Sung JJ, Chan-Yeung M. 2003. An outbreak of severe acute respiratory syndrome among hospital workers in a community hospital in Hong Kong. *Annals of Internal Medicine.* 139(7):564-7.

Hsieh Y-H, Chen CWS, Hsu S-B. 2004. SARS outbreak, Taiwan, 2003. *Emerging Infectious Diseases* [serial online]. 10(2). Available at: http://www.cdc.gov/ncidod/EID/vol10no2/03-0515.htm.

Hsueh P-R, Chen P-J, Hsiao C-H, Yeh S-H, Cheng W-C, Wang J-L, et al. 2004. Patient data, early SARS epidemic, Taiwan. *Emerging Infectious Diseases* [serial online]. 10(3). Available at: http://www.cdc.gov/ncidod/EID/vol10no3/03-0571.htm.

Isakbaeva ET, Khetsuriani N, Beard RS, Peck A, Erdman D, Monroe SS, et al. 2004. SARS-associated coronavirus transmission, United States. *Emerging Infectious Diseases* [serial online]. 10(2). Available at: http://www.cdc.gov/ncidod/EID/vol10no2/03-0734.htm.

Lau JTF, Lau M, Kim JH, Wong E, Tsui H-Y, Tsang T, et al. 2004. Probable secondary infections in households of SARS patients in Hong Kong. *Emerging Infectious Diseases* [serial online]. 10(2). Available at: http://www.cdc.gov/ncidod/EID/vol10no2/03-0626.htm.

Lipsitch M, Cohen T, Cooper B, Robins JM, Ma S, James L, Gopalakrishna G, Chew SK, Tan CC, Samore MH, Fisman D, Murray M. 2003. Transmission dynamics and control of severe acute respiratory syndrome. *Science.* 300(5627):1966-70.

Loeb M, McGeer A, Henry B, Ofner M, Rose D, Hlywka T, et al. 2004. SARS among critical care nurses, Toronto. *Emerging Infectious Diseases* [serial online]. 10(2). Available at: http://www.cdc.gov/ncidod/EID/vol10no2/03-0838.htm.

Meltzer MI. 2004. Multiple contact dates and SARS incubation periods. *Emerging Infectious Diseases* [serial online]. 10(2). Available at: http://www.cdc.gov/ncidod/EID/vol10no2/03-0426.htm.

Ng SK. 2003. Possible role of an animal vector in the SARS outbreak in Amoy Gardens. *Lancet.* 362(9383):570-2.

Olsen SJ, Chang HL, Cheung TY, Tang AF, Fisk TL, Ooi SP, Kuo HW, Jiang DD, Chen KT, Lando J, Hsu KH, Chen TJ, Dowell SF. 2003. Transmission of the severe acute respiratory syndrome on aircraft. *New England Journal of Medicine.* 349(25):2416-22.

Park BJ, Peck AJ, Kuehnert MJ, Newbern C, Smelser C, Comer JA, et al. 2004. Lack of SARS transmission among healthcare workers, United States. *Emerging Infectious Diseases* [serial online]. 10(2). Available at: URL: http://www.cdc.gov/ncidod/EID/vol10no2/03-0793.htm.

Peck AJ, Newbern EC, Feikin DR, Isakbaeva ET, Park BJ, Fehr JT, et al. 2004. Lack of SARS transmission and U.S. SARS case-patient. *Emerging Infectious Diseases* [serial online]. 10(2). Available at: http://www.cdc.gov/ncidod/EID/vol10no2/03-0746.htm.

Riley S, Fraser C, Donnelly CA, Ghani AC, Abu-Raddad LJ, Hedley AJ, Leung GM, Ho LM, Lam TH, Thach TQ, Chau P, Chan KP, Lo SV, Leung PY, Tsang T, Ho W, Lee KH, Lau EM, Ferguson NM, Anderson RM. 2003. Transmission dynamics of the etiological agent of SARS in Hong Kong: impact of public health interventions. *Science.* 300(5627):1961-6.

Shen Z, Ning F, Zhou W, He X, Lin C, Chin DP, et al. 2004. Superspreading SARS events, Beijing, 2003. *Emerging Infectious Diseases* [serial online]. 10(2). Available at: http://www.cdc.gov/ncidod/EID/vol10no2/03-0732.htm.

Varia M, Wilson S, Sarwal S, McGeer A, Gournis E , Galanis E, Henry B, Hospital Outbreak Investigation Team. 2003. Investigation of a nosocomial outbreak of severe acute respiratory syndrome (SARS) in Toronto, Canada. *Canadian Medical Association Journal.* 169(4):285-92.

WHO. Consensus document on the epidemiology of severe acute respiratory syndrome (SARS). 2003. Web Page. Available at: http://www.who.int/csr/sars/en/WHOconsensus.pdf.

Wilder-Smith A, Paton NI, Goh KT. 2003. Low risk of transmission of severe acute respiratory syndrome on airplanes: the Singapore experience. *Tropical Medicine & International Health.* 8(11):1035-7.

Wong T-W, Lee C-K, Tam W, Lau JTF, Yu T-S, Lui S-F, et al. 2004. Cluster of SARS among medical students exposed to single patient, Hong Kong. *Emerg-*

*ing Infectious Diseases* [serial online]. 10(2). Available at: http://www.cdc.gov/ncidod/EID/vol10no2/03-0452.htm.

Wu J, Xu F, Zhou W, Feikin DR, Lin C-Y, He X, et al. 2004. Risk factors for SARS among persons without known contact with SARS patients, Beijing, China. *Emerging Infectious Diseases* [serial online]. 10(2). Available at: http://www.cdc.gov/ncidod/EID/vol10no2/03-0730.htm.

Wu W, Wang JF, Liu PM, Jiang SP, Chen QY, Chen WX, Yin SM, Yan L, Zhan J, Chen XL, Li JG. 2004. Comparison of clinical course of patients with severe acute respiratory syndrome among the multiple generations of nosocomial transmission. *Chinese Medical Journal.* 117(1):14-8.

## SURVEILLANCE AND SCREENING

CDC. SARS: Surveillance and reporting. 2004. Web Page. Available at: http://www.cdc.gov/ncidod/sars/reporting.htm.

Chen SY, Su CP, Ma MH, Chiang WC, Hsu CY, Ko PC, Tsai KC, Yen ZS, Shih FY, Chen SC, Chen WJ. 2004. Predictive model of diagnosing probable cases of severe acute respiratory syndrome in febrile patients with exposure risk. *Annals of Emergency Medicine.* 43(1):1-5.

Desenclos J-C, van der Werf S, Bonmarin I, Levy-Bruhl D, Yazdanpanah Y, Hoen Beal. 2004. Introduction of SARS in France, March–April, 2003. *Emerging Infectious Diseases* [serial online]. 10(2). Available at: http://www.cdc.gov/ncidod/EID/vol10no2/03-0351.htm.

Heymann DL, Rodier G. 2004. Global surveillance, national surveillance, and SARS. *Emerging Infectious Diseases* [serial online]. 10(2). Available at: http://www.cdc.gov/ncidod/EID/vol10no2/03-1038.htm.

Jernigan JA, Low DE, Helfand RF. 2004. Combining clinical and epidemiologic features for early recognition of SARS. *Emerging Infectious Diseases* [serial online]. 10(2). Available at: http://www.cdc.gov/ncidod/EID/vol10no2/03-0741.htm.

Kaydos-Daniels SC, Olowokure B, Chang H-J, Barwick RS, Deng J-F, Lee M-L, et al. 2004. Body temperature monitoring and SARS fever hotline, Taiwan. *Emerging Infectious Diseases* [serial online]. 10(2). Available at: http://www.cdc.gov/ncidod/EID/vol10no2/03-0748.htm.

Pickles H. 2003. Screening international travellers in China for SARS. *Communicable Disease & Public Health.* 6(3):216-20.

Rainer TH, Cameron PA, Smit D, Ong KL, Hung AN, Nin DC, Ahuja AT, Si LC, Sung JJ. 2003. Evaluation of WHO criteria for identifying patients with severe acute respiratory syndrome out of hospital: prospective observational study. *BMJ.* 326(7403):1354-8.

Schrag SJ, Brooks JT, Van Beneden C, Parashar UD, Griffin PM, Anderson LJ, et al. 2004. SARS surveillance during emergency public health response, United States, March–July 2003. *Emerging Infectious Diseases* [serial online]. 10(2). Available at: http://www.cdc.gov/ncidod/EID/vol10no2/03-0752.htm.

Su CP, Chiang WC, Ma MH, Chen SY, Hsu CY, Ko PC, Tsai KC, Fan CM, Shih FY, Chen SC, Chen YC, Chang SC, Chen WJ. 2004. Validation of a novel severe acute respiratory syndrome scoring system. *Annals of Emergency Medicine.* 43(1):34-42.

Wang TL, Jang TN, Huang CH, Kao SJ, Lin CM, Lee FN, Liu CY, Chong CF, Lin CM, Dorji H, Teng HJ, Chang H. 2004. Establishing a clinical decision rule of severe acute respiratory syndrome at the emergency department. *Annals of Emergency Medicine.* 43(1):17-22.

WHO. WHO SARS international reference and verification laboratory network: Policy and procedures in the inter-epidemic period. 2004. Web Page. Available at: http://www.who.int/csr/sars/guidelines/en/WHOSARS ReferenceLab.pdf.

## CONTROL MEASURES

Abdullah AS, Tomlinson B, Cockram CS, Thomas GN. 2003. Lessons from the severe acute respiratory syndrome outbreak in Hong Kong. *Emerging Infectious Diseases* [serial online]. 9(9). Available at: http://www.cdc.gov/ncidod/eid/vol9no9/03-0366.htm.

Anonymous. 2003. Mechanical ventilation of SARS patients: safety issues involving breathing-circuit filters. *Health Devices.* 32(6):220-2.

Anonymous. 2003. Protecting against SARS during equipment maintenance. *Health Devices.* 32(6):213-9.

Castillo-Chavez C, Castillo-Garsow C, Yakuba A. 2003. Mathematical models of isolation and quarantine. *JAMA.* 290(21):2876-7.

CDC. 2003. Efficiency of quarantine during an epidemic of severe acute respiratory syndrome—Beijing, China, 2003. *Morbidity & Mortality Weekly Report.* 52(43):1037-40.

CDC. 2003. Use of quarantine to prevent transmission of severe acute respiratory syndrome—Taiwan, 2003. *Morbidity & Mortality Weekly Report.* 52(29): 680-3.

CDC. SARS: Infection control. 2004. Web Page. Available at: http://www.cdc.gov/ncidod/sars/ic.htm.

Chau PH, Yip PS. 2003. Monitoring the severe acute respiratory syndrome epidemic and assessing effectiveness of interventions in Hong Kong Special Administrative Region. *Journal of Epidemiology & Community Health.* 57(10):766-9.

Christian MD, Loutfy M, McDonald LC, Martinez KF, Ofner M, Wong T, et al. 2004. Possible SARS coronavirus transmission during cardiopulmonary resuscitation. *Emerging Infectious Diseases* [serial online]. 10(2). Available at: http://www.cdc.gov/ncidod/EID/vol10no2/03-0700.htm.

Derrick J.L. , Gomersall CD. 2004. Surgical helmets and SARS infection. *Emerging Infectious Diseases* [serial online]. 10(2). Available at: http://www.cdc.gov/ncidod/EID/vol10no2/03-0764.htm.

Dwosh HA, Hong HH, Austgarden D, Herman S, Schabas R . 2003. Identification and containment of an outbreak of SARS in a community hospital. *Canadian Medical Association Journal.* 168(11):1415-20.

Jiang S, Huang L, Chen X, Wang J, Wu W, Yin S, Chen W, Zhan J, Yan L, Ma L, Li J, Huang Z. 2003. Ventilation of wards and nosocomial outbreak of severe acute respiratory syndrome among healthcare workers. *Chinese Medical Journal.* 116(9):1293-7.

Kumar D, Tellier R, Draker R, Levy G, Humar A. 2003. Severe Acute Respiratory Syndrome (SARS) in a liver transplant recipient and guidelines for donor SARS screening. *American Journal of Transplantation.* 3(8):977-81.

Kwan A, Fok WG, Law KI, Lam SH. 2004. Tracheostomy in a patient with severe acute respiratory syndrome. *British Journal of Anaesthesia.* 92(2):280-2.

Lau JTF, Fung KS, Wong TW, Kim JH, Wong E, Chung S, et al. 2004. SARS transmission among hospital workers in Hong Kong. *Emerging Infectious Diseases* [serial online] 10(2). Available at: http://www.cdc.gov/ncidod/EID/vol10no2/03-0534.htm.

Lee A, Cheng FF, Yuen H, Ho M, Hong Kong Healthy Schools Support Group. 2003. How would schools step up public health measures to control spread of SARS? *Journal of Epidemiology & Community Health.* 57(12):945-9.

Lloyd-Smith JO, Galvani AP, Getz WM. 2003. Curtailing transmission of severe acute respiratory syndrome within a community and its hospital. *Proceedings of the Royal Society of London—Series B: Biological Sciences.* 270(1528):1979-89.

Ng PC, So KW, Leung TF, Cheng FW, Lyon DJ, Wong W, Cheung KL, Fung KS, Lee CH, Li AM, Hon KL, Li CK, Fok TF. 2003. Infection control for SARS in a tertiary neonatal centre. *Archives of Disease in Childhood Fetal & Neonatal Edition.* 88(5):F405-9.

Owolabi T, Kwolek S. 2004. Managing obstetrical patients during severe acute respiratory syndrome outbreak. *Journal of Obstetrics & Gynaecology Canada.* 26(1):35-41.

Pang X, Zhu Z, Xu F, Guo J, Gong X, Liu D, Liu Z, Chin DP, Feikin DR. 2003. Evaluation of control measures implemented in the severe acute respiratory syndrome outbreak in Beijing, 2003. *JAMA.* 290(24):3215-21.

Parmar HA, Lim TC, Goh JS, Tan JT, Sitoh YY, Hui F. 2004. Providing optimal radiology service in the severe acute respiratory syndrome outbreak: use of mobile CT. *American Journal of Roentgenology.* 182(1):57-60.

Seto WH, Tsang D, Yung RWH, Ching TY, Ng TK, Ho M, Ho LM, Peiris JSM. 2003. Effectiveness of precautions against droplets and contact in prevention of nosocomial transmission of severe acute respiratory syndrome (SARS). *Lancet.* 361(9368):1519-20.

Singh K, Hsu L, Villacian J, Habib A, Fisher D, Tambyah P. 2003. Severe acute respiratory syndrome: lessons from Singapore. *Emerging Infectious Diseases* [serial online]. 9(10). Available at: http://www.cdc.gov/ncidod/eid/vol9no10/ 03-0388.htm.

Tham KY. 2004. An emergency department response to severe acute respiratory syndrome: a prototype response to bioterrorism. *Annals of Emergency Medicine.* 43(1):6-14.

Tsou IY, Goh JS, Kaw GJ, Chee TS. 2003. Severe acute respiratory syndrome: management and reconfiguration of a radiology department in an infectious disease situation. *Radiology.* 229(1):21-6.

Twu SJ, Chen TJ, Chen CJ, Olsen SJ, Lee LT, Fisk T, Hsu KH, Chang SC, Chen KT, Chiang IH, Wu YC, Wu JS, Dowell SF. 2003. Control measures for severe acute respiratory syndrome (SARS) in Taiwan. *Emerging Infectious Diseases* [serial online]. 9(6). Available at: http://www.cdc.gov/ncidod/eid/ vol9no6/03-0283.htm.

WHO. WHO post-outbreak biosafety guidelines for handling of SARS-CoV specimens and cultures. 2003. Web Page. Available at: http://www.who.int/ csr/sars/biosafety2003_12_18/en/.

Wilder-Smith A, Paton NI, Goh KT. 2003. Experience of severe acute respiratory syndrome in Singapore: importation of cases, and defense strategies at the airport. *Journal of Travel Medicine.* 10(5):259-62.

## LAW, GOVERNMENT, AND ETHICS

Bernstein M. 2003. SARS and ethics. *Hospital Quarterly.* 7(1):38-40.

CDC. 2004. SARS: Community containment, including quarantine. Web Page. Available at: http://www.cdc.gov/ncidod/sars/quarantine.htm.

CDC. 2004. SARS: Legal authorities for isolation and quarantine. Web Page. Available at: http://www.cdc.gov/ncidod/sars/legal.htm.

Fidler DP. 2003. Emerging trends in international law concerning global infectious disease control. *Emerging Infectious Diseases* [serial online] 9(3). Available at: http://www.cdc.gov/ncidod/eid/vol9no3-02/ 0336.htm.

Gostin LO, Bayer R, Fairchild AL. 2003. Ethical and legal challenges posed by severe acute respiratory syndrome: implications for the control of severe infectious disease threats. *JAMA.* 290(24):3229-37.

Hopkins RS, Misegades L, Ransom J, Lipson L, Brink EW. 2004. SARS preparedness checklist for state and local health officials. *Emerging Infectious Diseases* [serial online]. 10(2). Available at: http://www.cdc.gov/ncidod/ EID/vol10no2/03-0729.htm.

Misrahi JJ, Foster JA, Shaw FE, Cetron MS. 2004. HHS/CDC legal response to SARS outbreak. *Emerging Infectious Diseases* [serial online]. 10(2). Available at: http://www.cdc.gov/ncidod/EID/vol10no2/03-0721.htm.

Parashar UD, Anderson LJ. 2004. SARS preparedness and response. *Emerging Infectious Diseases* [serial online]. 10(2). Available at: http://www.cdc.gov/ncidod/EID/vol10no2/03-0803.htm.

Richards EP, Rathburn KC. 2004. Making state public health laws work for SARS outbreaks. *Emerging Infectious Diseases* [serial online]. 10(2). Available at: http://www.cdc.gov/ncidod/EID/vol10no2/03-0836.htm.

Rothstein, MA, Alcalde, MG, Elster, NR, Majumder, MA, Palmer, LI, Stone, TH, and Hoffman, RE. 2003. Quarantine and isolation: Lessons learned from SARS. A report to the Centers for Disease Control and Prevention. Web Page. Available at: http://www.louisville.edu/medschool/ibhpl/publications/SARS%20REPORT.pdf.

Singer PA, Benatar SR, Bernstein M, Daar AS, Dickens BM, MacRae SK, Upshur RE, Wright L, Shaul RZ. 2003. Ethics and SARS: lessons from Toronto. *BMJ.* 327( 7427):1342-4.

## COMMUNICATION WITH THE PUBLIC

Arguin PM, Navin AW, Steele SF, Weld LH, Kozarsky PE. 2004. SARS travel alerts and advice. *Emerging Infectious Diseases* [serial online] 10(2). Available at: http://www.cdc.gov/ncidod/EID/vol10no2/03-0812.htm.

Lau JT, Yang X, Tsui H, Kim JH. 2003. Monitoring community responses to the SARS epidemic in Hong Kong: from day 10 to day 62. *Journal of Epidemiology & Community Health.* 57(11):864-70.

Leung GM, Lam TH, Ho LM, Ho SY, Chan BH, Wong IO, Hedley AJ. 2003. The impact of community psychological responses on outbreak control for severe acute respiratory syndrome in Hong Kong. *Journal of Epidemiology & Community Health.* 57(11):857-63.

Person B, Sy F, Holton K, Govert B, Liang A, NCID/SARS Emergency Outreach Team. 2004. Fear and stigma: the epidemic within the SARS outbreak. *Emerging Infectious Diseases* [serial online]. 10(2). Available at: http://www.cdc.gov/ncidod/EID/vol10no2/03-0750.htm.

Quah SR, Lee H-P. 2004. Crisis prevention and management during SARS outbreak, Singapore. *Emerging Infectious Diseases* [serial online]. 10(2). Available at: http://www.cdc.gov/ncidod/EID/vol10no2/03-0418.htm.

## CLINICAL FEATURES AND PATHOLOGY

Antonio GE, Wong KT, Chu WC, Hui DS, Cheng FW, Yuen EH, Chung SS, Fok TF, Sung JJ, Ahuja AT. 2003. Imaging in severe acute respiratory syndrome (SARS). *Clinical Radiology.* 58(11):825-32.

Avendano M, Derkach P, Swan S. 2003. Clinical course and management of SARS in health care workers in Toronto: a case series. *Canadian Medical Association Journal.* 168(13):1649-60.

Babyn PS, Chu WC, Tsou IY, Wansaicheong GK, Allen U, Bitnun A, Chee TS, Cheng FW, Chiu MC, Fok TF, Hon EK, Gahunia HK, Kaw GJ, Khong PL, Leung CW, Li AM, Manson D, Metreweli C, Ng PC, Read S, Stringer DA. 2004. Severe acute respiratory syndrome (SARS): chest radiographic features in children. *Pediatric Radiology.* 34(1):47-58.

Beijing Group of National Research Project for SARS. 2003. Dynamic changes in blood cytokine levels as clinical indicators in severe acute respiratory syndrome. *Chinese Medical Journal.* 116(9):1283-7.

Chan MS, Chan IY, Fung KH, Poon E, Yam LY, Lau KY. 2004. High-resolution ct findings in patients with severe acute respiratory syndrome: a pattern-based approach. *American Journal of Roentgenology.* 182(1):49-56.

Chao CC, Tsai LK, Chiou YH, Tseng MT, Hsieh ST, Chang SC, Chang YC. 2003. Peripheral nerve disease in SARS: report of a case. *Neurology.* 61(12): 1820-1.

Chen SY, Chiang WC, Ma MH, Su CP, Hsu CY, Chow-In Ko P, Tsai KC, Yen ZS, Shih FY, Chen SC, Lin SJ, Wang JL, Chang SC, Chen WJ. 2004. Sequential symptomatic analysis in probable severe acute respiratory syndrome cases. *Annals of Emergency Medicine.* 43(1):27-33.

Choi KW, Chau TN, Tsang O, Tso E, Chiu MC, Tong WL, Lee PO, Ng TK, Ng WF, Lee KC, Lam W, Yu WC, Lai JY, Lai ST, Princess Margaret Hospital SARS Study Group. 2003. Outcomes and prognostic factors in 267 patients with severe acute respiratory syndrome in Hong Kong. *Annals of Internal Medicine.* 139(9):715-23.

Ding Y, Wang H, Shen H, Li Z, Geng J, Han H, Cai J, Li X, Kang W, Weng D, Lu Y, Wu D, He L, Yao K . 2003. The clinical pathology of severe acute respiratory syndrome (SARS): a report from China. *Journal of Pathology.* 200(3): 282-9.

Fowler RA, Lapinsky SE, Hallett D, Detsky AS, Sibbald WJ, Slutsky AS, Stewart TE, Toronto SARS Critical Care Group. 2003. Critically ill patients with severe acute respiratory syndrome. *JAMA.* 290(3):367-73.

Franks TJ, Chong PY, Chui P, Galvin JR, Lourens RM, Reid AH, Selbs E, McEvoy CP, Hayden CD, Fukuoka J, Taubenberger JK, Travis WD. 2003. Lung pathology of severe acute respiratory syndrome (SARS): a study of 8 autopsy cases from Singapore. *Human Pathology.* 34(8):743-8.

Grinblat L, Shulman H, Glickman A, Matukas L, Paul N. 2003. Severe acute respiratory syndrome: radiographic review of 40 probable cases in Toronto, Canada. *Radiology.* 228(3):802-9.

Jang TN, Yeh DY, Shen SH, Huang CH, Jiang JS, Kao SJ. 2004. Severe acute respiratory syndrome in Taiwan: analysis of epidemiological characteristics in 29 cases. *Journal of Infection.* 48(1):23-31.

Lang ZW, Zhang LJ, Zhang SJ, Meng X, Li JQ, Song CZ, Sun L, Zhou YS, Dwyer D. 2003. A clinicopathological study of three cases of severe acute respiratory syndrome (SARS). *Pathology.* 35(6):526-31.

Lau K-K, Yu W-C, Chu C-M, Lau S-T, Sheng B, Yuen K-Y. 2004. Possible central nervous system infection by SARS coronavirus. *Emerging Infectious Diseases* [serial online]. 10(2). Available at: http://www.cdc.gov/ncidod/ EID/vol10no2/03-0638.htm.

Leung TF, Wong GW, Hon KL, Fok TF. 2003. Severe acute respiratory syndrome (SARS) in children: epidemiology, presentation and management. *Paediatric Respiratory Reviews.* 4(4):334-9.

Leung WK, To KF, Chan PK, Chan HL, Wu AK, Lee N, Yuen KY, Sung JJ. 2003. Enteric involvement of severe acute respiratory syndrome-associated coronavirus infection. *Gastroenterology.* 125(4):1011-7.

Lew TW, Kwek TK, Tai D, Earnest A, Loo S, Singh K, Kwan KM, Chan Y, Yim CF, Bek SL, Kor AC, Yap WS, Chelliah YR, Lai YC, Goh SK. 2003. Acute respiratory distress syndrome in critically ill patients with severe acute respiratory syndrome. *JAMA.* 290(3):374-80.

Li SS, Cheng CW, Fu CL, Chan YH, Lee MP, Chan JW, Yiu SF. 2003. Left ventricular performance in patients with severe acute respiratory syndrome: a 30-day echocardiographic follow-up study. *Circulation.* 108(15):1798-803.

Li T, Qiu Z, Han Y, Wang Z, Fan H, Lu W, Xie J, Ma X, Wang A. 2003. Rapid loss of both CD4+ and CD8+ T lymphocyte subsets during the acute phase of severe acute respiratory syndrome. *Chinese Medical Journal.* 116(7):985-7.

Li Z, Guo X, Hao W, Wu Y, Ji Y, Zhao Y, Liu F, Xie X. 2003. The relationship between serum interleukins and T-lymphocyte subsets in patients with severe acute respiratory syndrome. *Chinese Medical Journal.* 116(7):981-4.

Manocha S, Walley KR, Russell JA. 2003. Severe acute respiratory distress syndrome (SARS): a critical care perspective. *Critical Care Medicine.* 31(11): 2684-92.

Ooi CG, Khong PL, Lam B, Ho JC, Yiu WC, Wong WM, Wang T, Ho PL, Wong PC, Chan RH, Lam WK, Lai KN, Tsang KW. 2003. Severe acute respiratory syndrome: relationship between radiologic and clinical parameters. *Radiology.* 229(2):492-9.

Peiris JS, Chu CM, Cheng VC, Chan KS, Hung IF, Poon LL, Law KI, Tang BS, Hon TY, Chan CS, Chan KH, Ng JS, Zheng BJ, Ng WL, Lai RW, Guan Y, Yuen KY, HKU/UCH SARS Study Group. 2003. Clinical progression and viral load in a community outbreak of coronavirus-associated SARS pneumonia: a prospective study. *Lancet.* 361(9371):1767-72.

Robertson CA, Lowther SA, Birch T, Tan C, Sorhage F, Stockman L, et al. 2004. SARS and pregnancy: a case report. *Emerging Infectious Diseases* [serial online]. 10(2). Available at: http://www.cdc.gov/ncidod/EID/vol10no2/03-0736.htm.

Tan T, Tan B, Kurup A, Oon L, Heng D, Se Thoe S, et al. 2004. SARS and *Escherichia coli* bacteremia. *Emerging Infectious Diseases* [serial online]. 10(2). Available at: http://www.cdc.gov/ncidod/EID/vol10no2/03-0501.htm.

Tee AKH, Oh HML, Hui KP, Lien CTC, Narendran K, Heng BH, et al. 2004. Atypical SARS in geriatric patient. *Emerging Infectious Diseases* [serial online]. 10(2). Available at: http://www.cdc.gov/ncidod/EID/vol10no2/03-0322.htm.

Tiwari A, Chan S, Wong A, Tai J, Cheng K, Chan J, Tsang K, Nursing Task Force on Anti-SARS of Queen Mary Hospital. 2003. Severe acute respiratory syndrome (SARS) in Hong Kong: patients' experiences. *Nursing Outlook.* 51(5):212-9.

Tsang O, Chau T, Choi K, Tso E, Lim W, Chiu M, Tong W, Lee P, Lam B, Ng T, Lai J, Yu W, Lai S. 2003. Coronavirus-positive nasopharyngeal aspirate as predictor for severe acute respiratory syndrome mortality. *Emerging Infectious Diseases* [serial online]. 9(11). Available at: http://www.cdc.gov/ncidod/eid/vol9no11/03-0400.htm.

Tsui PT, Kwok ML, Yuen H, Lai ST. 2003. Severe acute respiratory syndrome: clinical outcome and prognostic correlates. *Emerging Infectious Diseases* [serial online]. 9(9). Available at: http://www.cdc.gov/ncidod/eid/vol9no9/03-0362.htm.

Vu HT, Leitmeyer KC, Le DH, Miller MJ, Nguyen QH, Uyeki TM, et al. 2004. Clinical description of a completed outbreak of severe acute respiratory syndrome (SARS) in Vietnam, February–May, 2003. *Emerging Infectious Diseases* [serial online]. 10(2). Available at: http://www.cdc.gov/ncidod/EID/vol10no2/03-0761.htm.

Wong KT, Antonio GE, Hui DS, Lee N, Yuen EH, Wu A, Leung CB, Rainer TH, Cameron P, Chung SS , Sung JJ, Ahuja AT. 2003. Severe acute respiratory syndrome: radiographic appearances and pattern of progression in 138 patients. *Radiology.* 228(2):401-6.

Wong KT, Antonio GE, Hui DS, Lee N, Yuen EH, Wu A, Leung CB, Rainer TH, Cameron P, Chung SS , Sung JJ, Ahuja AT. 2003. Thin-section CT of severe acute respiratory syndrome: evaluation of 73 patients exposed to or with the disease. *Radiology.* 228(2):395-400.

Wong PN, Mak SK, Lo KY, Tong GM, Wong Y, Watt CL, Wong AK. 2003. Clinical presentation and outcome of severe acute respiratory syndrome in dialysis patients. *American Journal of Kidney Diseases.* 42(5):1075-81.

Wong RS, Wu A, To KF, Lee N, Lam CW, Wong CK, Chan PK, Ng MH, Yu LM, Hui DS, Tam JS, Cheng G, Sung JJ. 2003. Haematological manifestations in patients with severe acute respiratory syndrome: retrospective analysis. *BMJ.* 326(7403):1358-62.

Yang G-G, Lin S-Z, Liao K-W, Lee J-J, Wang L-S. 2004. SARS-associated coronavirus infection in teenagers. *Emerging Infectious Diseases* [serial online]. 10(2). Available at: http://www.cdc.gov/ncidod/EID/vol10no2/03-0485.htm.

## DIAGNOSIS AND DETECTION OF THE SARS CORONAVIRUS

CDC. SARS: Evaluation and diagnosis. 2004. Web Page. Available at: http://www.cdc.gov/ncidod/sars/diagnosis.htm.

Chan KH, Poon LLLM, Cheng VCC, Guan Y, Hung IFN, Kong J, et al. 2004. Detection of SARS coronavirus in patients with suspected SARS. *Emerging Infectious Diseases* [serial online]. 10(2). Available at: http://www.cdc.gov/ncidod/EID/vol10no2/03-0610.htm.

Chong PY, Chui P, Ling AE, Franks TJ, Tai DY, Leo YS, Kaw GJ, Wansaicheong G, Chan KP, Ean Oon LL, Teo ES, Tan KB, Nakajima N, Sata T, Travis WD. 2004. Analysis of deaths during the severe acute respiratory syndrome (SARS) epidemic in Singapore: challenges in determining a SARS diagnosis. *Archives of Pathology & Laboratory Medicine*. 128 (2):195-204.

Emery SL, Erdman DD, Bowen MD, Newton BR, Winchell JM, Meyer RF, et al. 2004. Real-time reverse transcription–polymerase chain reaction assay for SARS-associated coronavirus. *Emerging Infectious Diseases* [serial online]. 10(2). Available at: http://www.cdc.gov/ncidod/EID/vol10no2/03-0759.htm.

Hui JY, Hon TY, Yang MK, Cho DH, Luk WH, Chan RY, Chan KS, Loke TK, Chan JC. 2004. High-resolution computed tomography is useful for early diagnosis of severe acute respiratory syndrome-associated coronavirus pneumonia in patients with normal chest radiographs. *Journal of Computer Assisted Tomography*. 28(1):1-9.

Jiang SS, Chen TC, Yang JY, Hsiung CA, Su IJ, Liu YL, Chen PC, Juang JL. 2004. Sensitive and quantitative detection of severe acute respiratory syndrome coronavirus infection by real-time nested polymerase chain reaction. *Clinical Infectious Diseases*. 38(2):293-6.

Lau LT, Fung YW, Wong FP, Lin SS, Wang CR, Li HL, Dillon N, Collins RA, Tam JS, Chan PK, Wang CG, Yu AC. 2003. A real-time PCR for SARS-coronavirus incorporating target gene pre-amplification. *Biochemical & Biophysical Research Communications*. 312(4):1290-6.

Mazzulli T, Farcas GA, Poutanen SM, Willey BM, Low DE, Butany J, Asa SL, Kain KC. 2004. Severe acute respiratory syndrome-associated coronavirus in lung tissue. *Emerging Infectious Diseases* [serial online] 10 (1). Available at: http://www.cdc.gov/ncidod/eid/vol10no1/03-0404.htm.

Ng EK, Hui DS, Chan KC, Hung EC, Chiu RW, Lee N, Wu A, Chim SS, Tong YK, Sung JJ, Tam JS, Lo YM. 2003. Quantitative analysis and prognostic implication of SARS coronavirus RNA in the plasma and serum of patients with severe acute respiratory syndrome. *Clinical Chemistry*. 49(12):1976-80.

Poon LL, Chan KH, Wong OK, Cheung TK, Ng I, Zheng B, Seto WH, Yuen KY, Guan Y, Peiris JS. 2004. Detection of SARS coronavirus in patients with severe acute respiratory syndrome by conventional and real-time quantitative reverse transcription-PCR assays. *Clinical Chemistry.* 50(1):67-72.

Shi Y, Yi Y, Li P, Kuang T, Li L, Dong M, Ma Q, Cao C. 2003. Diagnosis of severe acute respiratory syndrome (SARS) by detection of SARS coronavirus nucleocapsid antibodies in an antigen-capturing enzyme-linked immunosorbent assay. *Journal of Clinical Microbiology.* 41(12):5781-2.

Tang P, Louie M, Richardson SE, Smieja M, Simor AE, Jamieson F, Fearon M, Poutanen SM, Mazzulli T, Tellier R, Mahony J, Loeb M, Petrich A, Chernesky M, McGeer A, Low DE, Phillips E, Jones S, Bastien N, Li Y, Dick D, Grolla A, Fernando L, Booth TF, Henry B, Rachlis AR, Matukas LM, Rose DB, Lovinsky R , Walmsley S, Gold WL, Krajden S, The Ontario Laboratory Working Group for the Rapid Diagnosis of Emerging Infections. 2004. Interpretation of diagnostic laboratory tests for severe acute respiratory syndrome: the Toronto experience. *Canadian Medical Association Journal.* 170(1):47-54.

Wu HS, Chiu SC, Tseng TC, Lin SF, Lin JH, Hsu YF, et al. 2004. Serologic and molecular biologic methods for SARS-associated coronavirus infection, Taiwan. *Emerging Infectious Diseases* [serial online]. 10(2). Available at: http://www.cdc.gov/ncidod/EID/vol10no2/03-0731.htm.

Wu HS, Hsieh YC, Su IJ, Lin TH, Chiu SC, Hsu YF, Lin JH, Wang MC, Chen JY, Hsiao PW, Chang GD, Wang AH, Ting HW, Chou CM, Huang CJ. 2004. Early detection of antibodies against various structural proteins of the SARS-associated coronavirus in SARS patients. *Journal of Biomedical Science.* 11(1):117-26.

Zhai J, Briese T, Dai E, Wang X, Pang X, Du Z. 2004. Real-time polymerase chain reaction for detecting SARS coronavirus, Beijing, 2003. *Emerging Infectious Diseases* [serial online]. 10(2). Available at: http://www.cdc.gov/ncidod/EID/vol10no1/03-0799.htm.

Zhang J, Meng B, Liao D, Zhou L, Zhang X, Chen L, Guo Z, Peng C, Zhu B, Lee PP, Xu X, Zhou T, Deng Z, Hu Y, Li K. 2003. De novo synthesis of PCR templates for the development of SARS diagnostic assay. *Molecular Biotechnology.* 25(2):107-12.

## THERAPEUTICS

Cinatl J, Morgenstern B, Bauer G, Chandra P, Rabenau H, Doerr HW. 2003. Treatment of SARS with human interferons. *Lancet.* 362(9380):293-4. [Erratum appears in *Lancet.* 2003. 362(9385):748.]

Cooper A, Joglekar A, Adhikari N. 2003. A practical approach to airway management in patients with SARS. *Canadian Medical Association Journal.* 169(8):785-7.

De Groot AS. 2003. How the SARS vaccine effort can learn from HIV: speeding towards the future, learning from the past. *Vaccine.* 21(27-30):4095-104.

Ho JC, Ooi GC, Mok TY, Chan JW, Hung I, Lam B, Wong PC, Li PC, Ho PL, Lam WK, Ng CK, Ip MS, Lai KN, Chan-Yeung M, Tsang KW. 2003. High-dose pulse versus nonpulse corticosteroid regimens in severe acute respiratory syndrome. *American Journal of Respiratory & Critical Care Medicine.* 168(12):1449-56.

Knowles SR, Phillips EJ, Dresser L, Matukas L. 2003. Common adverse events associated with the use of ribavirin for severe acute respiratory syndrome in Canada. *Clinical Infectious Diseases.* 37(8):1139-42.

Loutfy MR, Blatt LM, Siminovitch KA, Ward S, Wolff B, Lho H, Pham DH, Deif H, LaMere EA, Chang M, Kain KC, Farcas GA, Ferguson P, Latchford M, Levy G, Dennis JW, Lai EK, Fish EN. 2003. Interferon alfacon-1 plus corticosteroids in severe acute respiratory syndrome: a preliminary study. *JAMA.* 290(24):3222-8.

Ooi CG, Khong PL, Ho JC, Lam B, Wong WM, Yiu WC, Wong PC, Wong CF, Lai KN, Tsang KW. 2003. Severe acute respiratory syndrome: radiographic evaluation and clinical outcome measures. *Radiology.* 229(2):500-6.

van Vonderen MG, Bos JC, Prins JM, Wertheim-van Dillen P, Speelman P. 2003. Ribavirin in the treatment of severe acute respiratory syndrome (SARS). *Netherlands Journal of Medicine.* 61(7):238-41.

Verbeek PR, Schwartz B, Burgess RJ. 2003. Should paramedics intubate patients with SARS-like symptoms? *Canadian Medical Association Journal.* 169(4): 299-300.

Wei WI, Tuen HH, Ng RW, Lam LK. 2003. Safe tracheostomy for patients with severe acute respiratory syndrome. *Laryngoscope.* 113(10):1777-9.

Zhaori G. 2003. Antiviral treatment of SARS: can we draw any conclusions? *Canadian Medical Association Journal.* 169(11):1165-6.

## MOLECULAR AND CELLULAR BIOLOGY

Anand K, Ziebuhr J, Wadhwani P, Mesters JR, Hilgenfeld R. 2003. Coronavirus main proteinase (3CLpro) structure: basis for design of anti-SARS drugs. *Science.* 300(5626):1763-7.

Cai QC, Jiang QW, Zhao GM, Guo Q, Cao GW, Chen T. 2003. Putative caveolin-binding sites in SARS-CoV proteins. *Zhongguo Yao Li Xue Bao/Acta Pharmacologica Sinica.* 24(10):1051-9.

Che XY, Hao W, Qiu LW, Pan YX, Liao ZY, Xu H, Chen JJ, Hou JL, Woo PC, Lau SK, Kwok YY, Huang Z. 2003. Antibody response of patients with severe acute respiratory syndrome (SARS) to nucleocapsid antigen of SARS-associated coronavirus. *Di Yi Junyi Daxue Xuebao.* 23(7):637-9.

Chou KC, Wei DQ, Zhong WZ. 2003. Binding mechanism of coronavirus main proteinase with ligands and its implication to drug design against SARS. *Biochemical & Biophysical Research Communications.* 308(1):148-51.

Fan K, Wei P, Feng Q, Chen S, Huang C, Ma L, Lai B , Pei J, Liu Y, Chen J, Lai L. 2004. Biosynthesis, purification, and substrate specificity of severe acute respiratory syndrome coronavirus 3C-like proteinase. *Journal of Biological Chemistry.* 279(3):1637-42.

Gao F, Ou HY, Chen LL, Zheng WX, Zhang CT. 2003. Prediction of proteinase cleavage sites in polyproteins of coronaviruses and its applications in analyzing SARS-CoV genomes. *FEBS Letters.* 553(3):451-6.

Goldsmith CS, Tatti KM, Ksiazek TG, Rollin PE, Comer JA, Lee WW, et al. 2004. Ultrastructural characterization of SARS coronavirus. *Emerging Infectious Diseases* [serial online]. 10(2). Available at: http://www.cdc.gov/ncidod/EID/vol10no2/03-0913.htm.

He R, Leeson A, Andonov A, Li Y, Bastien N, Cao J, Osiowy C, Dobie F, Cutts T, Ballantine M, Li X. 2003. Activation of AP-1 signal transduction pathway by SARS coronavirus nucleocapsid protein. *Biochemical & Biophysical Research Communications.* 311(4):870-6.

Hensley LE, Fritz EA, Jahrling PB, Karp CL, Huggins JW, Geisbert TW. 2004. Interferon-ß 1a and SARS coronavirus replication. *Emerging Infectious Diseases* [serial online]. 10(2). Available at: http://www.cdc.gov/ncidod/EID/vol10no2/03-0482.htm.

Ho TY, Wu SL, Cheng SE, Wei YC, Huang SP, Hsiang CY. 2004. Antigenicity and receptor-binding ability of recombinant SARS coronavirus spike protein. *Biochemical & Biophysical Research Communications.* 313(4):938-47.

Jenwitheesuk E, Samudrala R. 2003. Identifying inhibitors of the SARS coronavirus proteinase. *Bioorganic & Medicinal Chemistry Letters.* 13(22):3989-92.

Krokhin O, Li Y, Andonov A, Feldmann H, Flick R , Jones S, Stroeher U, Bastien N, Dasuri KV, Cheng K, Simonsen JN, Perreault H, Wilkins J, Ens W, Plummer F, Standing KG. 2003. Mass spectrometric characterization of proteins from the SARS virus: a preliminary report. *Molecular & Cellular Proteomics.* 2(5):346-56.

Navas-Martin S, Weiss SR. 2003. SARS: Lessons learned from other coronaviruses. *Viral Immunology.* 16(4):461-74.

Ng ML, Tan SH, See EE, Ooi EE, Ling AE. 2003. Proliferative growth of SARS coronavirus in Vero E6 cells. *Journal of General Virology.* 84(12):3291-303.

Spiga O, Bernini A, Ciutti A, Chiellini S, Menciassi N, Finetti F, Causarono V, Anselmi F, Prischi F, Niccolai N. 2003. Molecular modelling of S1 and S2 subunits of SARS coronavirus spike glycoprotein. *Biochemical & Biophysical Research Communications.* 310(1):78-83.

Tanner JA, Watt RM, Chai YB, Lu LY, Lin MC, Peiris JS, Poon LL, Kung HF, Huang JD. 2003. The severe acute respiratory syndrome (SARS) coronavirus NTPase/helicase belongs to a distinct class of 5' to 3' viral helicases. *Journal of Biological Chemistry.* 278(41):39578-82.

Wang J, Wen J, Li J, Yin J, Zhu Q, Wang H, Yang Y, Qin E, You B, Li W, Li X, Huang S, Yang R, Zhang X, Yang L, Zhang T, Yin Y, Cui X, Tang X, Wang L, He B, Ma L, Lei T, Zeng C, Fang J, Yu J, Wang J, Yang H, West MB, Bhatnagar A, Lu Y, Xu N, Liu S. 2003. Assessment of immunoreactive synthetic peptides from the structural proteins of severe acute respiratory syndrome coronavirus. *Clinical Chemistry.* 49(12):1989-96.

Xiao X, Chakraborti S, Dimitrov AS, Gramatikoff K, Dimitrov DS. 2003. The SARS-CoV S glycoprotein: expression and functional characterization. *Biochemical & Biophysical Research Communications.* 312(4):1159-64.

Xu X, Liu Y, Weiss S, Arnold E, Sarafianos SG, Ding J. 2003. Molecular model of SARS coronavirus polymerase: implications for biochemical functions and drug design. *Nucleic Acids Research.* 31(24):7117-30.

Yang H, Yang M, Ding Y, Liu Y, Lou Z, Zhou Z, Sun L, Mo L, Ye S, Pang H, Gao GF, Anand K, Bartlam M, Hilgenfeld R, Rao Z. 2003. The crystal structures of severe acute respiratory syndrome virus main protease and its complex with an inhibitor. *Proceedings of the National Academy of Sciences of the United States of America.* 100(23):13190-5.

Zhang R, Guo Z, Lu J, Meng J, Zhou C, Zhan X, Huang B, Yu X, Huang M, Pan X, Ling W, Chen X, Wan Z, Zheng H, Yan X, Wang Y, Ran Y, Liu X, Ma J, Wang C, Zhang B. 2003. Inhibiting severe acute respiratory syndrome-associated coronavirus by small interfering RNA. *Chinese Medical Journal.* 116(8):1262-4.

## GENOMICS

Campanacci V, Egloff MP, Longhi S, Ferron F, Rancurel C, Salomoni A, Durousseau C, Tocque F, BrA(C)mond N, Dobbe JC, Snijder EJ, Canard B, Cambillau C. 2003. Structural genomics of the SARS coronavirus: cloning, expression, crystallization and preliminary crystallographic study of the Nsp9 protein. *Acta Crystallographica Section D-Biological Crystallography.* 59(9):1628-31.

Chen LL, Ou HY, Zhang R, Zhang CT. 2003. ZCURVE_CoV: a new system to recognize protein coding genes in coronavirus genomes, and its applications in analyzing SARS-CoV genomes. *Biochemical & Biophysical Research Communications.* 307(2):382-8.

Chim SS, Tong YK, Hung EC, Chiu RW, Lo YM. 2004. Genomic sequencing of a SARS coronavirus isolate that predated the Metropole Hotel case cluster in Hong Kong. *Clinical Chemistry.* 50(1):231-3.

Chim SS, Tsui SK, Chan KC, Au TC, Hung EC, Tong YK, Chiu RW, Ng EK, Chan PK, Chu CM, Sung JJ, Tam JS, Fung KP, Waye MM, Lee CY, Yuen KY, Lo YM, CUHK Molecular SARS Research Group. 2003. Genomic characterisation of the severe acute respiratory syndrome coronavirus of Amoy Gardens outbreak in Hong Kong. *Lancet.* 362(9398):1807-8.

Hu LD, Zheng GY, Jiang HS, Xia Y, Zhang Y, Kong XY. 2003. Mutation analysis of 20 SARS virus genome sequences: evidence for negative selection in replicase ORF1b and spike gene. *Acta Pharmacologica Sinica.* 24(8):741-5.

Li L, Wang Z, Lu Y, Bao Q, Chen S, Wu N, Cheng S, Weng J, Zhang Y, Yan J, Mei L, Wang X, Zhu H, Yu Y, Zhang M, Li M, Yao J, Lu Q, Yao P, Bo X, Wo J, Wang S, Hu S. 2003. Severe acute respiratory syndrome-associated coronavirus genotype and its characterization. *Chinese Medical Journal.* 116(9):1288-92.

Marra MA, Jones SJ, Astell CR, Holt RA, Brooks-Wilson A, Butterfield YS, Khattra J, Asano JK, Barber SA, Chan SY, Cloutier A , Coughlin SM, Freeman D, Girn N, Griffith OL, Leach SR, Mayo M, McDonald H, Montgomery SB , Pandoh PK, Petrescu AS, Robertson AG, Schein JE, Siddiqui A, Smailus DE, Stott JM, Yang GS, Plummer F, Andonov A, Artsob H , Bastien N, Bernard K, Booth TF, Bowness D, Czub M, Drebot M, Fernando L, Flick R , Garbutt M, Gray M, Grolla A, Jones S, Feldmann H , Meyers A, Kabani A, Li Y, Normand S, Stroher U, Tipples GA, Tyler S, Vogrig R, Ward D, Watson B, Brunham RC, Krajden M, Petric M, Skowronski DM, Upton C, Roper RL. 2003. The Genome sequence of the SARS-associated coronavirus. *Science.* 300(5624):1399-404.

Rota PA, Oberste MS, Monroe SS, Nix WA, Campagnoli R, Icenogle JP, Penaranda S, Bankamp B, Maher K, Chen MH, Tong S, Tamin A, Lowe L, Frace M, DeRisi JL, Chen Q, Wang D, Erdman DD, Peret TC, Burns C, Ksiazek TG , Rollin PE, Sanchez A, Liffick S, Holloway B, Limor J, McCaustland K, Olsen-Rasmussen M, Fouchier R, Gunther S, Osterhaus AD, Drosten C, Pallansch MA, Anderson LJ, Bellini WJ. 2003. Characterization of a novel coronavirus associated with severe acute respiratory syndrome. *Science.* 300(5624):1394-9.

Ruan YJ, Wei CL, Ee AL, Vega VB, Thoreau H, Su ST, Chia JM, Ng P, Chiu KP, Lim L, Zhang T, Peng CK, Lin EO, Lee NM, Yee SL, Ng LF, Chee RE, Stanton LW, Long PM, Liu ET. 2003. Comparative full-length genome sequence analysis of 14 SARS coronavirus isolates and common mutations associated with putative origins of infection. *Lancet.* 361(9371):1779-85. [Erratum appears in *Lancet.* 2003. 361(9371):1832.]

Snijder EJ, Bredenbeek PJ, Dobbe JC, Thiel V, Ziebuhr J, Poon LL, Guan Y, Rozanov M, Spaan WJ, Gorbalenya AE. 2003. Unique and conserved features of genome and proteome of SARS-coronavirus, an early split-off from the coronavirus group 2 lineage. *Journal of Molecular Biology.* 331(5):991-1004.

Thiel V, Ivanov KA, Putics A, Hertzig T, Schelle B, Bayer S, Weissbrich B, Snijder EJ, Rabenau H, Doerr HW, Gorbalenya AE, Ziebuhr J. 2003. Mechanisms and enzymes involved in SARS coronavirus genome expression. *Journal of General Virology.* 84(Pt 9):2305-15.

Vicenzi E, Canducci F, Pinna D, Mancini N, Carletti S, Lazzarin A, et al. 2004. *Coronaviridae* and SARS-associated coronavirus strain HSR1. *Emerging Infectious Diseases* [serial online]. 10(3). Available at: http://www.cdc.gov/ncidod/EID/vol10no3/03-0683.htm.

Wang ZG, Li LJ, Luo Y, Zhang JY, Wang MY, Cheng SY, Zhang YJ, Wang XM, Lu YY, Wu NP, Mei LL, Wang ZX. 2004. Molecular biological analysis of genotyping and phylogeny of severe acute respiratory syndrome associated coronavirus. *Chinese Medical Journal.* 117(1):42-8.

Yan L, Velikanov M, Flook P, Zheng W, Szalma S, Kahn S. 2003. Assessment of putative protein targets derived from the SARS genome. *FEBS Letters.* 554(3):257-63.

Yap YL, Zhang XW, Danchin A. 2003. Relationship of SARS-CoV to other pathogenic RNA viruses explored by tetranucleotide usage profiling. *BMC Bioinformatics.* 4(1):43.

Yount B, Curtis KM, Fritz EA, Hensley LE, Jahrling PB, Prentice E, Denison MR, Geisbert TW, Baric RS. 2003. Reverse genetics with a full-length infectious cDNA of severe acute respiratory syndrome coronavirus. *Proceedings of the National Academy of Sciences of the United States of America.* 100(22):12995-3000.

Zeng FY, Chan CW, Chan MN, Chen JD, Chow KY, Hon CC, Hui KH, Li J, Li VY, Wang CY, Wang PY, Guan Y, Zheng B, Poon LL, Chan KH, Yuen KY, Peiris JS, Leung FC. 2003. The complete genome sequence of severe acute respiratory syndrome coronavirus strain HKU-39849 (HK-39). *Experimental Biology & Medicine.* 228(7):866-73.

## NATURAL HISTORY

Duan SM, Zhao XS, Wen RF, Huang JJ, Pi GH, Zhang SX, Han J, Bi SL, Ruan L, Dong XP, SARS Research Team. 2003. Stability of SARS coronavirus in human specimens and environment and its sensitivity to heating and UV irradiation. *Biomedical & Environmental Sciences.* 16(3):246-55.

Guan Y, Zheng BJ, He YQ, Liu XL, Zhuang ZX, Cheung CL, Luo SW, Li PH, Zhang LJ, Guan YJ, Butt KM, Wong KL, Chan KW, Lim W, Shortridge KF, Yuen KY, Peiris JSM, Poon LLM. 2003. Isolation and characterization of viruses related to the SARS coronavirus from animals in southern China. *Science.* 302(5643):276-8.

Martina BE, Haagmans BL, Kuiken T, Fouchier RA, Rimmelzwaan GF, Van Amerongen G, Peiris JS, Lim W, Osterhaus AD. 2003. Virology: SARS virus infection of cats and ferrets. *Nature.* 425(6961):915.

Rest JS, Mindell DP. 2003. SARS associated coronavirus has a recombinant polymerase and coronaviruses have a history of host-shifting. *Infection, Genetics & Evolution.* 3(3):219-25.

Stavrinides J, Guttman DS. 2004. Mosaic evolution of the severe acute respiratory syndrome coronavirus. *Journal of Virology.* 78(1):76-82.

Weingartl HM, Copps J, Drebot MA, Marszal P, Smith G, Gren J, Andonova M, Pasick J, Kitching P, Czub M. 2004. Susceptibility of pigs and chickens to SARS coronavirus. *Emerging Infectious Diseases* [serial online] 10(2). Available at: http://www.cdc.gov/ncidod/EID/vol10no2/03-0677.htm.

Zheng BJ, Guan Y, Wong KH, Zhou J, Wong KL, Young BWY, Lu LW, Lee SS. 2004. SARS-related virus predating SARS outbreak, Hong Kong. *Emerging Infectious Diseases* [serial online]. 10(2). Available at: http://www.cdc.gov/ncidod/EID/vol10no2/03-0533.htm.

# Appendix E

# Glossary and Acronyms

## GLOSSARY

**Adenovirus** any of a family (Adenoviridae) of DNA viruses shaped like a 20-sided polyhedron, originally identified in human adenoid tissue, causing respiratory diseases (as catarrh), and including some capable of inducing malignant tumors in experimental animals.

**Aerosolize** to disperse (as a medicine, bactericide, or insecticide) as an aerosol.

**Agalactia** the failure of the secretion of milk from any cause other than the normal ending of the lactation period.

**Agent** any power, principle, or substance capable of producing an effect, whether chemical, physical, or biological.

**AIDS** acquired immunodeficiency syndrome, the end stage of HIV disease.

**Airborne** the dissemination of microbial agents through a suitable portal of entry, usually the respiratory tract. Microbial aerosols are suspensions of particles in the air consisting partially or wholly of microorganisms.

**Algae** a plant or plantlike organism of any of several phyla, divisions, or classes of chiefly aquatic usually chlorophyll-containing nonvascular organisms of polyphyletic origin that usually include the green, yellow-green, brown, and red algae in the eukaryotes and the blue-green algae in the prokaryotes.

**Aminopeptidase** an enzyme (as one found in the duodenum) that hydrolyzes peptides by acting on the peptide bond next to a terminal amino acid containing a free amino group.

**Angiotensin** either of two forms of a kinin of which one has marked physiological activity and the other is its physiologically inactive precursor; a synthetic amide derivative of angiotensin II used to treat some forms of hypotension.

**Antibiotic** chemical substance produced by a microorganism which has the capacity to inhibit the growth of or to kill other microorganisms; antibiotics that are nontoxic to the host are used as chemotherapeutic agents in the treatment of infectious diseases.

**Antibody** a protein produced by the immune system in response to the introduction of a substance (an antigen) recognized as foreign by the body's immune system. Antibody interacts with the other components of the immune system and can render the antigen harmless, although for various reasons this may not always occur.

**Antigen** a usually protein or carbohydrate substance (as a toxin or enzyme) capable of stimulating an immune response.

**Antimicrobial** a drug for killing microorganisms or suppressing their multiplication or growth. For the purposes of this report, antimicrobials include antibiotics and antivirals.

**Antiretroviral** substance that stops or suppresses the activity of a retrovirus such as HIV.

**Antiviral** drugs, including interferon, which stimulate cellular defenses against viruses, reducing cell DNA synthesis and making cells more resistant to viral genes, enhancing cellular immune responses or suppressing their replication.

**Asymptomatic** presenting no symptoms of disease.

**Atypical pneumonia** any of a group of pneumonias (as Q fever and psittacosis) caused especially by a virus, mycoplasma, rickettsia, or Chlamydia.

**Autophagy** digestion of cellular constituents by enzymes of the same cell.

**Avian influenza** any of several highly variable diseases of domestic and wild birds that are caused by orthomyxoviruses and characterized usually by respiratory symptoms but sometimes by gastrointestinal, integumentary, and urogenital symptoms.

**Bioinformatics** the collection, classification, storage, and analysis of biochemical and biological information using computers especially as applied in molecular genetics and genomics.

**Biomedical** of, relating to, or involving biological, medical, and physical science.

**Biomolecule** an organic molecule and especially a macromolecule (as a protein or nucleic acid) in living organisms.

**Biosafety** safety with respect to the effects of biological research on humans and the environment.

**Biotechnology** applied biological science (as bioengineering or recombinant DNA technology).

**Bioterrorism** terrorism involving use of biological warfare agents (as disease-causing viruses or herbicides).

**Bronchodilator** relating to or causing expansion of the bronchial air passages.

**Bronchoscopy** the use of a bronchoscope in the examination or treatment of the bronchi.

**Cholera** any of several diseases of humans and domestic animals usually marked by severe gastrointestinal symptoms: as **a:** an acute diarrheal disease caused by an enterotoxin produced by a comma-shaped gram-negative bacillus of the genus *Vibrio* (*V. cholerae* syn. *V. comma*) when it is present in large numbers in the proximal part of the human small intestine.

**Cloaca** the common chamber into which the intestinal, urinary, and generative canals discharge especially in monotreme mammals, birds, reptiles, amphibians, and elasmobranch fishes **b:** the terminal part of the embryonic hindgut of a mammal before it divides into rectum, bladder, and genital precursors; a passage in a bone leading to a cavity containing a sequestrum.

**Colostrum** milk secreted for a few days after parturition and characterized by high protein and antibody content.

**Combinatorial chemistry** a branch of applied chemistry concerned with the rapid synthesis and screening of large numbers of different but related chemical compounds generated from a mixture of known building blocks in order to recover new substances optimally suited for a specific function.

**Communicable disease** an infectious disease transmissible (as from person to person) by direct contact with an affected individual or the individual's discharges or by indirect means (as by a vector).

**Computational chemistry** Computer-based modeling and prediction of the structure of chemical compounds most likely to bind a protein drug target. Known properties are used to calculate properties of new molecules and energy minimization is used to adjust the structure.

**Coronavirus** any of a family (Coronaviridae) of single-stranded RNA viruses that have a lipid envelope with club-shaped projections and include some causing respiratory symptoms in humans.

**Corticosteroid** any of various adrenal-cortex steroids (as corticosterone, cortisone, and aldosterone) that are divided on the basis of their major biological activity into glucocorticoids and mineralocorticoids.

**Cysteine** a sulfur-containing amino acid $C_3H_7NO_2S$ occurring in many proteins and glutathione and readily oxidizable to cystine.

**Cytokine** any of a class of immunoregulatory proteins (as interleukin, tumor necrosis factor, and interferon) that are secreted by cells especially of the immune system.

**Cytopathic** of, relating to, characterized by, or producing pathological changes in cells.

**Cytotoxic** toxic to cells.

**Dexamethasone** a synthetic glucocorticoid $C_{22}H_{29}FO_5$ used especially as an anti-inflammatory and antiallergic agent.

**Diphtheria** an acute febrile contagious disease marked by the formation of a false membrane especially in the throat and caused by a bacterium of the genus *Corynebacterium* (*C. diphtheriae*) which produces a toxin causing inflammation of the heart and nervous system.

**Dyspnea** difficult or labored respiration.

**Ebola** the hemorrhagic fever caused by the Ebola virus.

*E. Coli* a straight rod-shaped gram-negative bacterium (*Escherichia coli* of the family Enterobacteriaceae) that is used in public health as an indicator of fecal pollution (as of water or food) and in medicine and genetics as a research organism and that occurs in various strains that may live as harmless inhabitants of the human lower intestine or may produce a toxin causing intestinal illness.

**Enteric** of, relating to, or affecting the intestines.

**Enterovirus** any of a genus (*Enterovirus*) of picornaviruses (as the causative agent of poliomyelitis) that typically occur in the gastrointestinal tract but may be involved in respiratory ailments, meningitis, and neurological disorders.

**Epidemic** the occurrence in a community or region of cases of an illness (or outbreak) with a frequency clearly in excess of normal expectancy.

**Epidemiology** branch of science that deals with the incidence, distribution, and control of disease in a population; the sum of the factors controlling the presence or abundance of a disease or pathogen.

**Epithelial** of or relating to a membranous cellular tissue that covers a free surface or lines a tube or cavity of an animal body and serves especially to enclose and protect the other parts of the body, to produce secretions and excretions, and to function in assimilation.

**Etiology** a branch of medical science dealing with the causes and origin of diseases.

**Exonuclease** an enzyme that breaks down a nucleic acid by removing nucleotides one by one from the end of a chain.

**Fomite** an inanimate object (as a dish, toy, book, doorknob, or clothing) that may be contaminated with infectious organisms and serve in their transmission.

**Fungus** any of the major group Fungi of saprophytic and parasitic spore-producing organisms that lack chlorophyll, are often considered to be plants, and include the ascomyetes, basidiomycetes, phycomycetes, imperfect fungi, and slime molds.

**Gastroenteritis** inflammation of the lining membrane of the stomach and the intestines.

**Glycoprotein** a conjugated protein in which the nonprotein group is a carbohydrate.

**Gnotobiotic** of, relating to, living in, or being a controlled environment containing one or a few kinds of organisms ; free from other living organisms.

**Gross Domestic Product** measures the output produced by factors of production located in the domestic country regardless of who owns these factors.

**Guillain-Barré syndrome** French neurologists. Guillain published several significant neurological studies concerning the brain and the spinal column. An authority on the spinal column in particular, he made studies of the cerebrospinal fluid and the marrow of the spinal cord. Guillain and Barré published their description of the Guillain-Barré syndrome in 1916.

**Hantavirus** any of a genus (*Hantavirus*) of bunyaviruses (as the Hantaan virus) that are transmitted by rodent feces and urine and cause hantavirus pulmonary syndrome and hemorrhagic fevers marked by renal necrosis.

**Hemagglutinin** a molecule, such as an antibody or lectin, that agglutinates red blood cells.

**Hemorrhagic fever** an acute destructive disease of warm regions marked by sudden onset, prostration, fever, albuminuria, jaundice, and often hemorrhage and caused by a flavivirus (genus *Flavivirus*) transmitted especially by a mosquito of the genus *Aedes* (*A. aegypti*).

**Heterologous** derived from a different species; characterized by cross-reactivity.

**HIV disease** the broad spectrum of opportunistic infections and diseases that occur in an individual infected with the human immunodeficiency virus.

**Human metapneumovirus** a respiratory viral pathogen that causes a spectrum of illnesses, ranging from asymptomatic infection to severe bronchiolitis.

**Hyperplasia** an abnormal or unusual increase in the elements composing a part (as cells composing a tissue).

**Immunoassay** a technique or test (as the enzyme-linked immunosorbent assay) used to detect the presence or quantity of a substance (as a protein) based on its capacity to act as an antigen or antibody.

**Immunocompromised** a condition (caused, for example, by the administration of immunosuppressive drugs or irradiation, malnutrition, aging, or a condition such as cancer or HIV disease) in which an individual's immune system is unable to respond adequately to a foreign substance.

**Immunofluorescence** the labeling of antibodies or antigens with fluorescent dyes especially for the purpose of demonstrating the presence of a particular antigen or antibody in a tissue preparation or smear.

**Immunology** a science that deals with the immune system and the cell-mediated and humoral aspects of immunity and immune responses.

**Immunopathology** a branch of medicine that deals with immune responses associated with disease; the pathology of an organism, organ system, or disease with respect to the immune system, immunity, and immune responses.

**Immunosuppression** the retardation or cessation of an immune response as a result of, for example, anticancer drugs.

**Index case** an instance of a disease or a genetically determined condition that is discovered first and leads to the discovery of others in a family or population.

**Infectious** capable of causing infection; communicable by invasion of the body of a susceptible organism.

**Infectious agent** an organism (virus, rickettsia, bacteria, fungus, protozoan, or helminth) that is capable of producing infection or infectious disease.

**Influenza** an acute highly contagious virus disease that is caused by various strains of orthomyxoviruses belonging to three major types now considered as three separate genera and that is characterized by sudden onset, fever, prostration, severe aches and pains, and progressive inflammation of the respiratory mucous membrane—often used with the letter *A, B,* or *C* to denote disease caused by a virus of a specific one of the three genera; any human respiratory infection of undetermined cause—not used technically; any of numerous febrile usually virus diseases of domestic animals (as shipping fever of horses and swine influenza) marked by respiratory symptoms, inflammation of mucous membranes, and often systemic involvement.

**Interstitial pneumonia** any of several chronic lung diseases of unknown etiology that affect interstitial tissues of the lung without filling of the alveolae and that may follow damage to the alveolar walls or involve interstitial histological changes.

**Intubation** the introduction of a tube into a hollow organ (as the trachea or intestine) to keep it open or restore its patency if obstructed.

**Irradiate** to affect or treat by radiant energy (as heat); *specifically* to treat by exposure to radiation (as ultraviolet light or gamma rays).

**Lassa** a disease especially of Africa that is caused by the Lassa virus and is characterized by a high fever, headaches, mouth ulcers, muscle aches, small hemorrhages under the skin, heart and kidney failure, and a high mortality rate.

**Lethal** of, relating to, or causing death; capable of causing death.

**Lymphoproliferative** of or relating to the proliferation of lymphoid tissue.

**Malaria** an acute or chronic disease caused by the presence of sporozoan parasites of the genus *Plasmodium* in the red blood cells, transmitted from an infected to an uninfected individual by the bite of anopheline mosquitoes, and characterized by periodic attacks of chills and fever that coincide with mass destruction of blood cells and the release of toxic substances by the parasite at the end of each reproductive cycle.

**Mass spectrometry** an instrumental method for identifying the chemical constitution of a substance by means of the separation of gaseous ions according to their differing mass and charge—called also *mass spectroscopy.*

**Methyltransferase** any of several transferases that promote transfer of a methyl group from one compound to another.

**Microbe** any microorganism or biologic agent that can replicate in humans (including bacteria, viruses, protozoa, fungi, and prions); in other usage, any multicellular organism.

**Microbiology** a branch of biology dealing especially with microscopic forms of life.

**Morbidity** a diseased state or symptom; the incidence of disease : the rate of sickness.

**Mortality** the quality or state of being mortal; the number of deaths in a given time or place; the proportion of deaths to population.

**Mutation** a transmissible change in the genetic material of an organism, usually in a single gene.

**Nasopharyngeal** of, relating to, or affecting the nose and pharynx or the nasopharynx.

**Nebulise** to reduce to a fine spray.

**Neuraminidase** a substance used (as in detecting or measuring a component, in preparing a product, or in developing photographs) because of its chemical or biological activity.

**Nucleocapsid** the nucleic acid and surrounding protein coat of a virus.

**Nucleophile** a nucleophilic substance (as an electron-donating reagent).

**Oronasal** of or relating to the mouth and nose; *especially* : connecting the mouth and the nasal cavity.

**Outbreak** a sudden rise in the incidence of a disease.

**Pandemic** an epidemic that occurs worldwide.

**Parainfluenza** any of several paramyxoviruses (genus *Paramyxovirus*) that are associated with or responsible for some respiratory infections especially in children—called also *parainfluenza*.

**Pathogen** a specific causative agent (as a bacterium or virus) of disease.

**Pathogenesis** the origination and development of a disease.

**Pathogenic** capable of causing disease.

**PCR** see polymerase chain reaction.

**Pericardium** of, relating to, or affecting the conical sac of serous membrane that encloses the heart and the roots of the great blood vessels of vertebrates and consists of an outer fibrous coat that loosely invests the heart and is prolonged on the outer surface of the great vessels except the inferior vena cava and a double inner serous coat of which one layer is closely adherent to the heart while the other lines the inner surface of the outer coat with the intervening space being filled with pericardial fluid.

**Peritoneal** of, relating to, or affecting the smooth transparent serous membrane that lines the cavity of the abdomen of a mammal, is folded inward over the abdominal and pelvic viscera, and consists of an outer layer closely adherent to the walls of the abdomen and an inner layer that folds to invest the viscera.

**Peroxidation** the process of converting (a compound) into a peroxide for a chemical compound.

**Pharmacopoeia** a book describing drugs, chemicals, and medicinal preparations; *especially* : one issued by an officially recognized authority and serving as a standard; a collection or stock of drugs.

**Pharyngeal** relating to or located in the region of the pharynx; innervating the pharynx especially by contributing to the formation of the pharyngeal plexus; supplying or draining the pharynx.

**Phenotype** the visible properties of an organism that are produced by the interaction of the genotype and the environment.

**Phospholipid** any of numerous lipids (as lecithins and sphingomyelin) in which phosphoric acid as well as a fatty acid is esterified to glycerol and which are found in all living cells and in the bilayers of plasma membranes.

**Phylogenetic** of or relating to the evolutionary development of organisms.

**Physiochemical** of or relating to physiological chemistry.

**Picornavirus** any of a family (Picornaviridae) of small single-stranded RNA viruses that have an icosahedral virion with no envelope and that include the enteroviruses, rhinoviruses, and the causative agents of hepatitis A, foot-and-mouth disease, hand-foot-and-mouth disease, and encephalomyocarditis.

**Plague** an epidemic disease causing a high rate of mortality; a virulent contagious febrile disease that is caused by a bacterium of the genus *Yersinia* (*Y. pestis* syn. *Pasteurella pestis*), that occurs in bubonic, pneumonic, and septicemic forms, and that is usually transmitted from rats to humans by the bite of infected fleas (as in bubonic plague) or directly from person to person (as in pneumonic plague).

**Pleural** of or relating to the pleura or the sides of the thorax.

**Pneumonia** a disease of the lungs characterized by inflammation and consolidation followed by resolution and caused by infection or irritants.

**Polymerase chain reaction** a laboratory method of amplifying low levels of specific microbial DNA or RNA sequences.

**Polymicrobial** of, relating to, or caused by several types of microorganisms.

**Polypnea** rapid or panting respiration.

**Prophylactic** guarding from or preventing the spread or occurrence of disease or infection; tending to prevent or ward off.

**Proteolytic** of, relating to, or producing the hydrolysis of proteins or peptides with formation of simpler and soluble products (as in digestion).

**Public health** the art and science of dealing with the protection and improvement of community health by organized community effort and including preventive medicine and sanitary and social health.

**Quarantine** the enforced isolation or restriction of free movement imposed to prevent the spread a contagious disease.

**Reagent** a substance used (as in detecting or measuring a component, in preparing a product, or in developing photographs) because of its chemical or biological activity.

**Reovirus** any of a family (Reoviridae) of double-stranded RNA viruses that have an icosahedral structure, are 60 to 80 nanometers in diameter, have an inner core surrounded by several layers of protein, and include many plant or animal pathogens (as the orbiviruses and the rotaviruses).

**Respirator** a device (as a gas mask) worn over the mouth or nose for protecting the respiratory system; a device for maintaining artificial respiration.

**Respiratory syncytial virus** a paramyxovirus (genus *Pneumovirus*) that has numerous strains, forms syncytia in tissue culture, and is responsible for severe respiratory diseases (as bronchopneumonia and bronchiolitis) in children and especially in infants.

**Retrovirus** any of large family of RNA viruses that includes lentiviruses and oncoviruses, so called because they carry reverse transcriptase.

**Rhinitis** inflammation of the mucous membrane of the nose.

**Ribosome** any of the RNA- and protein-rich cytoplasmic organelles that are sites of protein synthesis.

**Serological** the use of immune serum in any number of tests (agglutination, precipitation, enzyme-linked immunosorbent assay, etc.) used to measure the response (antibody titer) to infectious disease; the use of serological reactions to detect antigen.

**Serology** a science dealing with serums and especially their reactions and properties.

**Seronegative** negative result in a serological test; that is, the inability to detect the antibodies or antigens being tested for.

**Seropositive** positive results in a serological test.

**Seroprevalence** the frequency of individuals in a population that have a particular element (as antibodies to HIV) in their blood serum.

**Serotype** the characterization of a microorganism based on the kinds and combinations of constituent antigens present in that organism; a taxonomic subdivision of bacteria based on the above.

**Smallpox** an acute contagious febrile disease characterized by skin eruption with pustules, sloughing, and scar formation and caused by a poxvirus (genus *Orthopoxvirus*) that is believed to exist now only in lab cultures.

**Superspreader** highly infective patient.

**Syncytial** of, relating to, or constituting a multinucleate mass of protoplasm (as in the plasmodium of a slime mold) resulting from fusion of cells.

**Thrombosis** the formation or presence of a blood clot within a blood vessel during life.

**Transmissible** capable of being transmitted (as from one person to another).

**Tropism** involuntary orientation by an organism or one of its parts that involves turning or curving by movement or by differential growth and is a positive or negative response to a source of stimulation.

**Tuberculosis** a usually chronic highly variable disease that is caused by the tubercle bacillus and rarely in the U.S. by a related mycobacterium (*Mycobacterium bovis*), is usually communicated by inhalation of the airborne causative agent, affects especially the lungs but may spread to other areas (as the kidney or spinal column) from local lesions or by way of the lymph or blood vessels, and is characterized by fever, cough, difficulty in breathing, inflammatory infiltrations, formation of tubercles, caseation, pleural effusion, and fibrosis.

**Vaccine** a preparation of purified polypeptide, protein or polysaccharide, or DNA or of killed microorganisms, living attenuated organisms, or living virulent or crude or purified organisms that is administered to produce or artificially in crease immunity to a particular disease.

**Viremia** the presence of virus in the blood of a host.

**Virology** a branch of science that deals with viruses.

**Virulence** the degree of pathogenicity of an organism as evidenced by the severity of resulting disease and the organisms's ability to invade the host tissues.

**West Nile virus** a flavivirus (genus *Flavivirus*) that causes an illness marked by fever, headache, muscle ache, skin rash, and sometimes encephalitis or meningitis, that is spread chiefly by mosquitoes, and that is closely related to the viruses causing Japanese B encephalitis and Saint Louis encephalitis.

**Westphalian system** "westphalian public health" refers to public health governance structured by Westphalian principles. "Post-Westphalian public health" describes public health governance that departs from the Westphalian template

**Yellow fever** an acute destructive disease of warm regions marked by sudden onset, prostration, fever, albuminuria, jaundice, and often hemorrhage and caused by a flavivirus (genus *Flavivirus*) transmitted especially by a mosquito of the genus *Aedes* (*A. aegypti*).

**Zoonotic** a disease communicable from animals to humans under natural conditions.

## ACRONYMS

| | |
|---|---|
| **3CL** | 3C-like |
| **ACH** | air changes per hour |
| **AG** | access grid |
| **AIDS** | acquired immunodeficiency syndrome |
| **AMRO/PAHO** | WHO Regional Office for the Americas |
| **APEC** | Asian Pacific Economic Community |
| **ASEAN** | Association of Southeast Asian Nations |
| **ASTM** | American Society for Testing and Materials |
| **ATP** | air transport |
| **BCoV** | bovine coronavirus |
| **BiPAP** | bi-level positive airway pressure |
| **BSL** | biosafety laboratory |
| **CBER** | Center for Biologics Evaluation and Research |
| **CDC** | Centers for Disease Control and Prevention |
| **cDNA** | complementary DNA |
| **CEACAM** | carcino-embryonic antigen-cell adhesion molecule |
| **CIA** | Central Intelligence Agency |
| **CNS** | central nervous system |
| **CoV** | coronavirus |
| **CSR** | Department of Communicable Disease Surveillance and Response |
| **DARPA** | Defense Advanced Research Projects Agency |
| **DHHS** | Department of Health and Human Services |

| | |
|---|---|
| **DMEM** | Dulbeco's Modified Eagle Medium |
| **DNA** | deoxyribonucleic acid |
| | |
| **EINET** | Emerging Infections Network |
| **EPA** | Environmental Protection Agency |
| **ERGIC** | endoplasmic-reticulum-golgi-intermediate compartment |
| | |
| **FAO** | Food and Agriculture Organization |
| **FASS** | FailSafe Air Safety Systems |
| **FDA** | Food and Drug Administration |
| **FCoV** | Group I Feline CoV |
| **FDI** | foreign direct investment |
| **FECoV** | feline enteric peritonitis virus |
| **FIPV** | feline infectious peritonitis virus |
| | |
| **GDP** | gross domestic product |
| **GHG** | global health governance |
| **GOARN** | Global Alert and Response Network |
| **GPGH** | global public goods for health |
| **GPHIN** | Global Public Health Information Network |
| | |
| **HAART** | Highly Active Antiretroviral Therapy |
| **HEPA** | high efficiency particulate air |
| **HIV** | human immunodeficiency virus |
| **IBV** | infectious bronchitis virus |
| | |
| **ICA** | intelligence community assessment |
| **IHR** | International Health Regulations |
| **IOM** | Institute of Medicine |
| **ITU** | International Telecommunications Union |
| | |
| **JCAHO** | Joint Commission on Accreditation of Health Care Organizations |
| | |
| **LPS** | lipopolysaccharides |
| | |
| **MAbs** | monoclonal antibodies |
| **MHV** | mouse hepatitis virus |
| **MoH** | Ministry of Health |
| | |
| **NGO** | nongovernmental organization |
| **NIAID** | National Institute for Allergy and Infectious Diseases |
| **NIC** | National Intelligence Council |

| | |
|---|---|
| **NIH** | National Institutes of Health |
| **NIOSH** | National Institute for Occupational Safety and Health |
| | |
| **OECD** | Organization for Economic Cooperation and Development |
| **OIE** | Office International des Epizooties |
| **OSHA** | Occupational Safety and Health Administration |
| **OTP** | land transport |
| | |
| **PCR** | polymerase chain reaction |
| **PRCV** | porcine respiratory coronavirus |
| **PEDV** | porcine epidemic diarrhea CoV |
| **PHE** | public health emergency |
| **PRCV** | porcine respiratory coronavirus |
| **PROMED** | Program for Monitoring Emerging Diseases |
| | |
| **RNA** | ribonucleic acid |
| **RSV** | respiratory syncytial virus |
| **RT-PCR** | reverse-transcription polymerase chain reaction |
| | |
| **SAIC** | Science Applications International Corporation |
| **SARS** | severe acute respiratory syndrome |
| **SCoV** | severe acute respiratory syndrome coronavirus |
| **SIV** | swine influenza virus |
| **SRP** | signal recognition particle |
| | |
| **TCID** | tissue culture infective dose |
| **TGEV** | transmissible gastroenteritis virus |
| **TIGER** | triangulation identification for genetic evaluation of risks |
| **TRD** | hotels and restaurants |
| **TRS** | transcriptional regulatory sequence |
| | |
| **UNAIDS** | Joint United National Program on HIV/AIDS |
| **USAMRIID** | United States Army Medical Research Institute for Infectious Diseases |
| **USDA** | United States Department of Agriculture |
| **UV** | ultraviolet |
| **UVGI** | ultraviolet germicidal irradiation |
| | |
| **VN** | virus neutralization |
| | |
| **WD** | winter dysentery |
| **WHO** | World Health Organization |
| **WPRO** | Western Pacific Regional Office of the World Health Organization |

# Appendix F

# Forum Member, Speaker, and
# Staff Biographies

**ADEL A.F. MAHMOUD, M.D., Ph.D.,** *(Chair),* is President of Merck Vaccines at Merck & Co., Inc. He formerly served Case Western Reserve University and University Hospitals of Cleveland as Chairman of Medicine and Physician-in-Chief from 1987 to 1998. Prior to that, Dr. Mahmoud held several positions, spanning 25 years, at the same institutions. Dr. Mahmoud and his colleagues conducted pioneering investigations on the biology and function of eosinophils. He prepared the first specific anti-eosinophil serum, which was used to define the role of these cells in host resistance to helminthic infections. Dr. Mahmoud also established clinical and laboratory investigations in several developing countries, including Kenya, Egypt, and The Philippines, to examine the determinants of infection and disease in schistosomiasis and other infectious agents. This work led to the development of innovative strategies to control those infections, which have been adopted by the World Health Organization (WHO) as selective population chemotherapy. In recent years, Dr. Mahmoud turned his attention to developing a comprehensive set of responses to the problems associated with emerging infections in the developing world. He was elected to membership of the American Society for Clinical Investigation in 1978, the Association of American Physicians in 1980, and the Institute of Medicine of the National Academy of Sciences in 1987. He received the Bailey K. Ashford Award of the American Society of Tropical Medicine and Hygiene in 1983, and the Squibb Award of the Infectious Diseases Society of America in 1984. Dr. Mahmoud currently serves as Chair of the Forum on Emerging Infections and is a member of the Board on

Global Health, both of the Institute of Medicine. He also chairs the U.S. Delegation to the U.S.-Japan Cooperative Medical Science Program.

**STANLEY M. LEMON, M.D.,** *(Vice-Chair),* is Dean of the School of Medicine at the University of Texas Medical Branch at Galveston. He received his undergraduate degree in biochemical sciences from Princeton University summa cum laude, and his M.D. with honors from the University of Rochester. He completed postgraduate training in internal medicine and infectious diseases at the University of North Carolina at Chapel Hill, and is board-certified in both. From 1977 to 1983, he served with the U.S. Army Medical Research and Development Command, directing the Hepatitis Laboratory at the Walter Reed Army Institute of Research. He joined the faculty of the University of North Carolina School of Medicine in 1983, serving first as Chief of the Division of Infectious Diseases, and then Vice Chair for Research of the Department of Medicine. In 1997, Dr. Lemon moved to the University of Texas Medical Branch as Professor and Chair of the Department of Microbiology & Immunology. He was subsequently appointed Dean *pro tem* of the School of Medicine in 1999, and permanent Dean of Medicine in 2000. Dr. Lemon's research interests relate to the molecular virology and pathogenesis of the positive-stranded RNA viruses responsible for hepatitis C and hepatitis A. He is particularly interested in the molecular mechanisms controlling replication of these RNA genomes and related mechanisms of disease pathogenesis. He has published over 180 papers, and numerous textbook chapters related to hepatitis and other viral infections, and has a longstanding interest in vaccine development. He has served previously as chair of the Anti-Infective Drugs Advisory Committee and the Vaccines and Related Biologics Advisory Committee of the U.S. Food and Drug Administration, and is past chair of the Steering Committee on Hepatitis and Poliomyelitis of WHO's Programme on Vaccine Development. He presently serves as Chairman of the U.S. Hepatitis Panel of the U.S.-Japan Cooperative Medical Sciences Program, and recently chaired an Institute of Medicine study committee related to vaccines for the protection of the military against naturally occurring infectious disease threats.

**DAVID ACHESON, M.D.,** is Chief Medical Officer at the Center for Food Safety and Applied Nutrition, U.S. Food and Drug Administration. He received his medical degree at the University of London. After completing internships in general surgery and medicine, he continued his postdoctoral training in Manchester, England, as a Wellcome Trust Research Fellow. He subsequently was a Wellcome Trust Training Fellow in Infectious Diseases at the New England Medical Center and at the Wellcome Research Unit in Vellore, India. Dr. Acheson was Associate Professor of Medicine, Division of Geographic Medicine and Infectious Diseases, New England Medical Center until 2001. He then joined the faculties of the Department of Epidemiology and Preventive Medicine and Department of Microbiology and Immunology at the University of Maryland Medical

School. Currently at the FDA, his research concentration is on foodborne pathogens and encompasses a mixture of molecular pathogenesis, cell biology, and epidemiology. Specifically, his research focuses on Shiga toxin-producing *E. coli* and understanding toxin interaction with intestinal epithelial cells using tissue culture models. His laboratory has also undertaken a study to examine Shiga toxin-producing *E. coli* in food animals in relation to virulence factors and antimicrobial resistance patterns. More recently, Dr. Acheson initiated a project to understand the molecular pathogenesis of *Campylobacter jejuni*. Other studies have undertaken surveillance of diarrheal disease in the community to determine causes, outcomes, and risk factors of unexplained diarrhea. Dr. Acheson has authored/coauthored over 72 journal articles, and 42 book chapters and reviews, and is coauthor of the book *Safe Eating* (Dell Health, 1998). He is reviewer of more than 10 journals and is on the editorial board of *Infection and Immunity* and *Clinical Infectious Diseases*. Dr. Acheson is a Fellow of the Royal College of Physicians, a Fellow of the Infectious Disease Society of America, and holds several patents.

**STEVEN J. BRICKNER, Ph.D.,** is Research Advisor, Antibacterials Chemistry, at Pfizer Global Research and Development. He received his Ph.D. in organic chemistry from Cornell University and was a NIH Postdoctoral Research Fellow at the University of Wisconsin–Madison. Dr. Brickner is a medicinal chemist with nearly 20 years of research experience in the pharmaceutical industry, all focused on the discovery and development of novel antibacterial agents. He is an inventor/co-inventor on 21 U.S. patents, and has published numerous scientific papers, primarily within the area of the oxazolidinones. Prior to joining Pfizer in 1996, he led a team at Pharmacia and Upjohn that discovered and developed linezolid, the first member of a new class of antibiotics to be approved in the last 35 years.

**NANCY CARTER-FOSTER, M.S.T.M.,** is Senior Advisor for Health Affairs for the U.S. Department of State, Assistant Secretary for Science and Health and the Secretary's Representative on HIV/AIDS. She is responsible for identifying emerging health issues and making policy recommendations for USG foreign policy concerns regarding international health, and coordinates the Department's interactions with the non-governmental community. She is a member of the National Academy of Sciences Institute of Medicine's Forum on Infectious Diseases, and a member of the Infectious Diseases Society of America (IDSA), and the American Association of the Advancement of Science (AAAS). She has helped bring focus to global health issues in U.S. foreign policy and brought a national security focus to global health. In prior positions as Director for Congressional and Legislative Affairs for the Economic and Business Affairs Bureau of the U.S. Department of State, and Foreign Policy Advisory to the Majority WHIP U.S. House of Representatives, Trade Specialist Advisor to the House of

Representatives Ways and Means Trade Subcommittee, and consultant to the World Bank, Asia Technical Environment Division, Ms. Carter-Foster has worked on a wide variety of health, trade and environmental issues amassing in-depth knowledge and experience in policy development and program implementation.

**GAIL H. CASSELL, Ph.D.,** is Vice President, Scientific Affairs, Distinguished Lilly Research Scholar for Infectious Diseases, Eli Lilly & Company. Previously, she was the Charles H. McCauley Professor and (since 1987) Chair, Department of Microbiology, University of Alabama Schools of Medicine and Dentistry at Birmingham, a department which, under her leadership, has ranked first in research funding from the National Institutes of Health since 1989. She is a member of the Director's Advisory Committee of the Centers for Disease Control and Prevention. Dr. Cassell is past president of the American Society for Microbiology (ASM) and is serving her third 3-year term as chairman of the Public and Scientific Affairs Board of ASM. She is a former member of the National Institutes of Health Director's Advisory Committee and a former member of the Advisory Council of the National Institute of Allergy and Infectious Diseases. She has also served as an advisor on infectious diseases and indirect costs of research to the White House Office on Science and Technology and was previously chair of the Board of Scientific Counselors of the National Center for Infectious Diseases, Centers for Disease Control and Prevention. Dr. Cassell served eight years on the Bacteriology-Mycology-II Study Section and served as its chair for three years. She serves on the editorial boards of several prestigious scientific journals and has authored over 275 articles and book chapters. She has been intimately involved in the establishment of science policy and legislation related to biomedical research and public health. Dr. Cassell has received several national and international awards and an honorary degree for her research on infectious diseases.

**JESSE L. GOODMAN, M.D., M.P.H.,** was professor of medicine and Chief of Infectious Diseases at the University of Minnesota, and is now serving as Deputy Director for the U.S. Food and Drug Administration's (FDA) Center for Biologics Evaluation and Research, where he is active in a broad range of scientific, public health, and policy issues. After joining the FDA commissioner's office, he has worked closely with several centers and helped coordinate FDA's response to the antimicrobial resistance problem. He was co-chair of a recently formed federal interagency task force which developed the national Public Health Action Plan on antimicrobial resistance. He graduated from Harvard College and attended the Albert Einstein College of Medicine followed by internal medicine, hematology, oncology, and infectious diseases training at the University of Pennsylvania and University of California Los Angeles, where he was also chief medical resident. He received his master's of public health from the University of Minnesota. He has been active in community public health activities, including creating an environmental health partnership in St. Paul, Minnesota. In recent years, his laboratory's research has focused on the molecular pathogenesis of tickborne diseases. His laboratory isolated the etiological intracellular agent of the emerging tickborne infection, human granulocytic ehrlichiosis, and identified its leukocyte receptor. He has also been an active clinician and teacher and has directed or participated in major multicenter clinical studies. He is a Fellow of the Infectious Diseases Society of America and, among several honors, has been elected to the American Society for Clinical Investigation.

**EDUARDO GOTUZZO, M.D.,** is Principal Professor and Director at the Instituto de Medicina Tropical "Alexander von Humbolt," Universidad Peruana Cayetan Heredia (UPCH), in Lima, Peru. As well as Chief of the Department of Infectious and Tropical Diseases at the Cayetano Heredia Hospital. As well as an Adjunct Professor of Medicine at the University of Alabama-Birmingham School of Medicine. Dr. Gotuzzo has proven to be an active member in numerous international societies such as President of the Latin America Society of Tropical Disease (2000-2003), Member of the Scientific Program of Infectious Diseases Society of America (2000-2003), Member of the International Organizing Committee of the International Congress of Infectious Diseases (1994-Present), President Elect of the International Society for Infectious Diseases (1996-1998), and President of the Peruvian Society of Internal Medicine (1991-1992). He has published over 230 articles and chapters as well as six manuals and one book. Recent honors and awards include being named an Honorary member of American Society of Tropical Medicine and Hygiene (since 2002), Associated Member of National Academy of Medicine (since 2002), Honorary Member of Society of Internal Medicine (since 2000), Distinguished Visitor, Faculty of Medical Sciences, University of Cordoba, Argentina (since 1999), and the Golden Medal for "Outstanding Contribution in the field of Infectious Diseases," awarded by the Trnava University, Slovakia (1998), among many others.

**MARGARET A. HAMBURG, M.D.,** is Vice President for Biological Programs at Nuclear Threat Initiative (NTI), a charitable organization working to reduce the global threat from nuclear, biological, and chemical weapons. Dr. Hamburg is in charge of the biological program area. Before taking on her current position, Dr. Hamburg was the Assistant Secretary for Planning and Evaluation, U.S. Department of Health and Human Services, serving as a principal policy advisor to the Secretary of Health and Human Services with responsibilities including policy formulation and analysis, the development and review of regulations and/or legislation, budget analysis, strategic planning, and the conduct and coordination of policy research and program evaluation. Prior to this, she served for almost six years as the Commissioner of Health for the City of New York. As chief health officer in the nation's largest city, Dr. Hamburg's many accomplishments included the design and implementation of an internationally recognized tuberculosis control program that produced dramatic declines in tuberculosis cases; the development of initiatives that raised childhood immunization rates to record levels; and the creation of the first public health bioterrorism preparedness program in the nation. She completed her internship and residency in Internal Medicine at the New York Hospital/Cornell University Medical Center and is certified by the American Board of Internal Medicine. Dr. Hamburg is a graduate of Harvard College and Harvard Medical School. She currently serves on the Harvard University Board of Overseers. She has been elected to membership in the Institute of Medicine, the New York Academy of Medicine, and the Council on Foreign Relations, and is a Fellow of the American Association for the Advancement of Science and the American College of Physicians.

**CAROLE A. HEILMAN, Ph.D.,** is Director of the Division of Microbiology and Infectious Diseases (DMID) of the National Institute of Allergy and Infectious Diseases (NIAID). Dr. Heilman received her bachelor's degree in biology from Boston University in 1972, and earned her master's degree and doctorate in microbiology from Rutgers University in 1976 and 1979, respectively. Dr. Heilman began her career at the National Institutes of Health as a postdoctoral research associate with the National Cancer Institute where she carried out research on the regulation of gene expression during cancer development. In 1986, she came to NIAID as the influenza and viral respiratory diseases program officer in DMID and, in 1988, she was appointed chief of the respiratory diseases branch where she coordinated the development of acellular pertussis vaccines. She joined the Division of AIDS as deputy director in 1997 and was responsible for developing the Innovation Grant Program for Approaches in HIV Vaccine Research. She is the recipient of several notable awards for outstanding achievement. Throughout her extramural career, Dr. Heilman has contributed articles on vaccine design and development to many scientific journals and has served as a consultant to the World Bank and WHO in this area. She is also a member of several professional societies, including the Infectious Diseases Society of America, the American Society for Microbiology, and the American Society of Virology.

**DAVID L. HEYMANN, M.D.,** is currently the Executive Director of the World Health Organization (WHO) Communicable Diseases Cluster. From October 1995 to July 1998 he was Director of the WHO Programme on Emerging and Other Communicable Diseases Surveillance and Control. Prior to becoming director of this program, he was the chief of research activities in the Global Programme on AIDS. From 1976 to 1989, prior to joining WHO, Dr Heymann spent 13 years working as a medical epidemiologist in sub-Saharan Africa (Cameroon, Ivory Coast, the former Zaire, and Malawi) on assignment from the Centers for Disease Control and Prevention (CDC) in CDC-supported activities aimed at strengthening capacity in surveillance of infectious diseases and their control, with special emphasis on the childhood immunizable diseases, African hemorrhagic fevers, pox viruses, and malaria. While based in Africa, Dr.

Heymann participated in the investigation of the first outbreak of Ebola in Yambuku (former Zaire) in 1976, then again investigated the second outbreak of Ebola in 1977 in Tandala, and in 1995 directed the international response to the Ebola outbreak in Kikwit. Prior to 1976, Dr. Heymann spent two years in India as a medical officer in the WHO Smallpox Eradication Programme. Dr. Heymann holds a B.A. from the Pennsylvania State University, an M.D. from Wake Forest University, and a Diploma in Tropical Medicine and Hygiene from the London School of Hygiene and Tropical Medicine, and completed practical epidemiology training in the Epidemic Intelligence Service (EIS) training program of the CDC. He has published 131 scientific articles on infectious diseases in peer-reviewed medical and scientific journals.

**JAMES M. HUGHES, M.D.,** received his B.A. in 1966 and M.D. in 1971 from Stanford University. He completed a residency in internal medicine at the University of Washington and a fellowship in infectious diseases at the University of Virginia. He is board-certified in internal medicine, infectious diseases, and preventive medicine. He first joined CDC as an Epidemic Intelligence Service officer in 1973. During his CDC career, he has worked primarily in the areas of foodborne disease and infection control in health care settings. He became Director of the National Center for Infectious Diseases in 1992. The center is currently working to address domestic and global challenges posed by emerging infectious diseases and the threat of bioterrorism. He is a member of the Institute of Medicine and a fellow of the American College of Physicians, the Infectious Diseases Society of America, and the American Association for the Advancement of Science. He is an Assistant Surgeon General in the Public Health Service.

**LONNIE KING, D.V.M.,** is Dean of the College of Veterinary Medicine, Michigan State University. Dr. King's previous positions include both Associate Administrator and Administrator of the USDA Animal and Plant Health Inspection Service (APHIS) and Deputy Administrator for USDA/APHIS/Veterinary Services. Before his government career, Dr. King was in private practice. He also has experience as a field veterinary medical officer, station epidemiologist, and staff member on assignments involving Emergency Programs and Animal Health Information. Dr. King has also directed the American Veterinary Medical Association's Office of Governmental Relations, and is certified in the American College of Veterinary Preventive Medicine. He has served as President of the Association of American Veterinary Medicine Colleges, and currently serves as Co-Chair of the National Commission on Veterinary Economic Issues, Lead Dean at Michigan State University for food safety with responsibility for the National Food Safety and Toxicology Center, the Institute for Environmental Toxicology, and the Center for Emerging Infectious Diseases. He is also co-developer and course leader for Science, Politics, and Animal Health Policy. Dr. King received his B.S. and D.V.M. degrees from The Ohio State University, and his M.S. degree in epidemiology from the University of Minnesota. He has also completed the Senior Executive Program at Harvard University, and received a M.P.A. from American University. Dr. King previously served on the Committee for Opportunities in Agriculture, the Steering Committee for a Workshop on the Control and Prevention of Animal Diseases, and the Committee to Ensure Safe Food from Production to Consumption.

**JOSHUA LEDERBERG, Ph.D.,** is Professor emeritus of Molecular Genetics and Informatics and Sackler Foundation Scholar at The Rockefeller University, New York, New York. His lifelong research, for which he received the Nobel Prize in 1958, has been in genetic structure and function in microorganisms. He has a keen interest in international health and was co-chair of a previous Institute of Medicine Committee on Emerging Microbial Threats to Health (1990–1992) and currently is co-chair of the Committee on Emerging Microbial Threats to Health in the 21st Century. He has been a member of the National Academy of Sciences since 1957 and is a charter member of the Institute of Medicine.

**JOSEPH MALONE, M.D.,** the director of the Department of Defense Global Emerging Infection System (DoD-GEIS), completed the Centers for Disease Control and Prevention's Epidemic Intelligence Service (EIS) program in June, 2003. He graduated from Boston University School of Medicine in 1980, and trained in internal medicine and infectious diseases at Naval Hospitals in San Diego, and Bethesda, MD leading to board certification. He was a staff physician at the Naval Hospitals in San Diego, CA and Bethesda, MD. He deployed to Guantanamo Bay, Cuba, in support of Operation Safe Harbor and was attached to Surgical Team 1 during Operation Desert Shield. He later directed the Infectious Disease Division and HIV unit at the Naval Medical Center at Portsmouth, VA, from 1996-1996. In 1999 he worked for the Disease Surveillance Program (in affiliation with DoD-GEIS) at the U.S. Naval Medical Research Unit No. 3 in Cairo, Egypt. While at CDC's EIS program he was deployed to New York City to assist in the emergency public health response after the September 11th 2001attacks, assisted in the public health response to documented anthrax contamination in Kansas City and was the acting state epidemiologist for the State of Missouri from February-June 2003. Capt. Malone has several military awards, including the HHS/USPHS Crisis Response Service Award. He is an Associate Professor at the Uniformed Services University of Health Sciences and holds the Certificate of Knowledge in Travelers' Health and Tropical Medicine from the American Society of Tropical Medicine and Hygiene. He has over 20 publications.

**LYNN MARKS, M.D.,** is board-certified in internal medicine and infectious diseases. He was on faculty at the University of South Alabama College of Medicine in the Infectious Diseases department focusing on patient care, teaching, and research. His academic research interest was on the molecular genetics of bacterial pathogenicity. He subsequently joined SmithKline Beecham's (now GlaxoSmithKline) anti-infectives clinical group and later progressed to global head of the Consumer Healthcare Division Medical and Regulatory Group. He then returned to pharmaceutical research and development as global head of the Infectious Diseases Therapeutic Area Strategy Team for GlaxoSmithKline.

**STEPHEN S. MORSE, Ph.D.,** is Director of the Center for Public Health Preparedness at the Mailman School of Public Health of Columbia University, and a faculty member in the Epidemiology Department. Dr. Morse recently returned to Columbia from 4 years in government service as Program Manager at the Defense Advanced Research Projects Agency (DARPA), where he co-directed the Pathogen Countermeasures program and subsequently directed the Advanced Diagnostics program. Before coming to Columbia, he was Assistant Professor (Virology) at The Rockefeller University in New York, where he remains an adjunct faculty member. Dr. Morse is the editor of two books, *Emerging Viruses* (Oxford University Press, 1993; paperback, 1996) (selected by *American Scientist* for its list of "100 Top Science Books of the 20th Century"), and *The Evolutionary Biology of Viruses* (Raven Press, 1994). He currently serves as a Section Editor of the CDC journal *Emerging Infectious Diseases* and was formerly an Editor-in-Chief of the Pasteur Institute's journal *Research in Virology*. Dr. Morse was Chair and principal organizer of the 1989 NIAID/NIH Conference on Emerging Viruses (for which he originated the term and concept of emerging viruses/infections); served as a member of the Institute of Medicine-National Academy of Sciences' Committee on Emerging Microbial Threats to Health (and chaired its Task Force on Viruses), and was a contributor to its report, *Emerging Infections* (1992); was a member of the IOM's Committee on Xenograft Transplantation; currently serves on the Steering Committee of the Institute of Medicine's Forum on Emerging Infections, and has served as an adviser to WHO, PAHO (Pan-American Health Organization), FDA, the Defense Threat Reduction Agency (DTRA), and other agencies. He is a Fellow of the New York Academy of Sciences and a past Chair of its Microbiology Section. He was the founding Chair of ProMED (the nonprofit international Program to Monitor Emerging Diseases) and was one of the originators of ProMED-mail, an international network inaugurated by ProMED in 1994 for outbreak reporting and disease monitoring using the Internet. Dr. Morse received his Ph.D. from the University of Wisconsin–Madison.

**MICHAEL T. OSTERHOLM, Ph.D., M.P.H.,** is Director of the Center for Infectious Disease Research and Policy at the University of Minnesota where he is also Professor at the School of Public Health. Previously, Dr. Osterholm was the state epidemiologist and Chief of the Acute Disease Epidemiology Section for the Minnesota Department of Health. He has received numerous research awards from the National Institute of Allergy and Infectious Diseases and the

Centers for Disease Control and Prevention (CDC). He served as principal investigator for the CDC-sponsored Emerging Infections Program in Minnesota. He has published more than 240 articles and abstracts on various emerging infectious disease problems and is the author of the best selling book, *Living Terrors: What America Needs to Know to Survive the Coming Bioterrorist Catastrophe*. He is past president of the Council of State and Territorial Epidemiologists. He currently serves on the National Academy of Sciences, Institute of Medicine (IOM) Forum on Emerging Infections. He has also served on the IOM Committee, Food Safety, Production to Consumption and the IOM Committee on the Department of Defense Persian Gulf Syndrome Comprehensive Clinical Evaluation Program, and as a reviewer for the IOM report on chemical and biological terrorism.

**GEORGE POSTE, Ph.D., D.V.M.,** is Director of the Arizona Biodesign Institute and Dell E. Webb Distinguished Professor of Biology at Arizona State University. From 1992 to 1999 he was Chief Science and Technology Officer and President, Research and Development of SmithKline Beecham (SB). During his tenure at SB he was associated with the successful registration of 29 drug, vaccine and diagnostic products. He is Chairman of diaDexus and Structural GenomiX in California and Orchid Biosciences in Princeton. He serves on the Board of Directors of AdvancePCS and Monsanto. He is an advisor on biotechnology to several venture capital funds and investment banks. In May 2003 he was appointed as Director of the Arizona Biodesign Institute at Arizona State University. This is a major new initiative combining research groups in biotechnology, nanotechnology, materials science, advanced computing and neuromorphic engineering. He is a Fellow of Pembroke College Cambridge and Distinguished Fellow at the Hoover Institution and Stanford University. He is a member of the Defense Science Board of the U.S. Department of Defense and in this capacity he Chairs the Task Force on Bioterrorism. He is also a member of the National Academy of Sciences Working Group on Defense Against Bioweapons. Dr. Poste is a Board Certified Pathologist, a Fellow of the Royal Society and a Fellow of the Academy of Medical Sciences. He was awarded the rank of Commander of the British Empire by Queen Elizabeth II in 1999 for services to medicine and for the advancement of biotechnology. He has published over 350 scientific papers, co-edited 15 books on cancer, biotechnology and infectious diseases and serves on the Editorial Board of multiple technical journals. He is invited routinely to be the keynote speaker at a wide variety of academic, corporate, investment and government meetings to discuss the impact of biotechnology and genetics on healthcare and the challenges posed by bioterrorism. Dr. Poste is married with three children. His personal interests are in military history, photography, automobile racing and exploring the wilderness zones of the American West.

**GARY A. ROSELLE, M.D.,** received his M.D. from Ohio State University School of Medicine in 1973. He served his residency at Northwestern University

School of Medicine and his Infectious Diseases fellowship at the University of Cincinnati School of Medicine. Dr. Roselle is the Program Director for Infectious Diseases for the VA Central Office in Washington, D.C., as well as the Chief of the Medical Service at the Cincinnati VA Medical Center. He is a professor of medicine in the Department of Internal Medicine, Division of Infectious Diseases at the University of Cincinnati College of Medicine. Dr. Roselle serves on several national advisory committees. In addition, he is currently heading the Emerging Pathogens Initiative for the Department of Veterans Affairs. Dr. Roselle has received commendations from the Cincinnati Medical Center Director, the Under Secretary for Health for the Department of Veterans Affairs, and the Secretary of Veterans Affairs for his work in the infectious diseases program for the Department of Veterans Affairs. He has been an invited speaker at several national and international meetings, and has published over 80 papers and several book chapters.

**JANET SHOEMAKER,** is director of the American Society for Microbiology's Public Affairs Office, a position she has held since 1989. She is responsible for managing the legislative and regulatory affairs of this 42,000-member organization, the largest single biological science society in the world. She has served as principal investigator for a project funded by the National Science Foundation (NSF) to collect and disseminate data on the job market for recent doctorates in microbiology and has played a key role in American Society for Microbiology (ASM) projects, including the production of the ASM *Employment Outlook in the Microbiological Sciences* and *The Impact of Managed Care and Health System Change on Clinical Microbiology*. Previously, she held positions as Assistant Director of Public Affairs for ASM, as ASM coordinator of the U.S./U.S.S.R. Exchange Program in Microbiology, a program sponsored and coordinated by the National Science Foundation and the U.S. Department of State, and as a freelance editor and writer. She received her baccalaureate, cum laude, from the University of Massachusetts, and is a graduate of the George Washington University programs in public policy and in editing and publications. She has served as commissioner to the Commission on Professionals in Science and Technology, and as the ASM representative to the ad hoc Group for Medical Research Funding, and is a member of Women in Government Relations, the American Society of Association Executives, and the American Association for the Advancement of Science. She has co-authored published articles on research funding, biotechnology, biological weapons control, and public policy issues related to microbiology.

**P. FREDERICK SPARLING, M.D.,** is J. Herbert Bate Professor Emeritus of Medicine, Microbiology and Immunology at the University of North Carolina (UNC) at Chapel Hill, and is Director of the North Carolina Sexually Transmitted Infections Research Center. Previously, he served as chair of the Department of Medicine and chair of the Department of Microbiology and Immunology at UNC.

He was president of the Infectious Disease Society of America in 1996-1997. He was also a member of the Institute of Medicine's Committee on Microbial Threats to Health (1991-1992). Dr. Sparling's laboratory research is in the molecular biology of bacterial outer membrane proteins involved in pathogenesis, with a major emphasis on gonococci and meningococci. His current studies focus on the biochemistry and genetics of iron-scavenging mechanisms used by gonococci and meningococci and the structure and function of the gonococcal porin proteins. He is pursuing the goal of a vaccine for gonorrhea.

## SPEAKERS

**ABU SALEH M ABDULLAH, M.D., M.P.H., Ph.D.,** is a Research Assistant Professor in the Department of Community Medicine, The University of Hong Kong. Trained as a family physician, he completed his Ph.D. in Community Medicine and specializes in Public Health Medicine. He is a Diplomat member of the Faculty of Public Health Medicine, the Royal College of Physicians, United Kingdom. He is a counsellor of the Asia Pacific Travel Health Society, a member of the Editorial Board of the Journal of Travel Medicine and the regional editor of the International Society of Travel Medicine Newsletter. He is a regular manuscript reviewer for several national and international journals. Currently, he is also the Director of the Hong Kong Smoking Cessation Health Centre at Ruttonjee Hospital and an active member of the Advisory Council on AIDS of the Government of the Hong Kong Special Administrative Region. He also serves as member to several other national and international organizations including International Society for Infectious Disease, Asia Pacific Travel Health Society, Asia Pacific AIDS Society and the Society for Research on Nicotine and Tobacco (USA). Dr. Abdullah has written few book chapters and his research work has been published in several prestigious journals including the Lancet, Emerging Infectious Disease, Sexually Transmitted Diseases, International Journal of STD & AIDS, Annals of Tropical Medicine & Parasitology and Preventive Medicine.

**ROBERT BREIMAN, M.D.,** is seconded since 2000 from the Centers for Disease Control and Prevention the International Centre for Diarrheal Disease Research, Bangladesh (ICDDR,B)—Centre for Health and Population Research where he is the head of the Programme on Infectious Diseases and Vaccine Sciences. Before joining ICDDR,B, Dr. Breiman was the Director of the United States National Vaccine Program Office from 1995-2000, and was the Chief of the Bacterial Respiratory Diseases Branch Epidemiology Section at CDC from 1989-1997. Dr. Breiman's research focus includes emerging and re-emerging infectious diseases, including respiratory infections, encephalitis, dengue, typhoid, tuberculosis, and leishmaniasis and the evaluation of new, promising vaccines to prevent disease in developing countries; currently, he is working on studies to evaluate new rotavirus, cholera, and influenza vaccines. In March and April 2003,

Dr. Breiman was the leader of a World Health Organization team of international expert consultants which provided assistance to WHO and the government of China on addressing the public health threat from severe acute respiratory disease (SARS); in January 2004, he returned to Beijing and Guangzhou, China, at the request of WHO to lead a team of experts in providing assistance in assessing the reappearance of SARS in Guangdong Province.

**MARTIN S. CETRON, M.D.,** received his B.A. from Dartmouth College in 1981, and his M.D. from Tufts University in 1985. He trained in Internal Medicine at the University of Virginia and Infectious Diseases at the University of Washington before becoming a Commissioned Officer in the U.S. Public Health Service (PHS) in 1992. Dr. Cetron is currently the Deputy Director for the Division of Global Migration and Quarantine (DGMQ) at the U.S. Centers for Disease Control and Prevention (CDC) whose mission is to prevent introduction and spread of infectious diseases in the U.S. and to prevent morbidity and mortality among immigrants, refugees, migrant workers, and international travelers. Dr Cetron holds faculty appointments in Division of Infectious Disease at the Emory University School of Medicine and Department of Epidemiology at Rollins School of Public Health. His primary research interest is international health and global migration with a focus on emerging infections, tropical diseases, and vaccine-preventable diseases in mobile populations. Dr. Cetron has worked at CDC since 1992 where he has lead numerous domestic and international outbreak investigations, conducted epidemiologic research throughout the world, and been involved in several domestic and international emergency responses to provide medical screening and disease prevention programs to refugees prior to U.S. resettlement. Recently, Dr Cetron has played a principal role in high profile CDC responses to intentional and naturally-acquired emerging infectious disease outbreaks including the anthrax bioterrorism incident in the Fall of 2001, the Global SARS epidemic in Spring 2003 and Monkeypox Outbreak in Summer 2003.

**PETER DRAGOVICH, Ph.D.,** is Senior Director, Head of Viral Diseases Drug Discovery at the La Jolla laboratories of Pfizer Global Research and Development. He was previously employed by Agouron Pharmaceuticals (1993-1999) and, via a corporate merger, the Warner-Lambert company (1999-2000). Prior to joining PGRD-La Jolla, Dr. Dragovich served in a number of capacities in the Agouron and Warner-Lambert organizations including Senior Scientist, Project Leader, and Group Leader (medicinal chemistry). Dr. Dragovich received a B.S. degree in Chemistry from the University of California, Berkeley in 1988 and a Ph.D. in Chemistry (Biology minor) from the California Institute of Technology in 1993.

**YANZHONG HUANG, Ph.D.,** is assistant professor in the John C. Whitehead School of Diplomacy and International Relations at Seton Hall University, where he directs the school's Center for Global Health Studies. His current research interests include health politics in post-Mao China, the impact of infectious diseases on state capacity, and SARS and the political economy of contagion in Pacific Rim. His most recent publications include a monograph "Mortal Peril: Public Health in China and Its Security Implications" (Chemical and Biological Arms Control Institute, 2003). In May of 2003, he appeared before the Congressional-Executive Commission on China to testify about the politics of SARS in China. Dr. Huang received a Ph.D. degree in political science from the University of Chicago.

**NATHANIEL HUPERT, M.D., M.P.H.,** is an Assistant Professor of Public Health and Medicine at Weill Medical College of Cornell University in New York City. In addition to maintaining a primary care internal medicine practice, Dr. Hupert has directed a number of federally funded studies since 2000 using computer modeling to improve public health response strategies for intentional and natural outbreaks of disease. Using tools developed by Dr. Hupert and colleagues such as the Weill/Cornell Bioterrorism and Epidemic Outbreak Response Model (BERM, available online at www.ahrq.gov/research/biomodel.htm), public health and emergency response planners from around the country can customize resource deployment strategies to suit local needs for mass prophylaxis or vaccination strategies. Dr. Hupert is a member of both local and national expert panels on bioterrorism response and has provided computer modeling support to the New York City Office of Emergency Management and to the NYC Department of Health and Mental Hygiene since the spring of 2001. He has served as a lecturer for the CDC Strategic National Stockpile Program and the US Public Health Service Commissioned Corps Readiness Force on antibiotic dispensing strategies. Currently he is a member of the New York Presbyterian Hospital Biological Pathogens Task Force.

**ANN MARIE KIMBALL, M.D., M.P.H.,** is currently Associate Professor, Health Services and Epidemiology, Adjunct in Medicine, University of Washington. She also serves as the Director and Graduate Program Coordinator, M.P.H. Program, School of Public Health and Community Medicine, University of Washington. Dr. Kimball has devoted her career to studying health issues and has worked in numerous positions in the United States and abroad. Her research interests are primarily in international health, HIV/AIDS, emerging infections, and maternal and child health. She has previously served as a panelist on the IOM Forum on Emerging Infections, as a member of the Department of Health Emerging and Reemerging Diseases Strategic Planning Task Force, as regional adviser for PAHO in HIV/AIDS, and as the Chair of the National Alliance of State and Territorial AIDS Directors in the United States.

**JAMES W. LEDUC, Ph.D.,** is the Director, Division of Viral and Rickettsial research activities, prevention initiatives and outbreak investigations for viral and rickettsial pathogens of global importance, including viral hemorrhagic fevers, influenza and other respiratory infections, childhood viral diseases, and newly emerging diseases such as SARS. Prior to becoming Director of the Division, he served as the Associate Director for Global Health (1996-2000) in the Office of the Director, National Center for Infectious Diseases at CDC, and was a Medical Officer in charge of arboviruses and viral hemorrhagic fevers at the World Health Organization in Geneva, Switzerland (1992-1996). He also held leadership positions during a 23-year career as a U.S. Army officer in the medical research and development command, with assignments in Brazil, Panama and at various locations in the United States, including the Walter Reed Army Medical Center and the U.S. Army Medical Research Institute of Infectious Diseases. He is a native of southern California and earned his doctoral degree from the University of California at Los Angeles.

**DONALD E. LOW, M.D., F.R.C.P.C.,** holds a Fellowship in Medical Microbiology, Internal Medicine and Infectious Diseases. He is a Professor of Laboratory Medicine and Pathobiology and Medicine at the University of Toronto where he is the Head of the Division of Microbiology in the Department of Laboratory Medicine and Pathobiology. He is Chief of the Toronto Medical Laboratories and Mount Sinai Hospital Department of Microbiology; a laboratory which provides diagnostic services to eleven hospitals in the Toronto area. He is also Chair of the National Advisory Committee on Chemical, Biological, Radio-nuclear Safety, Security and Research, Health Canada; and Member of the National Committee on Clinical Laboratory Standards. Dr. Low's primary research interests are in the study of epidemiology and the mechanisms of antimicrobial resistance in community and hospital pathogens. Other research interests include the epidemiology, pathogenesis, and treatment of severe invasive streptococcal diseases.

**JOHN MACKENZIE, Ph.D.,** is presently Professor of Microbiology (from 1995) and Professor of Tropical Infectious Diseases (from 1999), University of Queensland, Australia. He was previously Professor (1994), Associate Professor (1980-1994), and Senior Lecturer (1973-1999) at the University of Western Australia, Perth, Australia, Head of Genetics Department at the Animal Virus Research Institute, Pirbright, England (1990-1992), and Research Fellow at the Public Health Research Institute, New York (1969-1970). He was appointed to a short-term consultancy as Professional Officer at the World Health Organization (WHO) in 2003-2004 to convene the WHO International SARS Research Advisory Committee, and to chair the WHO SARS Laboratory Network. Honorary and elected positions have included Secretary-General, International Union of Microbiological Societies (IUMS) (1999-2005); Member-at-Large, Executive Board of IUMS (1994-1999); Member of the WHO Global Outbreak Alert and Response Network Steering Committee (since 2000); Member of the WHO Scientific Advisory Committee for Global Health Security (since 2001); President of the Asian-Pacific Society for Medical Virology (2000-2003); President of the Australian Society for Microbiology (1992-1994). He was leader of the first WHO mission into China in March 2003 to investigate cases of atypical pneumonia in Guangdong Province, and the etiological relationship of these cases to SARS. Recent research has been concerned with the ecology, epidemiology, and molecular phylogeny of mosquito-borne viruses, especially Japanese encephalitis virus, and emergent zoonotic viruses. He received the award of Officer in the Order of Australia (AO) in 2001.

**GENE MATTHEWS, J.D.,** as the Legal Advisor to CDC in Atlanta and, as the manager of the legal staff there for 25 years, has handled a wide range of public health law issues. His initial work at CDC coincided with the beginning of the HIV/AIDS epidemic. His experience has included questions of patient confidentiality, access to records, liability for vaccine-related injuries, occupational health protection, environmental concerns, and chronic disease prevention strategies. He has litigated important public health lawsuits and civil discovery questions. Mr. Matthews is widely published and is frequently called upon to lecture on cutting-edge legal issues facing CDC, such as AIDS, livable communities, and bioterrorism preparedness. Most recently, Mr. Matthews has also provided leadership for CDC's development of a newly created Public Health Law Program designed to improve the understanding of the use of laws as tools of public health in the 21st century. He has guided this exciting initiative to reach out both to the legal community and to public health practitioners through research, training, information, and partnerships. Mr. Matthews is a graduate of the University of North Carolina School of Law and is an avid distance swimmer.

**PROFESSOR WARWICK J. MCKIBBIN, Ph.D.,** is Professor of International Economics and Convenor of the Economics Division in the Research School of Pacific and Asian Studies at the Australian National University. He is also a Professorial Fellow at the Lowy Institute for International Policy; a nonresident Senior Fellow at the Brookings Institution in Washington D.C. and President of McKibbin Software Group. He is a member of the Board of the Reserve Bank of Australia. Professor McKibbin has worked at the Reserve Bank of Australia, Japanese Ministry of Finance, US Congressional Budget office and World Bank. He has been a consultant for many international agencies and a range of governments on issues of macroeconomic policy, international trade and finance and greenhouse policy issues. Professor McKibbin has published widely in technical journals and the popular press including the book "Global Linkages: Macroeconomic Interdependence and Cooperation in the World Economy" written with Professor Jeffrey Sachs of Harvard University and the new book "Climate Change Policy after Kyoto: A Blueprint for a Realistic Approach" with Professor Peter Wilcoxen of the University of Texas. He received his B.Com. (Honours 1) and University of the University of Texas. He received his B.Com. (Honours 1) and University Medal from University of NSW (1980) and his A.M. (1984) and a Ph.D. (1986) from Harvard University. He is a Fellow of the Australian Academy of Social Sciences and a founding member of the Harvard University Asian Economic Panel. He was awarded the Centenary medal in 2003 "For Service to Australian Society through Economic Policy and Tertiary Education."

**KAREN J. MONAGHAN,** joined the National Intelligence Council as the Deputy National Intelligence Officer for Economics and Global Issues in May 2002. She was named Acting NIO in September 2002. Prioir to her assignment with the NIC, she served in the Department of State and in the Central Intelligence Agency's Directorate of the Intelligence (DI) in a variety of managerial and analytic positions. Most recently she supervised current and long-term analysis of Asian Economic developments. Ms. Monaghan also spearheaded a corporate outreach program, tapping into corporate and financial sector expertise to help bolster financial vulnerability analysis and the impact of international capital flows on national and regional stability among emerging market countries. Ms. Monaghan is a graduate of Vassar College and undertook graduate studies in international relations and economics at St. Antony's College, Oxford University, where she earned an M.Phil. degree in 1982. Currently, Ms. Monaghan is an adjunct professor at the School of Foreign Service at Georgetown University. She has published extensively on issues of economic development and global issues.

**AMY PATICK, Ph.D.,** is Senior Director, Head of Virology, at Pfizer Global Research and Development, La Jolla (formerly Agouron Pharmaceuticals, Inc.). Amy earned her Ph.D. in Medical Microbiology from the University of Wisconsin in 1987. She has been involved in antiviral drug research since 1990 initially at Bristol-Myers Squibb Co. and subsequently (1994–present) at Pfizer Global Research and Development, La Jolla. Her research efforts are currently focused on antiviral chemotherapy and the emergence of resistance to antiviral agents. She has published more than 100 articles and abstracts in prominent scientific journals in the area of antiviral research. She is the Secretary for the International Society for Antiviral Research and has served as a member on the HIV Intercompany Collaborative Committee, HIV Resistance Collaborative Group, and the Scientific Subcommittee, International Workshop on HIV Resistance and Treatment Strategies. Amy is a regular ad hoc reviewer for several journals including *Antimicrobial Agents and Chemotherapy*, *AIDS Research and Human Retroviruses*, and *Antiviral Therapy*.

**LINDA J. SAIF, Ph.D.,** is Professor and Researcher at the Ohio State University's Ohio Agricultural Research and Development Center (OARDC). Dr. Saif brings to the committee her contributions to the study of virology, disease pathogenesis, and immunity, in both animal and human health, and mechanisms viruses, including rotaviruses, caliciviruses, and coronaviruses, which cause mortality and morbidity in both food-producing animals and humans. During the past 30 years, she has identified new intestinal viruses and developed diagnostic tests and research methods for working with them in the laboratory. Furthermore, she discovered viruses that cause intestinal diseases in livestock, and developed methods for their control. She is also credited with discovering the potential of enteric viral infections in animals to infect human populations in epidemic proportions. One example is Dr. Saif's ongoing effort to develop safe and effective vaccines for rotavirus diarrhea, which kills nearly a half million children every year. In 2002, Dr. Saif became the first Ohio State researcher not based on the Columbus campus to be recognized as a Distinguished University Professor, and was awarded an honorary doctorate by Belgium's Ghent University. She was elected a member of the National Academy of Sciences in 2003. Dr. Saif earned her bachelor's degree from the College of Wooster in 1969, and received her master's degree (1971) and doctorate (1976) in microbiology/immunology from the Ohio State University.

**RANGA SAMPATH, Ph.D.,** is the Director of Genomics and Computational Biology at Ibis Therapeutics, a division of Isis Pharmaceuticals. He leads Ibis's genomics efforts, both in RNA-based drug discovery and in microbial detection and diagnosis. Dr. Sampath has over 7 years of experience in the pharmaceutical industry and has been the lead genomics investigator on several DARPA programs related to bioinformatics, drug discovery and biological warfare agent detection and treatment. He has several publications and patents in RNA structure and target discovery, computational algorithms for RNA structure prediction, and pathogen and infectious agent diagnostics. Prior to joining Ibis Therapeutics, Dr. Sampath was a postdoctoral fellow at the Indiana University School of Medicine. He received his Ph.D. in chemical engineering from Rice University (Houston, Texas), and bachelor's in chemical engineering from the Indian Institute of Technology (Chennai, India).

**JEROME J. SCHENTAG, Pharm.D.,** is Professor of Pharmaceutical Sciences and Pharmacy, at the University at Buffalo School of Pharmacy and Pharmaceutical Sciences. He is also Chief Executive Officer at CPL Associates LLC, a private CRO. His Research emphasis has been in the clinical applications of pharmacokinetic/pharmacodynamic models to anti-infectives and other classes of pharmaceuticals used in seriously ill patients. Earlier work established correlations between pharmacokinetic parameters and biologic response to disease, drug efficacy and toxicity and managing antimicrobial resistance. Dr. Schentag received his Pharm.D. degree from the Philadelphia College of Pharmacy and Science and postdoctoral fellowship in clinical pharmacokinetics from SUNY Buffalo School of Pharmacy. A member of numerous professional societies, including the American Society for Microbiology and American Society of Hospital Pharmacists, Dr. Schentag is a

Fellow of American College of Clinical Pharmacy and the American College of Clinical Pharmacology. He has authored over 300 original research papers in prestigious journals, including the *Journal of Antimicrobial Chemotherapy*, *Pharmacotherapy*, *Antimicrobial Agents and Chemotherapy*, *Annals of Pharmacotherapy* and *Journal of the American Medical Association*. He has lectured extensively, both nationally and internationally, on a wide variety of topics, notably the clinical application of PK/PD and managing antimicrobial resistance.

**ALAN R. SHAW, Ph.D.**, is the Executive Director of Virus & Cell Biology at Merck Research Laboratories, and is responsible for all aspects of live virus vaccine research, as well as technical aspects of development and production. He is also responsible for research and early development of recombinant protein-based vaccines. Prior to joining Merck, Dr. Shaw worked on vaccines for hepatitis B and *Plasmodium falciparum* as well as cytokines and natural inhibitors of interleukin-1 at Biogen, SA in Geneva, Switzerland. Dr. Shaw received a B.A. from Rice University, a M.S. in molecular biology from the University of Texas at Dallas, and a Ph.D. in molecular biology at the Medical College of Ohio. He had postdoctoral fellowships at the International Institute of Cellular Pathology in Brussels and the Rockefeller University. Dr. Shaw is the past Chairman of the International Federation of Pharmaceutical Manufacturers Association Biologicals Committee.

**ROBERT G. WEBSTER, Ph.D.**, is Professor in the Division of Virology, Department of Infectious Diseases at St. Jude Children's Research Hospital. A native of New Zealand, Dr. Webster received his B. Sc. and M. Sc. in Microbiology from Otago University in New Zealand. In 1962, he earned his Ph.D. from the Australian National University and spent the next two years as a Fullbright Scholar working on influenza in the Department of Epidemiology at the University of Michigan, Ann Arbor. Since 1968, Dr. Webster has been with St. Jude Children's Research Hospital, Memphis, Tennessee. In 1988, he was appointed to the Rose Marie Thomas Chair in Virology. In 1989, he was admitted to the Royal Society of London in recognition for his contribution to influenza virus research. In 1998 he was appointed to the National Academy of Sciences of the United States. In 2002 he received the Twelfth Annual Bristol-Myers Squibb Award for Distinguished Achievement in Infectious Disease Research. Dr. Webster is Director of the World Health Organization Collaborating Center for Studies on the Ecology of Influenza in Animals and Birds. His interests include the structure and function of influenza virus proteins and the development of new vaccines and antivirals. The major focus of his research is the importance of influenza viruses in wild aquatic birds as a major reservoir of influenza viruses and their role in the evolution of new pandemic strains for humans and lower animals. His curriculum vitae contains over 450 original articles and reviews on influenza viruses.

animals. His curriculum vitae contains over 450 original articles and reviews on influenza viruses.

## FORUM STAFF

**STACEY L. KNOBLER,** is Director of the Forum on Microbial Threats at the Institute of Medicine (IOM) and a senior program officer for the Board on Global Health (BGH). She has served as the director of the BGH study, *Neurological, Psychiatric, and Developmental Disorders in Developing Countries* and as a research associate for the Board's earlier studies on *The Assessment of Future Scientific Needs for Live Variola (Smallpox) Virus and Cardiovascular Disease in Developing Countries.* Previously, Ms. Knobler has held positions as a Research Associate at the Brookings Institution, Foreign Policy Studies Program and as an Arms Control and Democratization Consultant for the Organization for Security and Cooperation in Europe in Vienna and Bosnia-Herzegovina. She has also worked as a research and negotiations analyst in Israel and Palestine. Ms. Knobler received her baccalaureate, summa cum laude, in political science and molecular genetics from the University of Rochester, and her M.P.A from Harvard University. She has conducted research and published on issues that include, biological and nuclear weapons control, foreign aid, health in developing countries, poverty and public assistance, and the Arab-Israeli peace process.

**KARL GALLE, Ph.D.,** is a research associate for the president's office at the Institute of Medicine. He received his Ph.D. in the history and philosophy of science from the University of London in 2002, prior to joining the National Academies through the Christine Mirzayan internship program in science and technology policy. He has worked at the Institute of Medicine since 2003 and also holds a B.A. in international development from Williams College, an M.A. in the conceptual foundations of science from the University of Chicago, and an M.Sc. in the history of science and medicine from the University of London.

**KATHERINE A. OBERHOLTZER,** is research assistant for the Institute of Medicine's Board on Global Health. She recently played a key role in the development and production of the BGH study, *Microbial Threats to Health: Emergence, Detection, and Response.* Katherine received her B.S. in Integrated Science and Technology with a concentration in Biotechnology from James Madison University in 2000. She is currently pursuing her Professional Editing Certificate at the George Washington University. Katherine has worked as the Meeting Coordinator for the Maryland AIDS Education and Training Center of the Institute of Human Virology at the University of Maryland, Baltimore. Katherine joined the staff at the Institute of Medicine in December 2000.

**LAURA SIVITZ, M.S.J.,** joined the staff of the Institute of Medicine in 2002 as

November 2003, she joined the staff of the Forum on Microbial Threats in the Board on Global Health at IOM. Previously, Ms. Sivitz had served as a technology reporter for *Washington Techway* magazine; as the science-writer intern for *Science News;* as the Washington correspondent for the *York Daily Record* of Pennsylvania; and as a science, legal, and business reporter for the Medill News Service of Chicago. She won a National Science Foundation fellowship in 1994 to conduct research at the University of Pennsylvania on piezoelectric ceramics for use in mammography systems. Ms. Sivitz received her bachelor of arts in physics from Bryn Mawr College in 1996 and her master of science in journalism from Northwestern University in 2001.